Aesthetic Surgery
of the Eyelids

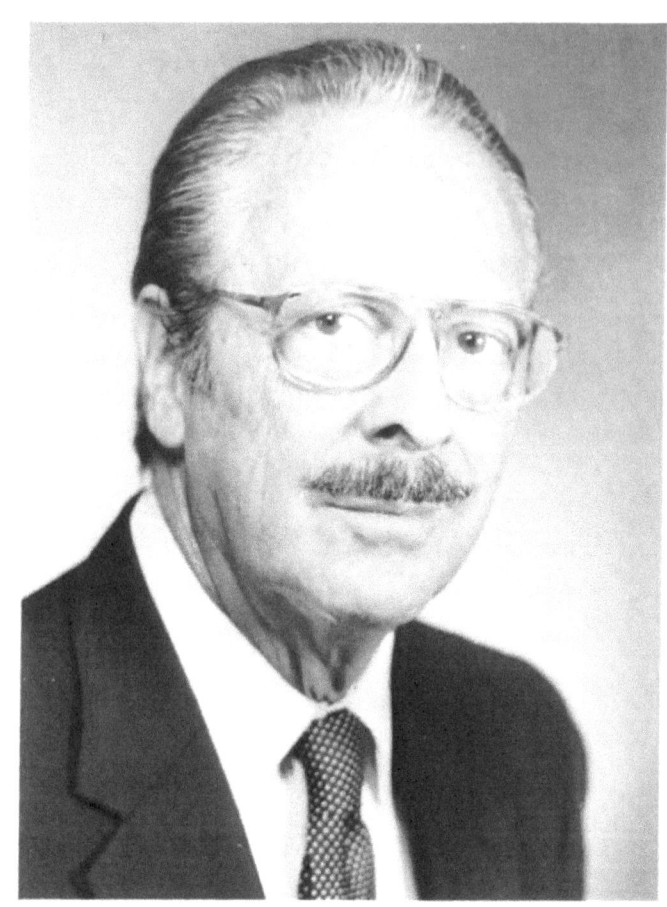

Raul Loeb

Raul Loeb

Aesthetic Surgery of the Eyelids

Translated from the Portuguese by Silas Braley

With 167 Illustrations in 474 Parts, Including 260 in Color

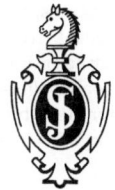

Springer-Verlag
New York Berlin Heidelberg
London Paris Tokyo Hong Kong

RAUL LOEB, M.D.
Associate Professor, Escola Paulista de Medicina, Federal University of São Paulo,
São Paulo, Brazil
International Society of Aesthetic Plastic Surgery, São Paulo, Brazil

Translator

SILAS BRALEY
1427 East Stuart Avenue, Fresno, CA 93710, USA

Library of Congress Cataloging-in-Publication Data
Loeb, Raul.
  Aesthetic surgery of the eyelids / Raul Loeb ; translated from the
Portuguese by Silas Braley.
    p. cm.
  Includes index.
  ISBN-13: 978-1-4612-8173-3
  1. Blepharoplasty. I. Title.
  [DNLM: 1. Eyelids-surgery. 2. Surgery, Plastic. WW 205 L825a]
RD119.5.E94L64 1989
617.7'71-dc19
DNLM/DLC
for Library of Congress   89-6100

Printed on acid-free paper.

Typeset, printed, and bound by Universitätsdruckerei H. Stürtz AG, Würzburg, Federal Republic of
Germany.

9 8 7 6 5 4 3 2 1

ISBN-13: 978-1-4612-8173-3   e-ISBN-13: 978-1-4612-3600-9
DOI: 10.1007/978-1-4612-3600-9

Foreword

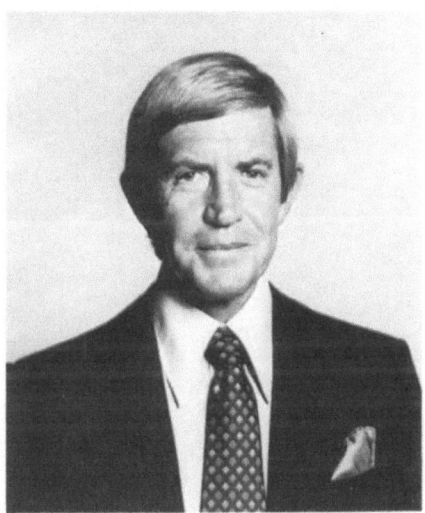

Dr. Loeb is a seasoned and respected plastic surgeon who has gained a reputation throughout the world. His special interest is blepharoplasty. A subject of which he has for many years been an intense student. I was delighted when I learned of this book on the subject.

It is not the routine that challenges us, but all of the special variations, problems, and complications that can occur. It is important that each plastic surgeon who performs blepharoplasty becomes aware of the many nuances of technique that will improve his or her results. It is even more important that each of us be aware of the pitfalls and how to avoid them in so far as possible.

The reader of this book will find a great deal of important information on the subject that he might not find elsewhere. The chapters on scleral show, anatomical variants, and the replacement of fat are especially intriguing, since these problems plague the results of the surgery. The correction of depression deformities that occur as a natural morphological feature or, as the result of fat removal feature, by fat flaps, is original with Dr. Loeb. His management of these problems in particular has been a very significant contribution. The anatomical analysis of the problems of depression and the management thereof are detailed in this excellent work. Such a thorough treatment of such deformities is not to be found elsewhere.

The treatment of complications is of prime importance, and Dr. Loeb shares with the reader his extensive experience of the important complications of blepharoplasty.

It gives me special pleasure to write the foreword to this book, since I have known Dr. Loeb since 1955, and have been in constant touch with him since that time. We have often shared our experience, especially as it has related to problems and the process of problem solving. I have learned much from him. I congratulate Dr. Loeb on this timely publication and enthusiastically recommend it to plastic surgeons everywhere.

THOMAS D. REES, M.D., F.A.C.S.

Preface

*Youth has an obligation to please
and the old not to offend*

These words were said to us by a patient on whom we had performed a blepharoplasty in the 1960s. He was an intelligent man whom we admired greatly, and his words stirred our imagination and affected us deeply.

Over the years, with daily experience in plastic surgery, we came to have a better understanding of some of the basic human feelings that are so clearly reflected in the face, and that are echoed in the expression of the eyes by the movements of the lids and the periorbital regions.

We then decided to learn everything possible about what happens when, with advancing age, a person's eyes lose their expression and become so altered that the individual scarcely recognizes him/herself. Defects become more pronounced and former beauty disappears. A patient may discover, in his or her own face, the aged physiognomy of a mother or father, or of some other ancestor.

Now the stage is set for the consideration of an esthetic blepharoplasty, the most routinely performed of cosmetic facial procedures. As a general rule, what people who decide to undergo this type of surgery actually desire is a return to the past, with a face that does not show the characteristics of old age. Obviously, although this may be questioned, camouflaged, or even denied, vanity also plays an important role in this decision.

Ethnic and racial factors are extremely important, as these naturally imprint their particular racial characteristics on the lid structure. In one ethnic group, certain anatomic standards may be considered beautiful, while in another the same appearance can be regarded as strange.

For example, in Orientals a flat upper eyelid is natural and therefore attractive, but in Caucasians, it is not a standard of beauty, and it seems strange to them that Orientals could want a flat sulcus in the upper eyelid. Our mentalities are different, and the facial expression of the Oriental gives a westerner the impression of constant self-satisfaction. On the other hand, why then do some Orientals want to change this facial aspect? Could it be due to admiration for a western type of beauty, for a famous personality, an admired acquaintance?

Apart from beauty, what encites admiration and causes one to want to imitate another? Could it be the character or some other unforgettable trait of a person, or perhaps a personality, or some other attribute that remains indelibly engraved on one's memory?

It is certain that all of us have our own ideas of what constitutes beauty. Thus a slight bulging of the lower lid is sometimes acceptable, since it conveys an air of nostalgia. But this does not preclude a reduction of these bulges when they are excessive. Also, in some youths a smile causes a thickening of the obicularis muscle of the lower eyelid, which imparts an air of happiness; even so, some cases need a reduction of the muscle. A slight "scleral show" may possibly enhance the beauty of the eyes, but when excessive it should be corrected.

The principal aim of the plastic surgeon is not only to effect the necessary alterations in the external morphology of his patient, but also to react relative to something much greater, something that is imponderable in its brilliant variety: the human mind. This has its rights, and we, the plastic surgeons, are here to attend to it.

Confidence in blepharoplasty procedures is based on quality. The results are there for all to see. A bad blepharoplasty cannot be concealed, whereas a good one will be so natural as to be unnoticed, and the surgeon will have fulfilled his obligation to his patient.

Surgery is never totally absent from risks, we can only seek to reduce them. Surprisingly, incisions next to the ciliary border are used by many surgeons, even though they are aware that this leaves them open to ectropion, or scleral show. These and other details in the planning of blepharoplasties are analyzed in this book, always with the success of the surgical procedure in mind.

In Chapters 1, 2, and 4, we will demonstrate the surgical precautions needed to prevent ectropion and/or scleral show. Each of these chapters also includes comments on the possible consequences of not following these recommendations. Chapter 5 presents useful techniques for the correction of scleral show and for looseness of the upper quadrant of the face (a temporal face lift), as well as for the splitting and elevation of the orbicular muscle of the eye. Chapter 6 is concerned with other possible blepharoplasty complications.

We do not intend, in this work, to discuss all the techniques or ideas recommended by other authors, as much as we recognize their value. After 30 years of experience in palpebral surgery, we present here only our own techniques, original or modified, along with those others with which we have obtained satisfactory results, thereby demonstrating to us their validity.

In this book we have adopted the nomenclature recommended by the IANC, the International Anatomical Nomenclature Committee.

São Paulo, Brazil

RAUL LOEB

Acknowledgments

The writing of this book was made possible by my family life. Thanks to the understanding and love of my wife, Elsie, and our daughters, Tania, Katia, Cynthia, and Sheila, I have been able to work happily. I dedicate this book to them. I am grateful to my beloved parents, Felix and Jessie Loeb, for the marvelous ideals and principles that they showed me by example. Their memory supports me in all my endeavors.

I want to thank Professor Sebastiao Hermeto, dedicated surgeon, outstanding scientist, and unfailing friend, for his guidance in the early days of my medical career. To Professor Antonio Prudente, one of the pioneers in Latin American plastic surgery, I express my thanks, my respect, and my admiration. I remember his words: "Esthetic surgery patients almost always confront us with two complex problems: money and vanity. It is always difficult to handle these. However, the scientific part of the specialty can be gratifying, and even compensate somewhat for these problems." His integrity, as well as that of his wife, Carmen Annes Dias Prudente, who still today dedicates herself to the Instituto Central da Fundacao Antonio Prudente, will always be engraved in my memory. Dr. James Barret Brown of the Barnes Hospital in St. Louis in the United States, through his scientific ethics and creative spirit, was of fundamental importance in my training. I am grateful to him, and to his co-workers, for teaching me the basic principles of plastic surgery, as well as for the special friendships that they extended to me while I interned there. The outstanding personality of Dr. Gustave Aufricht of New York is deeply engraved on my memory. His personal refinement and the artistry with which he did his work, as well as his care of and extreme respect for his patients, will never be forgotten. Special thanks go to Dr. Thomas Rees for his encouragement. His unique person is always noted and admired, whether in scientific, social, or sports events. To see Professor Rees operate, especially in his own milieu in the Manhatten Eye and Ear Hospital in New York, is a privilege. To exchange ideas with him always results in new knowledge. Not only is he a great surgeon technically, but also his clear mind and pleasing manner of explanation are always welcome. Professor Eros A. Erhart of the Faculty of Medicine of the University of São Paulo, Brazil, was a tireless reviewer of the manuscript of this book. He was always with me in difficult moments, particularly when I was concerned with the minutia of anatomical description. With patience and an iron will, he eliminated those trivial terms that do not belong in International Anatomical Nomenclature, at times even against my desire to use them. I am grateful for his pleasant and constant presence and dedication.

I am grateful for the work of Ana Maria Bolant, who has worked with me in the double occupation of secretary and surgical nurse for 20 years. Only her excellent knowledge of the surgery performed during all these years allowed us to make the studies that resulted in this book. In these last 30 months she was of outstanding help in the compilation and mounting of the scattered material.

I also thank my secretaries, Marilena Moreira de Carvalho and Rosana Favilla, for their efficient help in the dictation and typing of the manuscript.

Innumerable assistants aided in the surgery; Dr. Nelson Augusto Letizio and Marcio Michel Nassif were most often with us during these years, and deserve thanks for their help and dedication.

I am extremely grateful to my patients, who are the principal motivation for my work, for granting permission to publish their photographs in this book.

The São Paulo Anesthesia Clinic was most valuable to me. Many times the surgery would not have been possible without the tranquility that they conveyed. To them, I express my profound gratitude. Dr. Carlos Pereira de Magalhaes was of great help in the preparation of the topic on anesthesia.

The majority of the photographs in this book are the work of Miguel Paschoal, a distinguished professional in São Paulo, whose dedication and talent helped me greatly. He was tireless during all these years, giving of his precious time, seeking to standardize and perfect the documentation. My gratitude.

With the exception of a few figures by Jose Goncalves, the anatomical figures and drawings were all made by Lucia Moreira Machado de Oliveira, to whom I owe my gratitude.

To Paulo Marti of the Instituto Brasiliero de Edicoes Pedagogicas, I express profound thanks for the confidence that he has had in my work. His strong support, and that of his graphic production team, encouraged me and accelerated the production of this book greatly. The entire undertaking can be attributed in large measure to the selflessness and generosity of Paulo Marti.

In an effort to repay the efforts of all those who in one way or another have helped me, I pray that this book may bring benefit to its readers, be they plastic surgeons, ophthalmologists, or other specialists. To them all go my wishes for a thriving career.

Contents

1

Anatomical Considerations

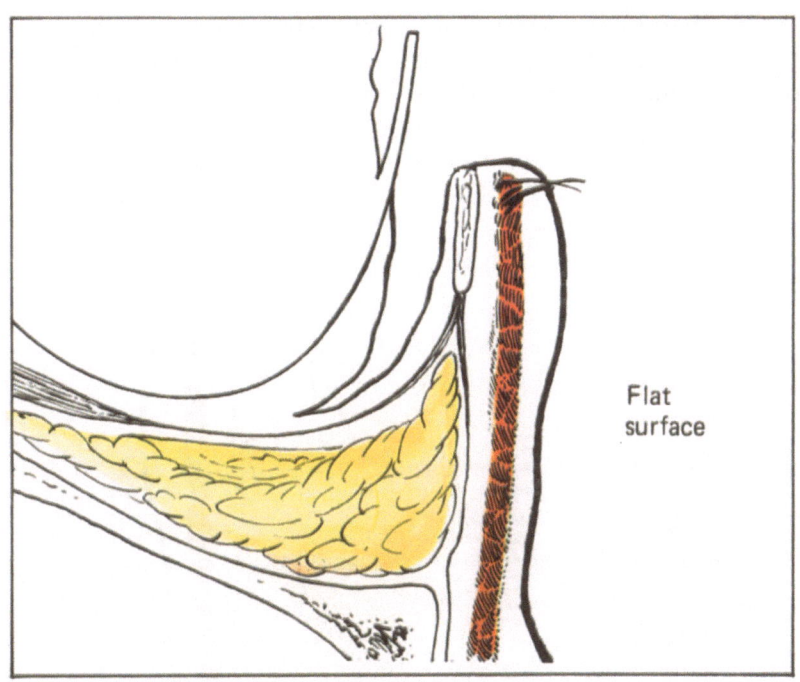

Flat
surface

Introduction

Blepharoplasty is routinely accomplished by removing excess skin, muscle or fatty tissue and, more recently, by the building up of sunken areas with small fat grafts. The purpose is to beautify and/or rejuvenate the patient's appearance while maintaining the functional integrity of the eyelids. The eyelids are specialized anatomical structures that protect the eye from trauma, limit the amount of entering light, and distribute tears over the surface of the globe by constant blinking.

In this chapter we will study the palpebral and parapalpebral anatomical structures that are significant for a successful blepharoplasty. Knowledge of the anatomy of this area enables the surgeon to make an accurate diagnosis of the aesthetic palpebral problems as well as to choose among the various types of treatments available.

The orbital region, however, is subject to great surgical risks during blepharoplasty. Any technical error by the surgeon can result in functional and/or morphological changes whose consequences are most varied and unpredictable, the most common being ectropions and "scleral show." Obviously, surgery that proposes to beautify should not be the cause of other major problems.

We will also analyze the anatomical structures that result in palpebral bulges and depressions, which when excessive, can appreciably jeopardize the aesthetics of the area, as well as the techniques used to eliminate them. We will seek to create *"flat surfaces,"* where and when they should exist in the eyelids. This ideal concept of beauty is a useful parameter that serves as the base for the planning of blepharoplasty.

Flat Surfaces

In the aesthetic ideal, the upper and lower eyelids should show areas of "flat surfaces," with a minimum of bulges and depressions (Fig. 1.1). The flat surface can occupy the whole surface of the lid or only a sector of it.

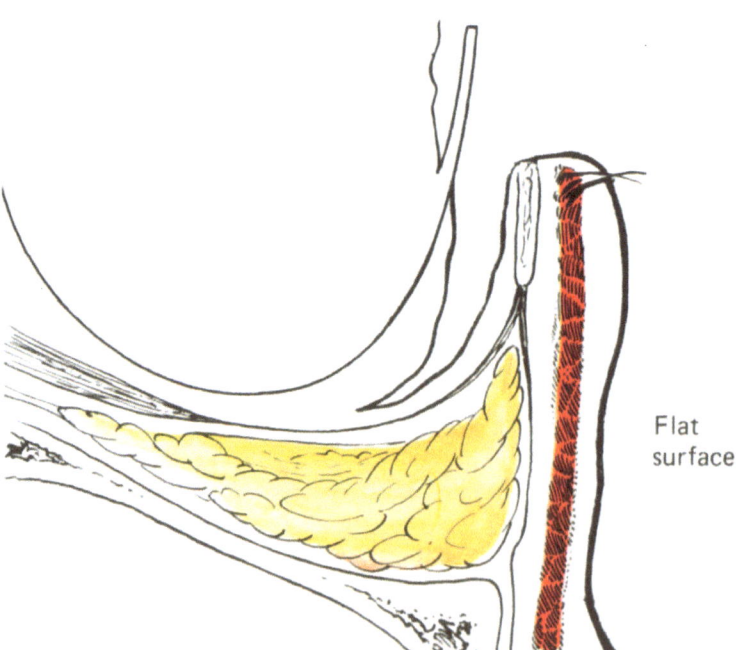

Flat
surface

FIGURE 1.1. Flat surface of the lower lid, with a minimum of bulges or depressions. The aesthetic ideal. (From Loeb R: Improvements in blepharoplasty: Creating a flat surface for the lower lid, in: *Transactions of the Seventh International Congress of Plastic and Reconstructive Surgery.* São Paulo, Sociedade Brasileira de Cirurgia Plástica, 1979, pp 390–393).

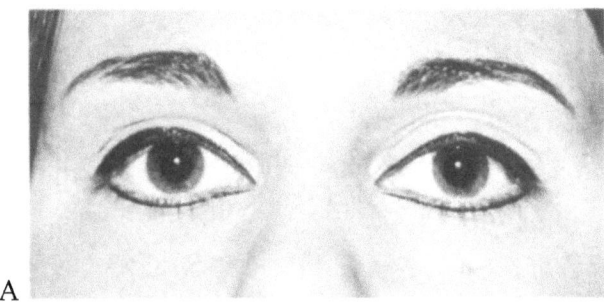

A

FIGURE 1.2. The "flat surface." *A*. Occupying the entire extension of the lid. *B*. Sectorial, that is, occupying only part of the lid (in this case the septal portion).

B

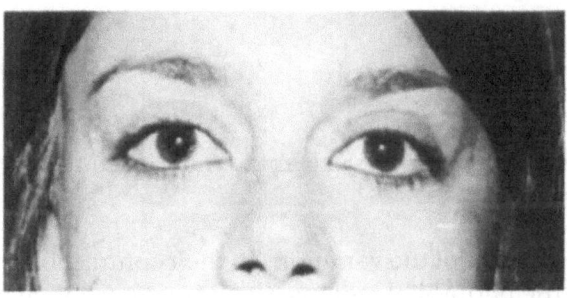

FIGURE 1.3. Flat surface of the lower lid in a young white woman.

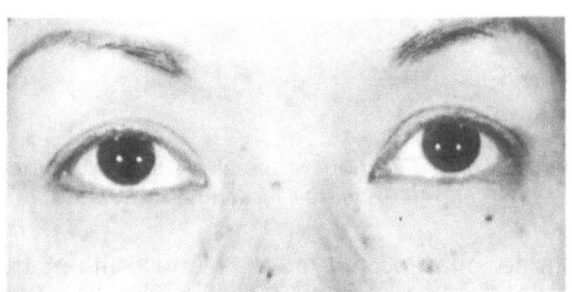

FIGURE 1.4. Flat surface of the lower lid in a young Oriental.

The Lower Eyelid

The flat surface in the lower eyelid can be one of two forms (Fig 1.2):

1. The "flat surface" occupies the whole extension of the lid (Fig. 1.2A). In this case the lower eyelid is totally flat, from the palpebral border to the nasojugal and the palpebromalar sulci. No noticeable bulges of the orbicularis oculi muscle or of the fat compartments can be observed in either the tarsal or septal portions. The palpebral sulci show their normal slight depressions. This is the aesthetic ideal. This concept is valid for both whites and Orientals when the orbicularis oculi muscle is relaxed (Figs. 1.3 and 1.4).

When this muscle is contracted, however, its volume increases with the formation of a tarsal bulge and a marked change in the flat surface (Fig. 1.5B).

2. The flat surface occupies only a portion of the lid; it is sectorial. In Figure 1.2B the flat surface is situated in the septal portion. The lower palpebral and nasojugal sulci present normal retraction. The orbicularis oculi muscle in the pretarsal portion may be normal or augmented.

The Upper Eyelid

In Orientals, where the supratarsal sulcus is lacking because of racial characteristics, the flat

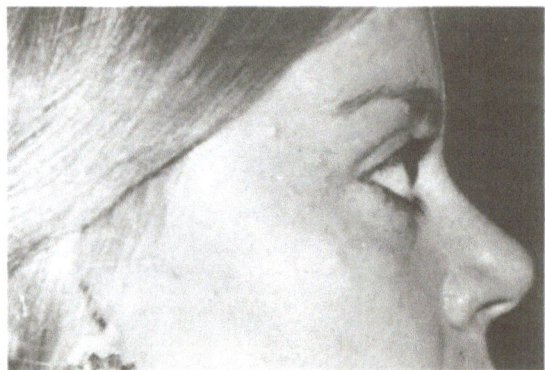
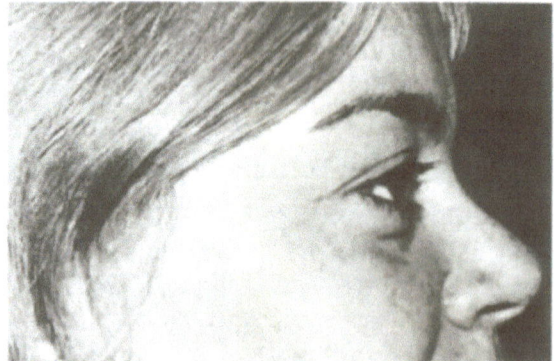

FIGURE 1.5. Patient showing change in the lower eyelid surface A. Flat surface when the face is in repose. B. Hypertrophy of the tarsal portion when smiling.

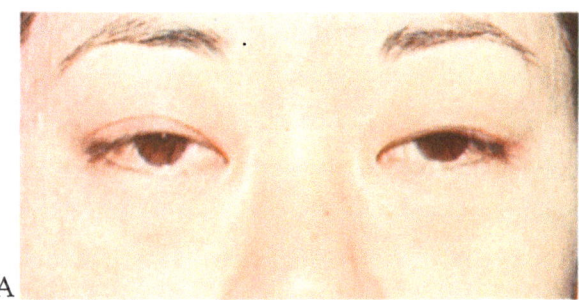
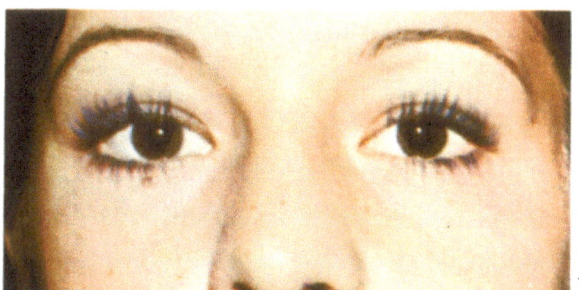

FIGURE 1.6. Flat surfaces of the upper lid. A. In Orientals, the flat surface occupies the entire extension of the upper eyelid. B. In whites it occupies only the septal portion.

surface may occupy all, or almost all, of the extension of the upper lid. In whites in which the tarsal portion is convex, the flat surface is sectorial. It exists only in the septal portion. This flat surface of the septal portion can almost disappear when skin, muscle, and fat bulges are present (Fig. 1.6).

The flat surfaces are altered through the natural morphological changes that occur with aging. These changes can also be iatrogenic in nature. The resultant bulges and/or depressions must be surgically corrected to restore the original flatness. The structures that contribute the most to this loss of flatness are the skin, the septum orbitale, the orbicularis oculi muscle, and the fat pockets. Also contributing are the principal sulci of the lid: the superior and inferior palpebral sulci and the nasojugal and palpebromalar sulci.

In addition, the lacrimal gland can vary in size and cause different types of bulges. Müller's muscle and the levator palpebrae superioris muscles influence the bulkiness of the upper lid

because of the variations in their contractions. In the periorbital regions, the frontal portion of the occipitofrontal muscle and the corrugator, procerus, and angular muscles are important (Fig. 1.7).

For a better understanding of the factors that interfere with the presence of flat surfaces, we will consider the "septum orbitale" and the principal sulci of the lids separately. The orbicularis muscle and the fat pockets are better analyzed in Chapter 3.

Orbital Septum

It is necessary to know the anatomical significance of the orbital septum in order to understand the etiology of bulges and of the main sulci of the lid. The subfascial tissues of the lids follow the trajectory of the orbital septum, and thus influence the formation of bulges and depressions of the eyelids.

The orbital septum serves to separate the eyelids from the deep orbital portions, as well as

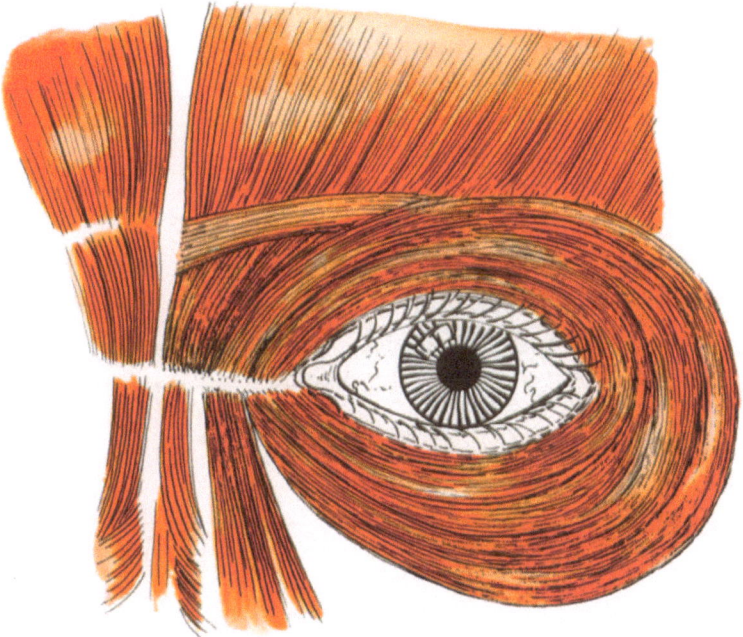

FIGURE 1.7. The orbital and periorbital musculature.

from the periorbital portions, and acts as a barrier to hemorrhages, infections, inflammations, and other pathologies.

The thickness of the "septum orbitale" changes from person to person and can vary even in the same eyelid. The latter explains the differences in the size of bulges in the fat pockets in the same eyelid (see Chapter 3).

The orbital septum inserts into the orbital arch in an enlarged portion called the arcus marginalis. This arch is generally thicker in the lateral portions of the upper and lower eyelids. In the medial portion, the orbital septum inserts directly into the orbital rim (Fig. 1.8).

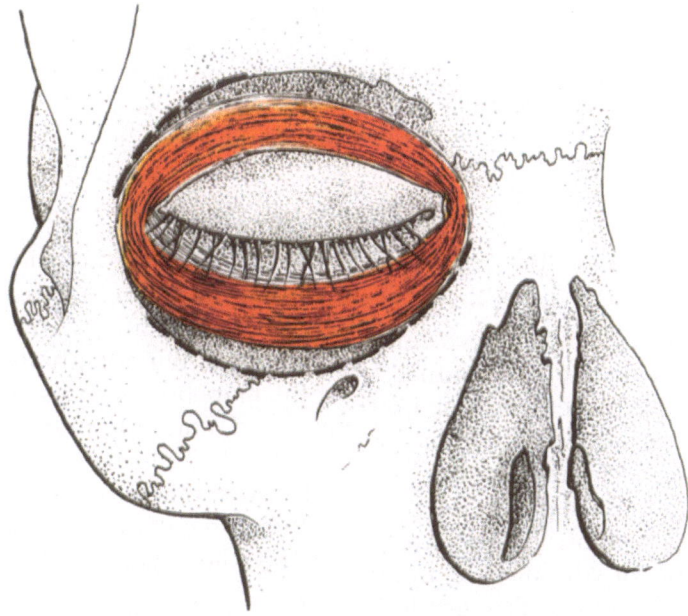

FIGURE 1.8. The orbital septum inserts into the arcus marginalis and into the rim of the upper and lower orbital archs.

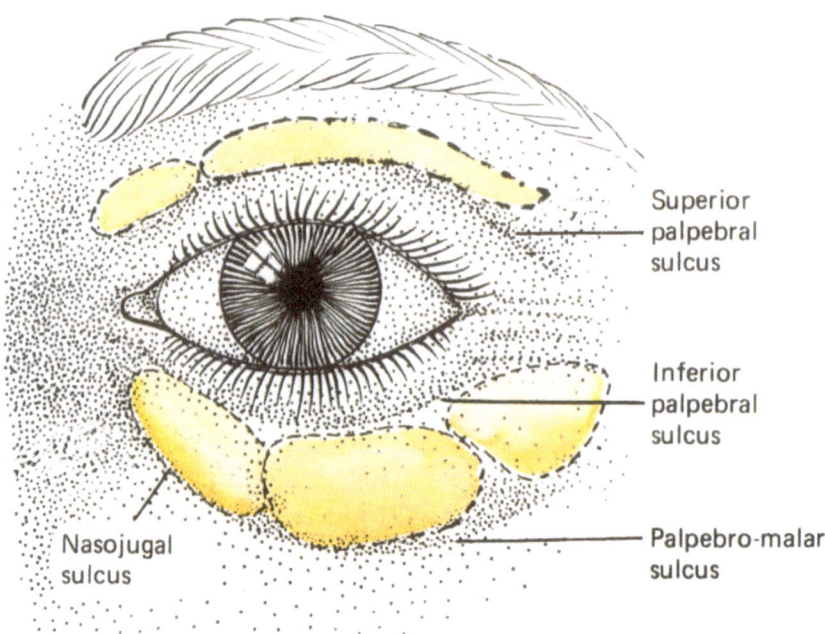

FIGURE 1.9. Principal sulci of the eyelids. The fat pockets are also indicated.

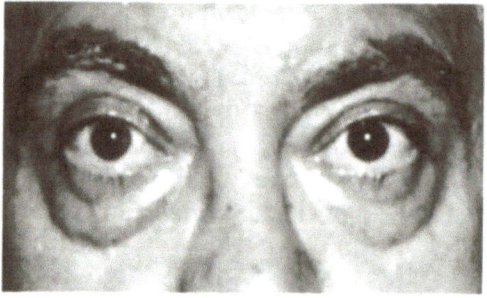

FIGURE 1.10. Nasojugal, lower, and upper palpebral sulci, and palpebro-malar sulcus, made more evident by the presence of hypertrophied fat pockets.

Principal (Natural) Sulci of the Eyelids

These are so named because they are true sulci in the skin of the lids and are not to be confused with deep wrinkles, which sometimes look like true sulci. The sulci are also called folds or grooves. These principal sulci demarcate the various parts of the lids and also separate the lids from their neighboring regions. For example, the nasojugal sulcus separates the lower lid from the nasal and the cheek regions. Exaggerated depth of the sulcus can create aesthetic problems.

Because of their direct linkage with the orbital septum, the skin retraction that corresponds to the sulci of the lids maintains its fixation in the deep plane. It is accentuated by the movements of the palpebral muscles. These sulci should be analyzed and interpreted correctly to understand their significance.

The *sulci* that we consider the most important to the correction of lid depressions and bulges are the following (Fig. 1.9):

1. Superior palpebral sulcus (better known as the supratarsal fold) in the upper lid;
2. Inferior palpebral sulcus in the lower lid;

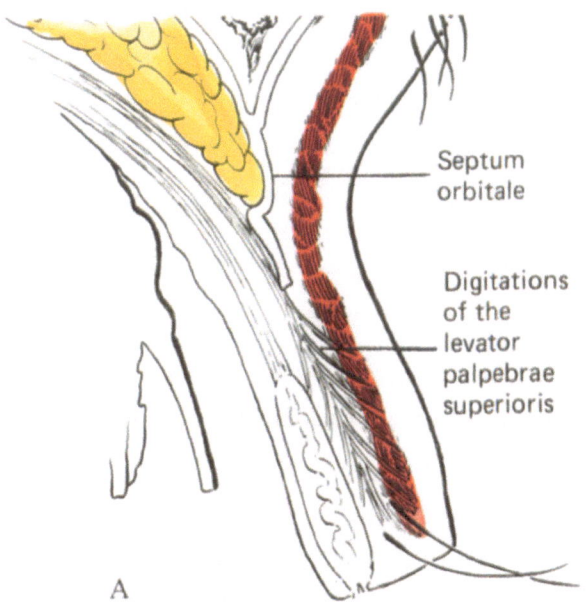
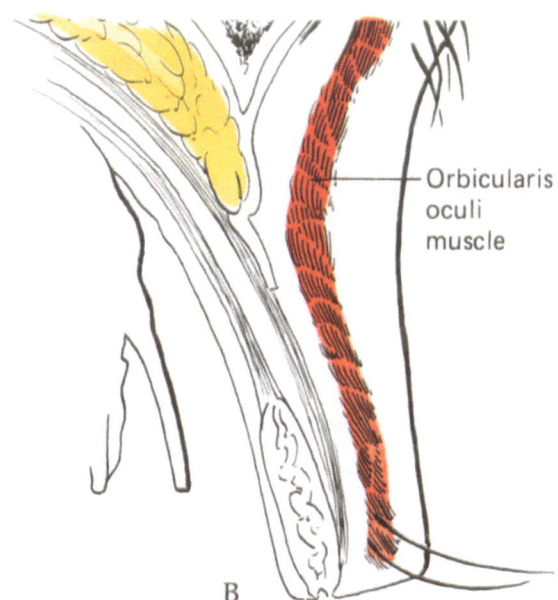

FIGURE 1.11. Parasagittal section of the upper eyelid. *A.* The Occidental eyelid: the levator muscle of the upper eyelid has its digitations inserted into the dermis of the lid. Together with the Müller muscle it helps to enhance the supratarsal fold. *B.* The Oriental upper eyelid. The levator muscle does *not* have digitations inserted into the dermis, and therefore there is no supratarsal fold, thus producing the flat surface of the Oriental upper lid.

3. Nasojugal sulcus between the lower lid and the nasal and cheek regions;
4. Palpebro-malar sulcus between the lower lid and the malar region.

All these sulci vary with age and with the racial characteristics and particular morphology of each individual. They are most evident when they are found in conjunction with the septal fat pockets or with the hypertrophied pretarsal portions of the orbicularis oculi muscle (Fig. 1.10). The sulci can also seem more accentuated because of an increase in the volume of the cheek region.

The Superior Palpebral Sulcus

In the upper eyelid the orbital septum inserts at the level of the Müller muscle, near the highest portion of the tarsal cartilage. It thus forms a retraction that contributes to the formation of the superior palpebral sulcus (Fig. 1.11).

A knowledge of the superior palpebral sulcus is important during blepharoplasty since there are procedures to make it more evident, to create it, or to make it less evident.

Making the Sulcus More Evident. When a skin resection is performed to correct looseness in the upper lid, the suture can be intentionally placed between the tarsal and septal regions, where, anatomically, the sulcus is situated. Then, because of the normal retraction of the resultant scar, the sulcus becomes more evident.

Creating a Superior Palpebral Sulcus (Millard, 1955). In many cases the Oriental eye has a totally flat surface on the upper lid owing to the absence of the superior palpebral sulcus (Fig. 1.12). Some Orientals prefer to have Western-type eyes, and in these cases the "occidentalization of the Oriental eye" is performed. This consists of the creation of the superior palpebral sulcus through a tarsal fixation. Basically it is the surgical removal of a layer of the orbicularis oculi muscle, plus some of the hypertrophied adipose (oversized fat) tissue underlying it. Following this, the skin is anchored to the tarsal cartilage, thus creating the sulcus (Fig. 1.13).

Making the Superior Palpebral Sulcus Less Evident. The sulcus can be made shallower in cases of exaggerated depressions (Fig. 1.14). See page 95 in Chapter 4, "Depressions of the Eyelids."

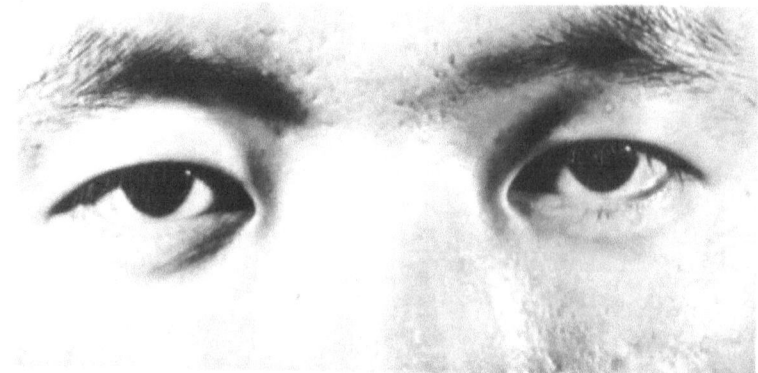

FIGURE 1.12. Oriental patient showing absence of the superior palpebral sulcus. Presence of epicanthus.

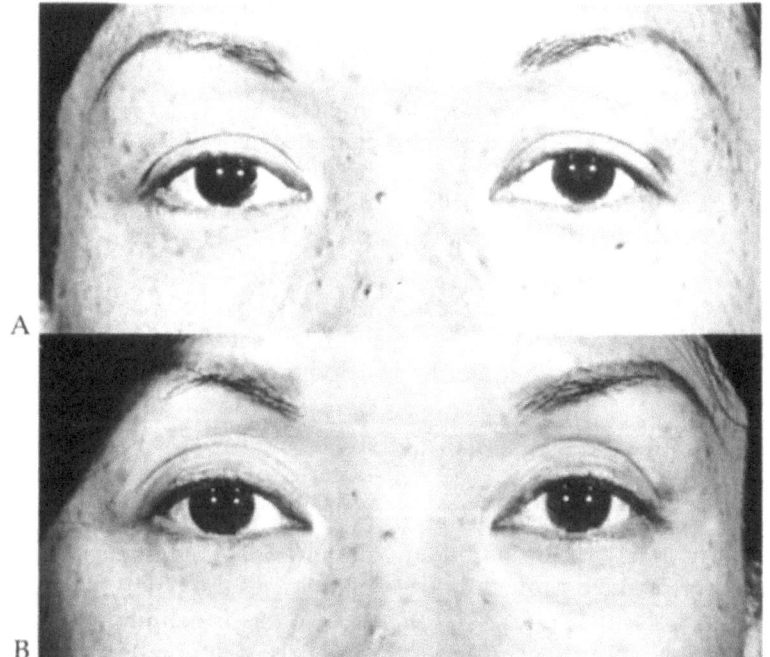

FIGURE 1.13. Occidentalization of the Oriental eye through tarsal fixation. *A.* Preoperative view; *B.* Postoperative view.

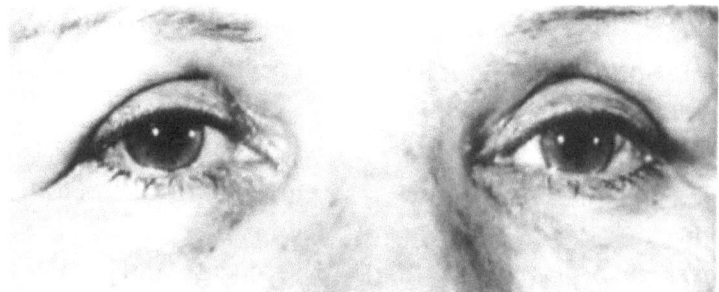

FIGURE 1.14. Exaggerated retraction of the supratarsal fold, needing correction. (See technique on page 96).

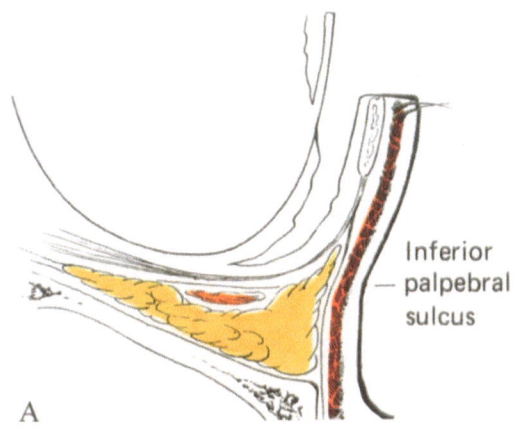

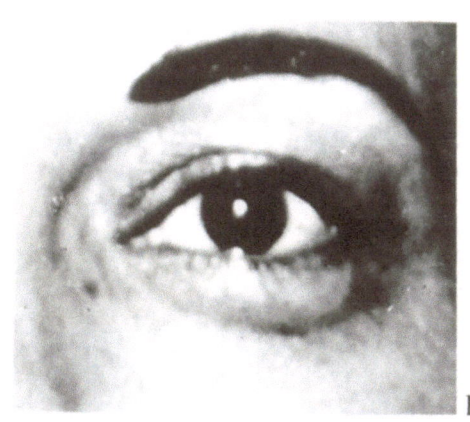

FIGURE 1.15. The inferior palpebral sulcus is situated between the pretarsal portion (more voluminous) and the preseptal protion (less voluminous) of the orbicularis oculi muscle. *A.* Parasagittal section of the eyelid showing the inferior palpebral sulcus. *B.* Patient in whom the sulcus is noticeable.

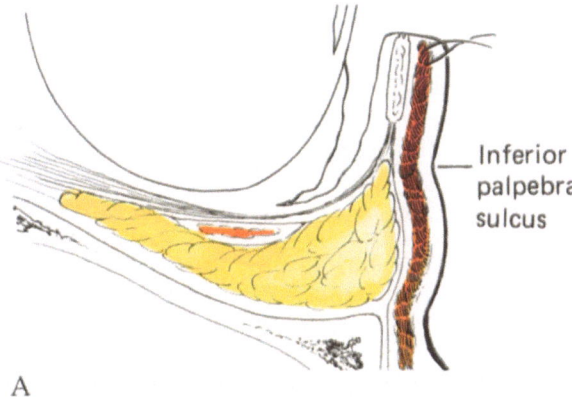

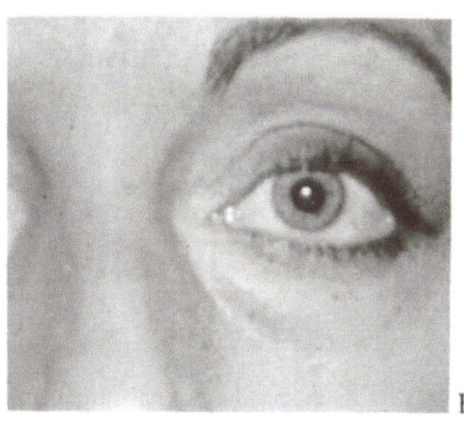

FIGURE 1.16. Influence of the fat pockets on the morphology of the sulcus. When the palpebral pockets are somewhat larger than normal, the inferior palpebral sulcus becomes more marked and visible. *A.* Parasagittal section of the eyelid. *B.* Clinical case.

The Inferior Palpebral Sulcus

This represents the projection on the skin of the deep reflection line of the palpebral and bulbar conjunctivae. Its etiology is based on the abrupt differences in volume between the tarsal and septal portions of the lower eyelid (Zide and McCarthy, 1981). The pretarsal portion of the orbicularis oculi muscle is at times more voluminous than the preseptal portion, and the thickness of the tarsal cartilage also contributes to the increase in volume of this part of the eyelid. These two volumes are additive. The deepest plane of the "septum orbitale" is fixed at the level of the lower border of the tarsus and constitutes the anterior border of the preaponeurotic adipose space (Fig. 1.15).

The morphology of the lower palpebral sulcus is directly influenced by the amount of fat in the septal portion of the lid. It is accentuated when the fat is of moderate volume and tends to disappear when the fat is very bulky (Figs. 1.16 and 1.17).

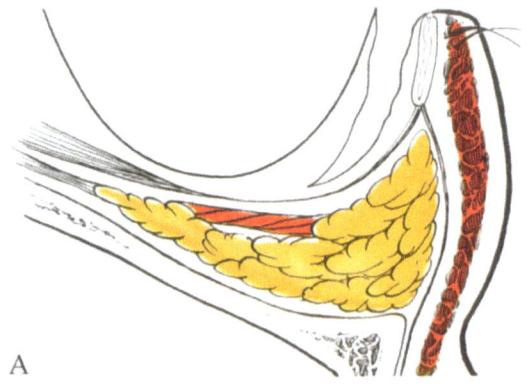

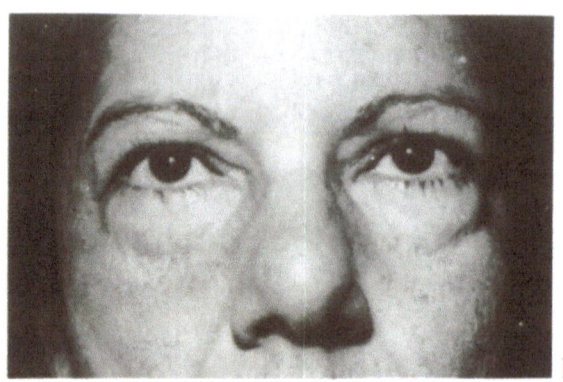

FIGURE 1.17. Influence of marked hypertrophy of the fat pockets on the morphology of the lower palpebral sulcus. When the fat pockets of the lower lids are bulky, they may conceal the inferior palpebral sulcus. *A*. Parasagittal section showing absence of the sulcus. *B*. Clinical case.

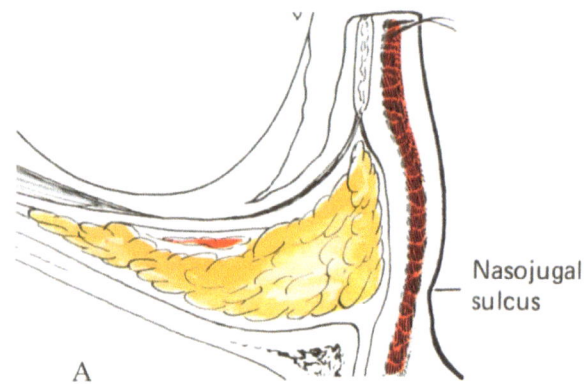

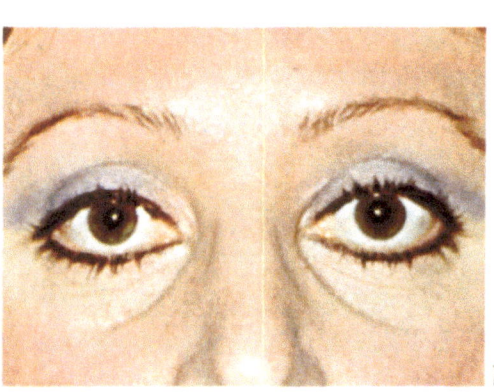

Nasojugal sulcus

FIGURE 1.18. An exacerbated nasojugal sulcus. *A.* Parasagittal section showing the nasojugal sulcus. *B.* Clinical case. (From Loeb R: Improvements in blepharoplasty: creating a flat surface for the lower lid, in: *Transactions of the Seventh International Congress of Plastic and Reconstructive Surgery.* São Paulo, Sociedade Brasileira de Cirurgia Plástica, 1979, pp 390-393).

The Nasojugal Sulcus

The nasojugal sulcus is situated at the inferior-medial limits of the lower lid (Elder and Wybar, 1961). We believe that it is caused by two factors, whose effects are additive:

1. The fixation of the septum orbitale at the level of the inferior-medial portion of the arcus marginalis, and
2. The existence of a triangular gap limited by the superior-lateral border and the inferior-lateral portion of the angular muscle on one side and the inferior-medial portion of the orbicularis oculi muscle on the other (Fig. 1.7).

With aging, the nasojugal sulcus becomes relatively deeper because of the growth of neighboring fat pockets, both medial and central. These pockets, on growing, do not invade the depression of the nasojugal sulcus because the septum orbitale prevents it at this level (Fig. 1.18).

The Palpebral-Malar Sulcus

The palpebral-malar sulcus separates the inferior-lateral portion of the orbit from the malar region. In young people this sulcus is usually not very accentuated, generally being imperceptible. However, with age, the growth

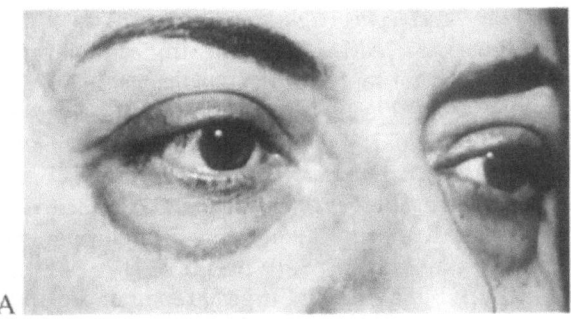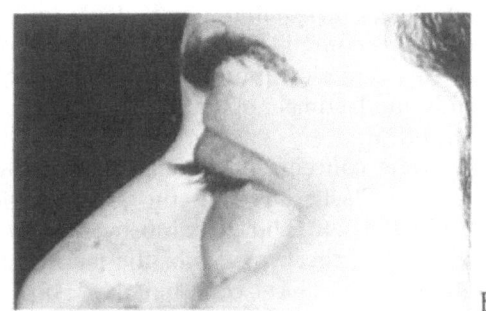

A   B

FIGURE 1.19. Typical example of a marked depression of the palpebral-malar sulcus.

of the lateral fat pocket causes a relative depression in the area where the projection ceases, that is, at the point of fixation of the septum orbitale in the inferior–lateral portion of the orbital arch. This pocket has a rather fixed position because of its connection with the septum orbitale (Fig. 1.19).

Additional Reading

General Considerations

BERRY EP: Planning and evaluating blepharoplasty. *Plast Reconstr Surg* 1974; 54:257.

CALLAHAN A: *Surgery of the Eye: Diseases*. Springfield Ill, Charles C Thomas Published, 1956.

CONELL B: Symposium on the ageing face. Dalinde Hospital, Mexico, DF, October, 1978.

CONVERSE JM, SMITH B et al: Deformities of the eyelid and adnexa, orbit and the zygoma, in Converse JM (ed): *Reconstructive Plastic Surgery*. Philadelphia, WB Saunders Co, 1977.

COURTISS EH: Selection of alternatives in esthetic blepharoplasty. *Clin Plast Surg* 1981; 8:739.

DUPUIS C, RESS TD: Historical notes on blepharoplasty. *Plast Reconstr Surg* 1971; 47:246.

ELDER DS and WYBAR KC: System of Ophthalmology: The anatomy of the Visual System, Vol.2, London, Henry Kimpton 1961.

GONZALEZ-ULLOA M: An update on blepharoplasty. *Aesthetic Plast Surg* 1983; 7:1.

GONZALEZ-ULLOA M, MEYER R et al: *Aesthetic Plastic Surgery*, vol 2. Padova, Italy, Piccin Nuova Libraria, 1987.

GRAY's Anatomy: ed 35. Longman, 1975.

GUY CL, CONVERSE JM et al: Esthetic surgery for the aging face, in Converse JM (ed): Reconstructive Plastic Surgery. ed 2. Philadelphia, WB Saunders, 1977.

HINDERER UT: Aging of the palpebral and periorbital regions, in Gonzalez-Ulloa M, Meyer R (eds): *Aesthetic Plastic Surgery* vol II. Padova, Italy, Piccin Nuova Libraria, 1987. p.64.

KUWABARA I, COGAN, D et al: Structure of the muscles of the upper eyelid. *Arch. Ophthalmol.*, 1975; 93:1189.

LEWIS JR Jr: A comparison of blepharoplasty techniques, In Masters WF, Lewis JR Jr (eds): *Symposium on Aesthetic Surgery of Face, Eyelid and Breast*. St. Louis, CV Mosby Co, 1972.

MACOMBER WB: Symposium on orbital and eyelid surgery. *Clin Plast Surg* 1978; 5:4

PUTTERMAN AM: Surgical treatment of dysthyroid eyelid retraction and orbital fat hernia. *Otolaryngol Clin North Am* 1980; 13:39–51.

SMITH JW, NEWMAN F: Blepharoplasty: Technical details, in Gonzalez-Ulloa M, and Meyer R M (eds): Aesthetic Plastic Surgery Vol. II. Padova, Italy, Piccin Nuova Libraria, 1987. p.95.

Anatomical Considerations

ANDERSON RL, BEARD C: The levator aponeurosis: Attachments and their clinical significance. *Arch Ophthalmol* 1977; 95:1437.

BEARD C, QUICKERT M: Anatomy of the Orbit, ed 2. Birmingham, Alabama, *Aesculepius Publishing Company*, 1977.

BOO-CHAI K: Plastic construction of the superior palpebral fold. *Plast Reconstr Surg* 1963; 31:74.

DUKE-ELDER S: *The Anatomy of the Visual System. System of Ophthalmology Series*, vol 2. St. Louis, CV Mosby Co, 1961.

HOLLINGSHEAD WH: Anatomy for Surgeons, vol 1 – The Head and Neck, ed 3. Harper and Row Publishers Inc, 1982.

Hugo NE, Stone E: Anatomy of a blepharoplasty. *Plast Reconstr Surg* 1974; 53:381.

Jones TL: An anatomical approach to problems of the eyelids and lacrimal apparatus. *Arch Ophthalmol* 1961; 66:111.

Jones TL: New concepts of orbital anatomy. Symposium on Plastic Surgery in the Orbital Region. Tessier P (eds). St. Louis, CV Mosby Co, 1976.

Le-Quang C: The cheek plexus of the facial nerve: Anatomy and clinical consequences. *Ann Chir Plast* 1976, 21:5. (in French)

Lodovici O, Psillakis JM: The upper orbito-palpebral sulcus in the oriental eyes. *Rev Paul Med* 1963; 62:257. (in Portuguese)

Marchac D: Relationship of the orbits to the upper eyelids. *Clin Plast Surg* 1981; 8:717.

Millard DR: Oriental Peregrinations. *Plast Reconstr Surg*, 1955; 16:319.

Mustardé JC, Jones TL et al: Ophthalmic Plastic Surgery – Up To Date. Birmingham: Alabama, *Aesculepius Publishing Company* 3-4, 1970.

Putterman AM, Urist MJ: Surgical anatomy of the orbital septum. *Ann Ophthalmol* 1974; 6:290.

Sayoc BT: Plastic construction of the superior palpebral fold. *Am J. Ophthalmol* 1954; 38:556.

Scherz W, Dohlman CH: Is the lacrimal gland dispensable? *Arch Ophthalmol* 1975; 93:281.

Siegel R: – Surgical anatomy of the upper eyelid fascia. *Ann Plast Surg* 1984; 13:263.

Smith B, Petrelli R: Surgical repair of prolapsed lacrimal glands. *Arch Ophthalmol* 1978; 96:113.

Warwick R: Eugene Wolff's Anatomy of the Eye and Orbit. ed 7. Philadelphia, Saunders Co, 1976.

Zide BM, and McCarthy J.Gr. et al: The medial canthus revisited – an anatomical basis for canthopexy. *Ann Plast Surg* 1983; 11:1

Zide BM, Jelks GW: *Surgical Anatomy of the Orbit*. New York, Raven Press, 1985.

Zubiri JS: Correction of the oriental eyelid. *Clin Plast Surg* 1981; 8:725.

2
Scleral Show

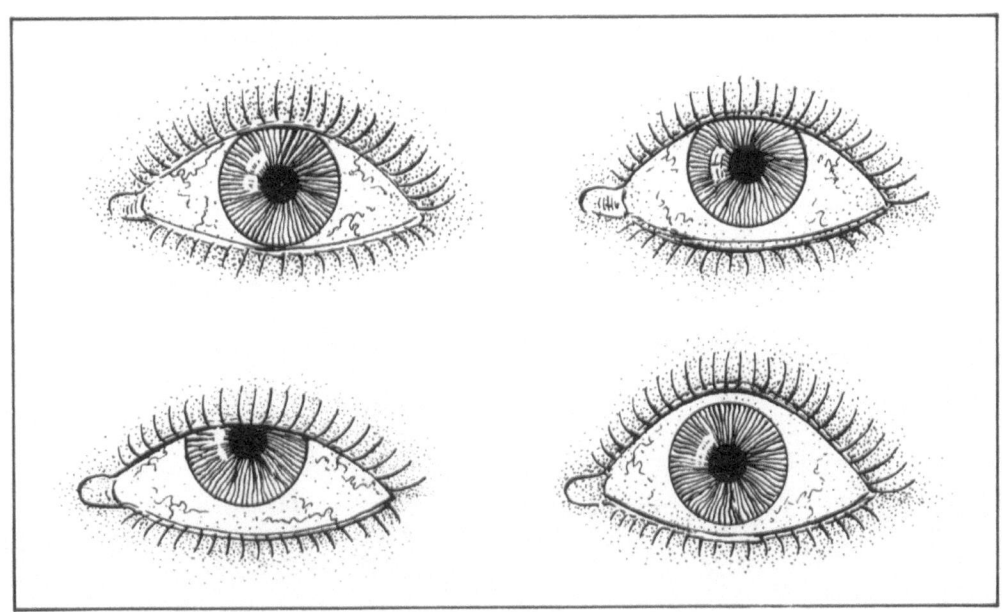

Introduction

The ocular globe is covered anteriorly by the eyelids, which, when closed, occlude the palpebral rim. When the lids are open to their normal position, the whole iris is visible through the cornea except for a small portion of its upper ciliary margin. The upper border of the lower lid is practically tangential to the lower ciliary margin of the iris, with no sclera showing between the two (Fig. 2.1A). At times the upper border of the lower lid can cover a portion of the iris (Fig. 2.1B).

When an area of the sclera is visible between the lower ciliary margin of the iris and the border

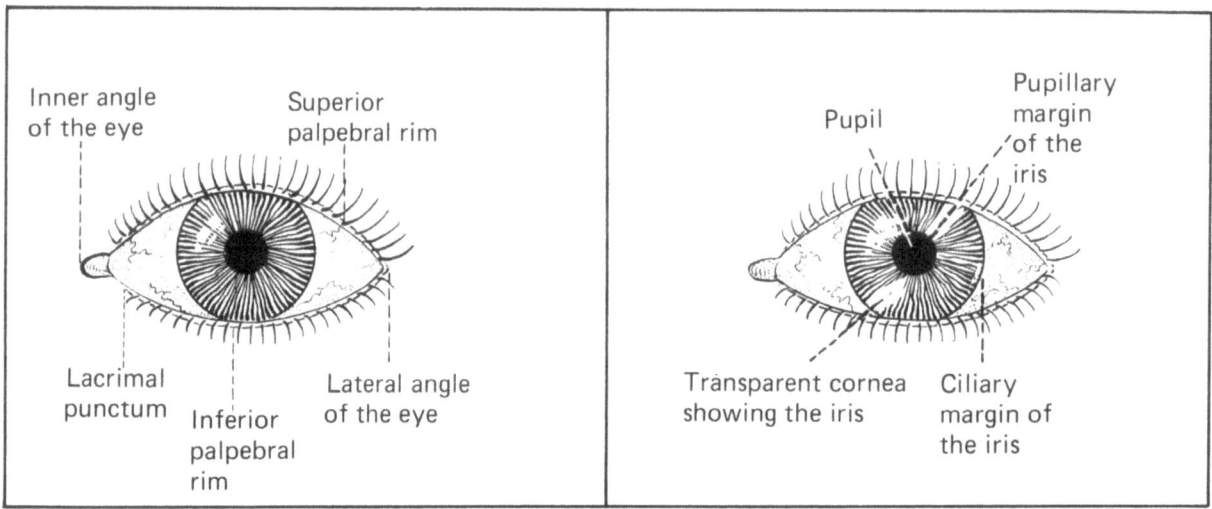

A   B

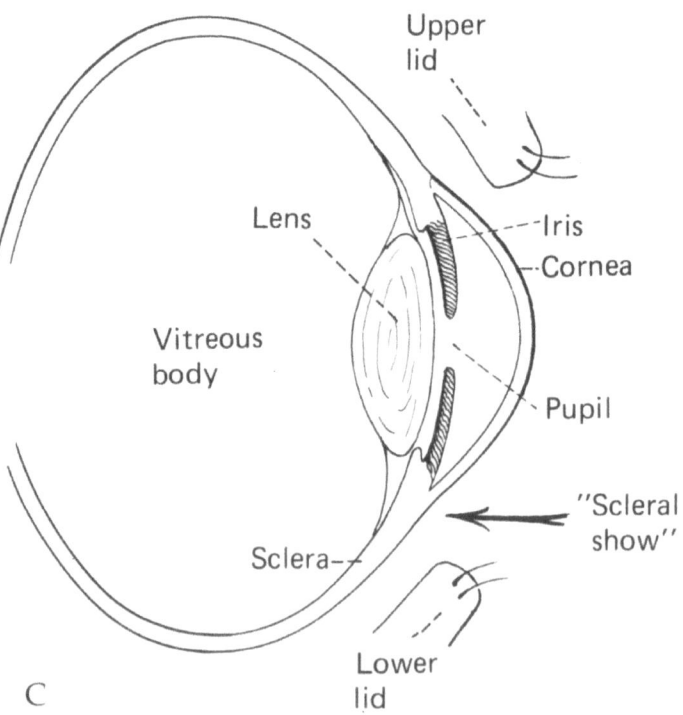

C

FIGURE 2.1. Details of palpebral and global anatomy. *A.* The lids. *B.* The globe. *C.* Saggital section of the globe and lids, demonstrating scleral show.

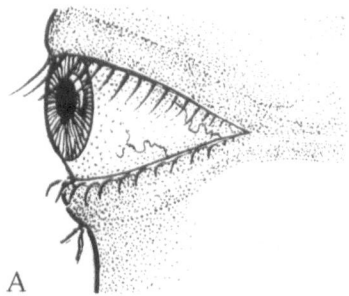

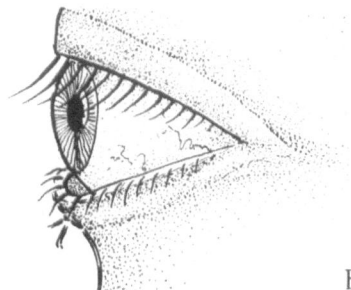

A

B

FIGURE 2.2. *A.* Scleral show. The palpebral border has been pulled caudally, but there is still contact between it and the global conjunctiva.

B. Ectropion. A somewhat greater force has been exerted on the palpebral border so that it has become everted.

of the lower lid, it is called "scleral show." The same term is used to describe an exaggerated amount of sclera visible above the iris or above the lateral third of the lower lid.

Although they have some details in common, scleral show should not be confused with ectropion. The word "ectropion" comes from the Greek *ektrepein,* meaning "to turn out," a condition that does not occur in scleral show (Fig. 2.2A). Obviously, in both these conditions there is an exaggerated amount of sclera visible in the lower portion of the globe, but only in ectropion is there an eversion of the lower lid (Fig. 2.2B).

This chapter details the condition of scleral show, its etiology, prevention, and treatment. We will also consider the anterior-posterior positioning of the ocular globe, as related to the lids, since its protrusion can cause scleral show.

Basic Differences Between Scleral Show and Ectropion

The ocular globe has little variation in size from individual to individual. What varies is the position of the lids in relation to the globe. Obviously, the basic difference between scleral show and ectropion is that in ectropion there is eversion of the lid, and in "scleral show" there is not. In addition, in ectropion there is epiphora or tearing because of lack of contact between the scleral conjunctiva and the lid. In scleral show, epiphora does not normally occur, and if it does, it is mild.

According to some authors, scleral show is the first stage of ectropion, the second stage being a slight eversion, and the third stage severe eversion, including the appearance of the fornix. We believe that scleral show cannot be categorically linked to ectropion, since the former can occur as an isolated condition – sometimes even of congenital origin – independent of any ectropion.

Patients can tolerate the presence of scleral show, since it is only an aesthetic problem and rarely causes alterations in the normal physiology of the lids or the globe. Ophthalmologists believe that even in patients with advanced myopia, despite proptosis, optical problems caused by an exaggerated exposure of the sclera rarely occur. It is only when the amount of sclera exposed is large enough to cause aesthetic problems that correction becomes necessary. In contrast, because of the eversion of the palpebral border, ectropion generally causes intolerable functional problems in addition to aesthetic distress. At times there is a natural improvement in the eversion, but the scleral show frequently remains, sometimes permanently.

Scleral show is curious. It can appear as a beautifying factor, as in the case of a person with large eyes. At other times it appears as a defect, with a display of excessive sclera and diverse asymetries. Of all the complications occurring as the result of a blepharoplasty, scleral show is one of the most complex because of its multiple causes, its questionable progress, and its poor response to treatment.

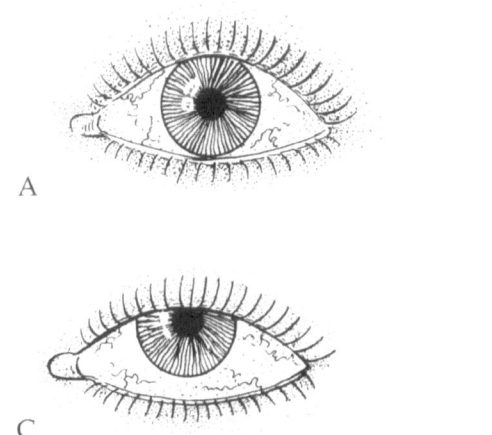

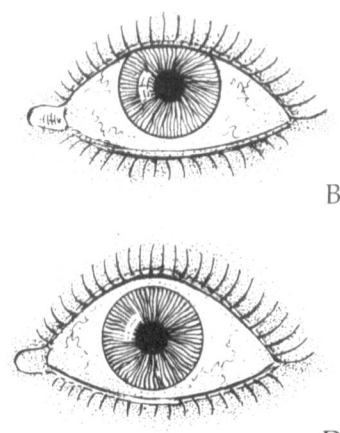

FIGURE 2.3. Variations in the positioning of the lids in relation to the ocular globe. *A.* Normal position. The upper border of the lower lid is practically tangential to the lower margin of the iris. *B.* Constitutional scleral show. This is not always a defect. The sclera is slightly visible below the lower limbus. *C.* Developmental scleral show. Because of the loss of tonicity of the orbicularis oculi muscle, there is some scleral show below the lower limbus and a slight ptosis of the upper eyelid, which covers part of the cornea and the upper ciliary margin of the iris. *D.* Endocrine scleral show. The sclera can be seen below the lower limbus and above the upper.

Etiology

Scleral show can be of constitutional, developmental, or endocrine origin. It can also occur iatrogenically (Fig. 2.3).

Candidates for a blepharoplasty who show signs of one of the three abnormal positions of the lids, as illustrated in Figure 2.3, run the risk of having the defect aggravated iatrogenically, and special care should be taken with such patients.

Scleral Show – Constitutional Origin

This is due to heredity and family characteristics and is not always considered a defect (Fig. 2.4). Persons with large eyes are usually cases of constitutional scleral show. This condition gives the impression that the lids are too small to contain the ocular globe (Fig. 2.5). It can also occur in young persons with congenital hypotonicity of the orbicularis oculi muscle. With aging the defect becomes more noticeable (Fig. 2.6).

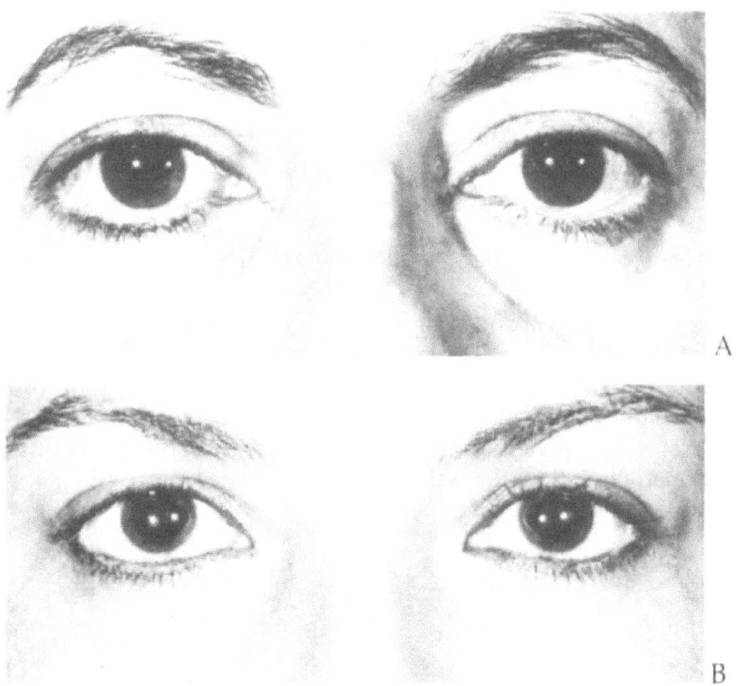

FIGURE 2.4. Slight constitutional scleral show. This is not always seen as a defect and may even be considered a mark of beauty by some.

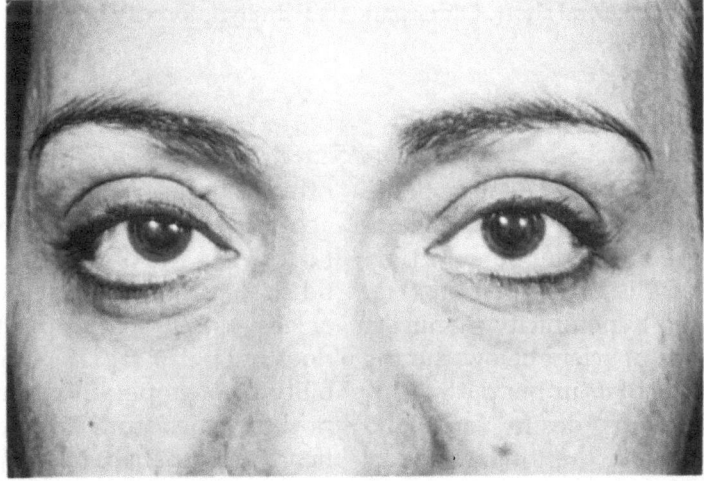

FIGURE 2.5. Constitutional scleral show in a patient with proptosis. This is an aesthetic defect.

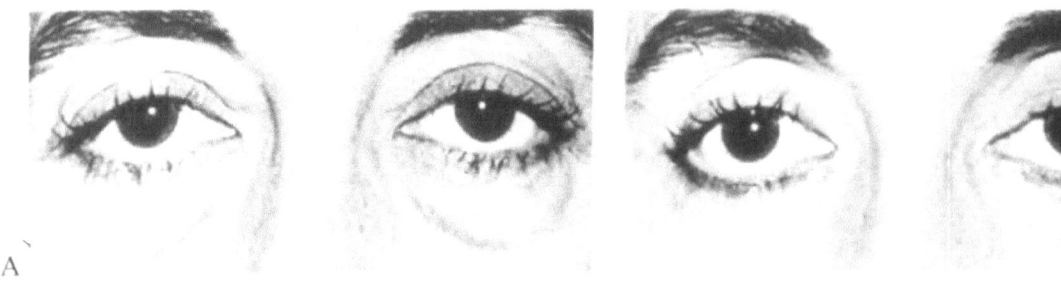

A   B

FIGURE 2.6. Serious constitutional scleral show iatrogenically aggravated by a wrongly performed blepharoplasty. The patient had "drooping eyelids" since infancy. There is blepharochalasis and marked fat pockets in the lower lids. *A.* Preoperative view. *B.* Postoperative view demonstrating that the scleral show was exacerbated, with unaesthetic results. (From Loeb R: Esthetic blepharoplasties with special reference to the ectropion of the lateral and central thirds of the lower lid. *Rev Col Brasileiro de Cirurgiões.* Sept-Oct, 1976, pp 177–187, Brazil; in Portuguese).

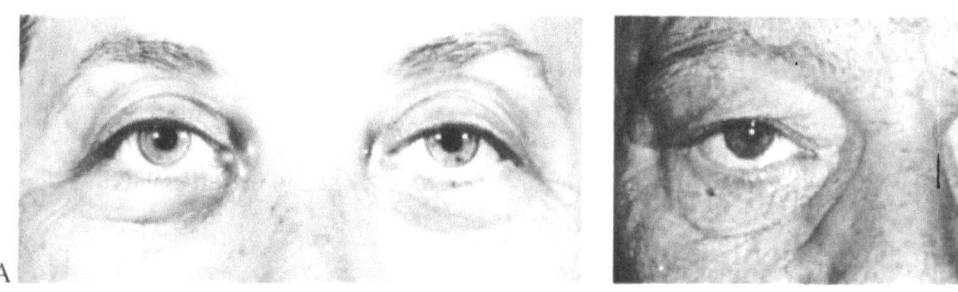

A   B

FIGURE 2.7. Developmental scleral show. Older patients with hypotonicity of the orbicularis oculi muscle.

Scleral Show – Developmental Origin

This type of scleral show is observed in patients with significant hypotonicity of the orbicularis oculi muscle, usually seen in older persons (Fig. 2.7) in whom the levator is also hypotonic (Fig. 2.8). In these cases the hypotonicity manifests itself in the appearance of sclera below the iris and by a partial covering of its upper part.

Elderly patients who desire aesthetic blepharoplasty should have the tonicity of the orbicular muscle tested before surgery. This is accomplished by pulling the border of the lower lid forward and down, and then releasing it. The lid should return rapidly to its normal position, at least within two or three blinks. If the recovery does not occur rapidly, one must face the possibility of postoperative scleral show. This prognosis is frustrating for the surgeon and is difficult for the patient to accept (Figs. 2.9 and 2.10).

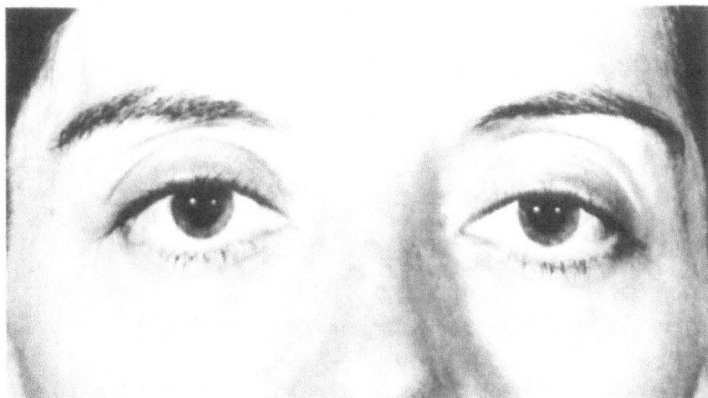

FIGURE 2.8. Developmental scleral show. This patient reported that her scleral show appeared with age.

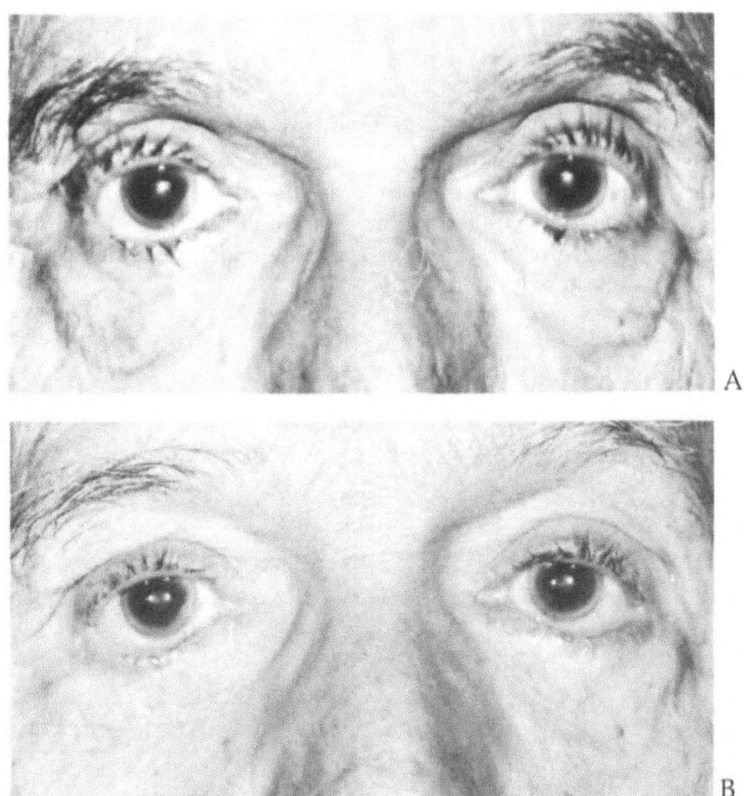

FIGURE 2.9. Slight exacerbation of scleral show after a blepharoplasty in an older person. The patient presented hypertrophied fat pockets and looseness of the lower lids. The upper lids did not show evidence of looseness, nor were there enlarged fat pockets – surprising findings in a man of 70. The sclera is very evident near the lateral angle of the eye above the lower lids. Because of the hypotonicity of the orbicularis oculi muscle characteristic of older persons, we considered this case to be at great risk if we were to resect tissue from the lower lids, given the possibility of exacerbation of the scleral show, or of causing ectropion. We reduced the fat pockets in the lower eyelids and performed a moderate skin ressection. A. Preoperative view. B. Postoperative view after reduction of the fat pockets and moderate skin resection of the lower lids.

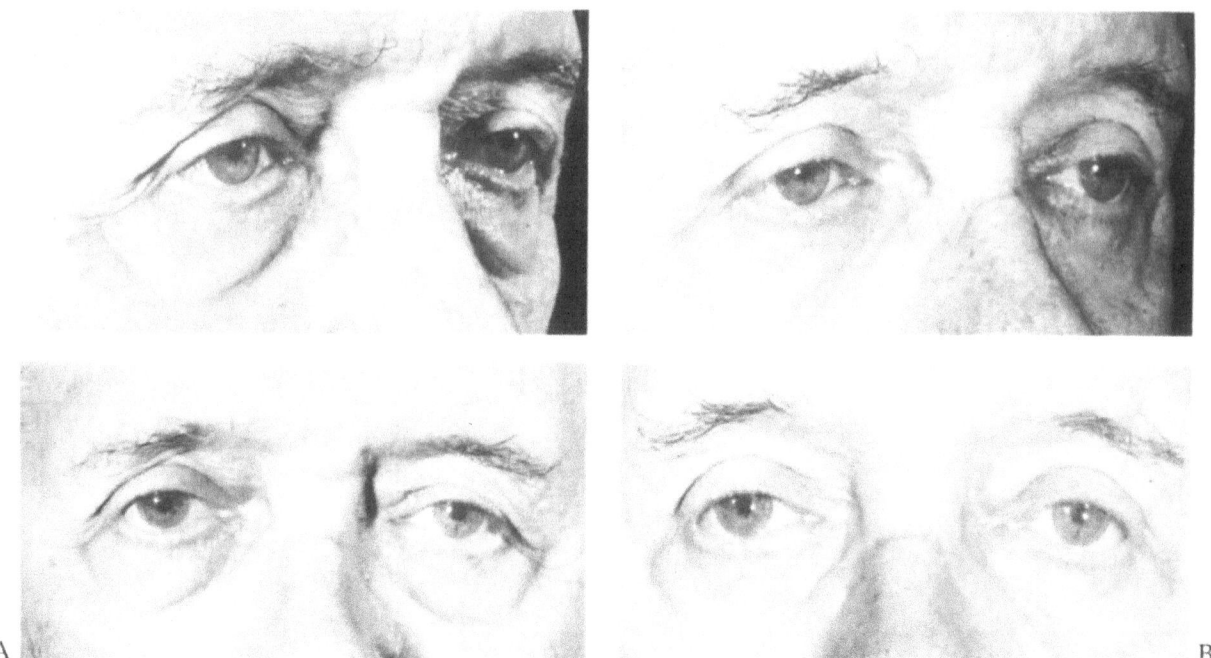

A   B

FIGURE 2.10. Elderly patient with skin looseness and hypertrophic fat pockets in both the upper and lower lids. *A.* Preoperative view. The senile drop of both lower palpebral rims is accentuated on the left side. *B.* Postoperative view after conservative resection of excess skin and fat. Observe that there is no increase in the distance between the lower palpebral border and the iris. A major drop in the lower palpebral border has also been avoided. In these cases one should eventually perform a blepharocanthoplasty next to the lateral angle of the eye.

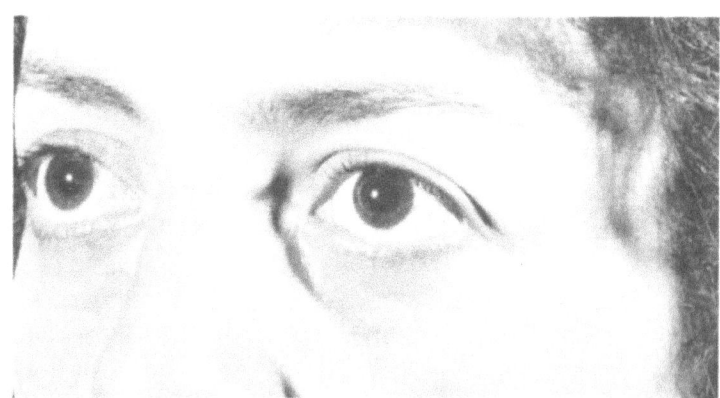

FIGURE 2.11. Endocrine scleral show. These cases do not always show sclera above the superior limbus, as demonstrated here. However, scleral show above the superior limbus is common in these endocrine cases.

Scleral Show – Endocrine Origin

A slight forward protrusion of the ocular globe, known as proptosis, can be an inherited family trait causing scleral show below the corneoscleral limbus.

However, this positioning of the globe can also be caused by hyperthyroid-related thyrotoxicosis (Fig. 2.11). In this condition there is

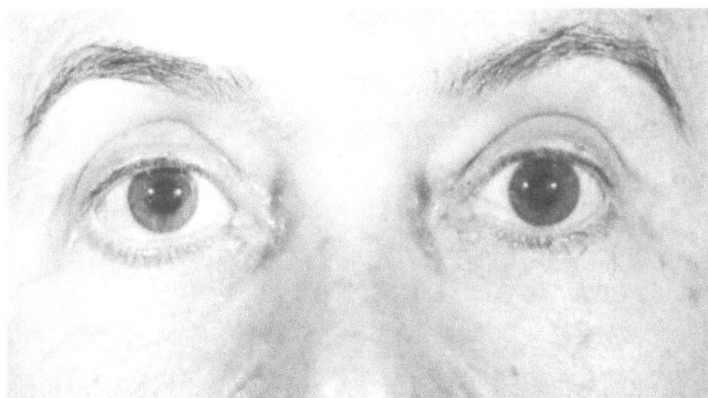

FIGURE 2.12. Patient with iatrogenic scleral show after an aesthetic blepharoplasty.

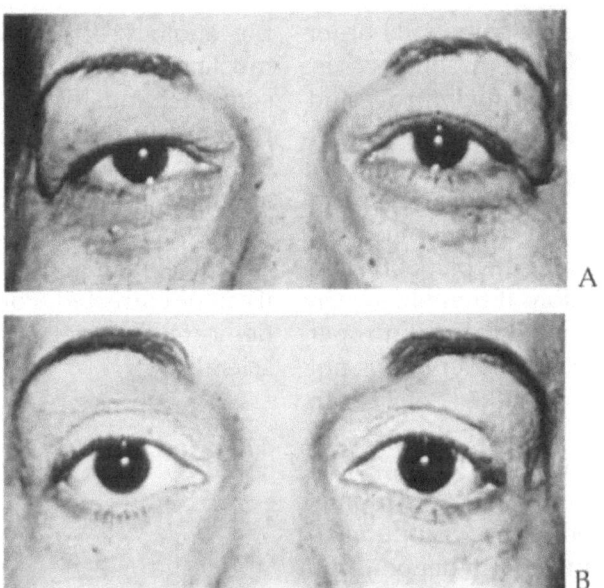

FIGURE 2.13. Iatrogenic scleral show subsequent to a blepharoplasty. *A.* Preoperative view. Patient presenting with wrinkles and palpebral pockets. *B.* Postoperative view. The wrinkles and palpebral pockets were corrected, but scleral show has appeared and is accentuated in the lateral third of the lower palpebral borders. (From Loeb R: Esthetic blepharoplasties with special reference to the ectropion of the lateral and central thirds of the lower lid. *Rev Col Brasileiro de Cirurgiões.* Sept-Oct, 1976, pp 177–187, Brazil; in Portuguese).

usually a spasm of the Müller's muscle and consequent retraction of the upper lid, causing scleral show above the limbus as well. Retrobulbar edema can occur in both hypo- and hyperthyroidism.

For all these reasons, great care must be taken with cases of scleral show of endocrine origin. Blepharoplasty on these patients is apt to further aggravate existing problems.

Scleral Show – Iatrogenic Origin

After a blepharoplasty, iatrogenic scleral show can range in severity from incipient to serious (Figs. 2.12 and 2.13). The possibility of such an occurrence is always present in those patients who show congenital developmental or endocrine tendencies for scleral show. The error is seen immediately after surgery, but is not

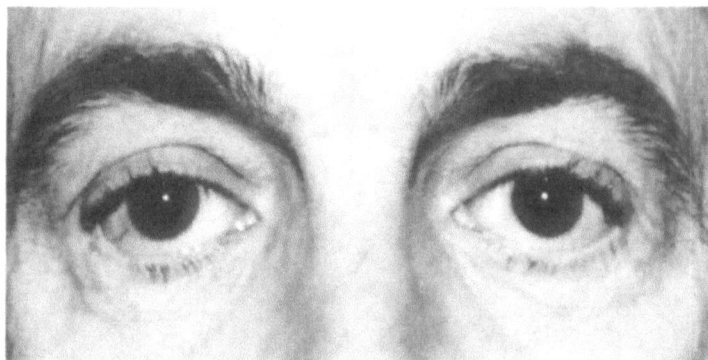

FIGURE 2.14. Iatrogenic scleral show subsequent to a blepharoplasty in patient without aparent tendency for scleral show. In this patient the defect appears extremely exacerbated.

always cause for alarm, since the defect can disappear spontaneously and the palpebral border return to its normal position. In some cases, however, the scleral show does not improve and can even become worse, depending on the cause of the problem (Fig. 2.14).

Iatrogenic scleral show will correct itself if it has been caused by edema or hematoma. With healing, these disappear, and the palpebral rim returns to its normal position. If there has been too much skin resected, or if there is improper suturing of the orbital fascia, recovery does not necessarily take place, and the defect can become permanent. Similarly, after exaggerated adipose or muscular resection, scleral show often appears and can become worse with time. The worsening is explained by the postoperative disappearance of the edema, which deepens the depression and pulls the lower lid down, causing a drop in the palpebral border. Damage to the zygomatic branch of the facial nerve, altough not common in blepharoplasty, can cause a reduction in or abscence of tonicity of the orbicularis oculi muscle and thus should not be rejected as a possible cause of scleral show.

It is surprising how unpredictable scleral show can be, and surgeons frequently ask themselves what could be causing or exacerbating it. It can occur even when marked resection of skin and fat has been avoided. We want to emphasize that in doing blepharoplasties, one must become accustomed to the difficulties that can arise, one after the other. It can sometimes seem that every routine step of blepharoplasty is a trap prepared for just this type of iatrogenicity.

One univeral trap is gravity, which is basic to the etiology of scleral show and ectropion. It must be treated as a major factor. It is always present, insidiously pulling the lid down whenever the head is upright. With any technical error on the part of the surgeon, gravity will promote or aggravate scleral show.

When faced with this defect, the surgeon will have to explain to the patient its cause, and how it can be corrected. For all these reasons, we have dedicated special attention to the problem of scleral show.

Prevention

In Chapter 3 we explain how scleral show can be avoided by judicious undermining and skin or skin-muscle resection. Also, in the analysis of fat and muscular bulges (pages 47 and 48), we demonstrate the criteria we use when performing these procedures.

Excessive skin resection during a blepharoplasty can cause scleral show. The undermining is more often performed using skin-muscle flaps, which are frequently initiated through a subciliary incision. With these incisions, the orbicularis oculi muscle is sectioned perpendicularly to the tarsal cartilage (Fig. 2.15A). The undermining continues caudally, above the tarsus, to the septal orbital fascia. The flap now includes the larger portion of the orbicularis oculi muscle, with only a small portion of it

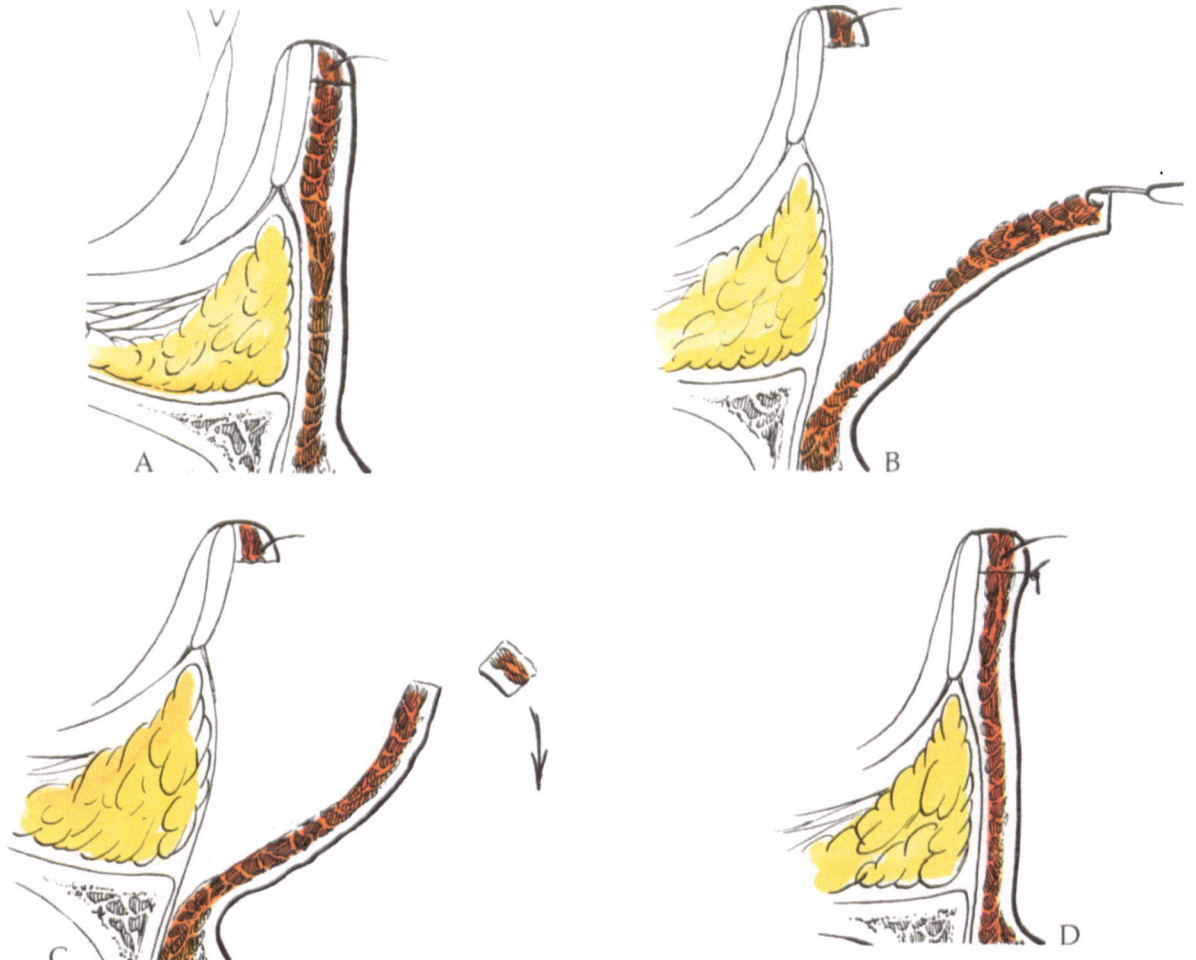

FIGURE 2.15. *A.* The orbicularis oculi muscle is sectioned perpendicularly through a periciliar incision, up to the tarsal cartilage. *B.* Because of its small size, the remaining portion of the orbicularis oculi muscle next to the palpebral border cannot maintain the tonus of the lid. *C.* The myocutaneous flap is shortened, but remains attached to the lower part of the palpebral tarsus. *D.* The shortened flap is elevated and returned to the pretarsal region, where it is sutured in contact with the remaining part of the orbicularis oculi muscle.

remaining at the palpebral border (Fig. 2.15B). The routine surgical steps that follow are the shortening of the undermined flap (Fig. 2.15C), and its elevation and reinsertion at its original site in the tarsal region (Fig. 2.15D).

It is apparent that the remaining pretarsal portion of the muscle of the palpebral border has reduced tonicity and therefore is not able to maintain the normal level of the border (Fig. 2.15).

Any traction, small as it may be, can cause scleral show at this point. No matter how careful the surgeon has been in resecting only a small amount of the flap, the weight of the attached flap itself, sutured in the tarsal portion, can provoke a traction. It should also be mentioned that this flap contains the orbicularis oculi muscle, which was formerly attached to the preseptal region, and whose capacity to contract has now been substantially reduced. All of these factors can act together to cause excess sclera to become visible in the middle third of the eye.

In view of the above, it must be emphasized that excessive reductions of the orbicular muscle from the tarsal portion of the lower lid can cause scleral show.

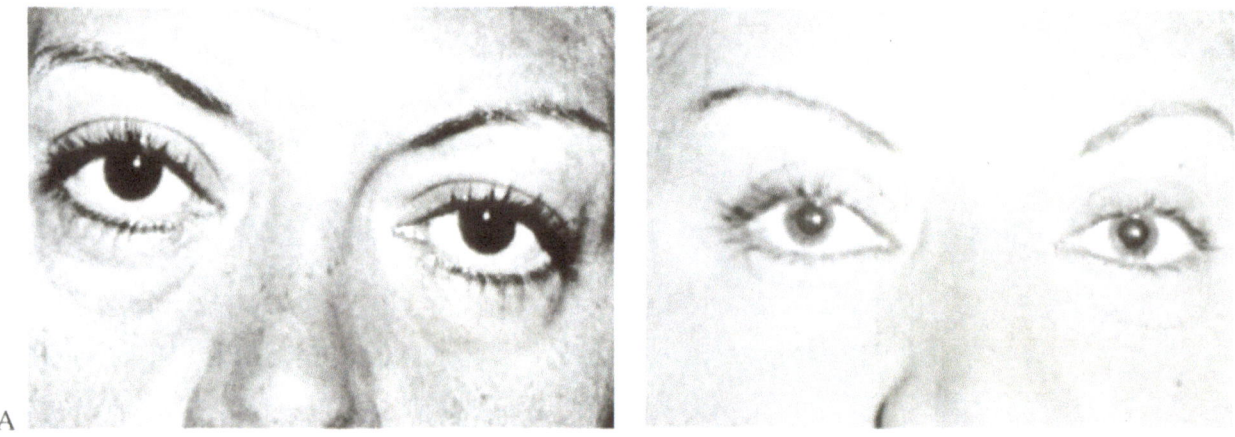

FIGURE 2.16. Reduction of scleral show by means of a temporal lift. This technique elevates the external angle of the eye, distending the tissue in the lateral third of the lids.

Treatment

When indicated, some extreme cases of scleral show can be treated secondarily. Some improvement can be obtained by means of a temporal lift (see Chapter 5, page 100 and 101), which increases the tension on the lower lid and elevates the lateral angle of the eye. Another technique is the division and suspension of the orbicularis oculi muscle. This reduces the opening of the palpebral rim by the elevation of the lateral third of the lid (Fig. 2.16) (Aston, 1980). A blepharocanthoplasty can be useful (Hinderer, 1975). Also, a wedge resection can be applied (Kuhnt and Szymanowski, 1948).

In some cases, correction must be done by the use of skin grafts similar to those used to repair an ectropion (Fig. 2.17).

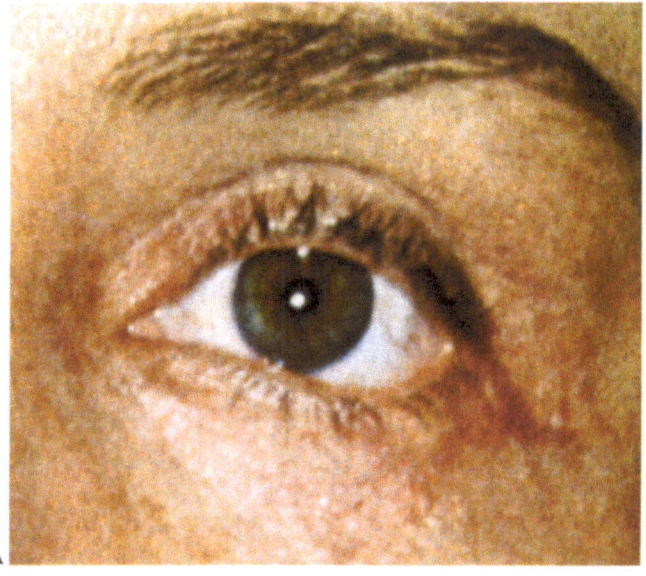

FIGURE 2.17. At times the exposed portion of the sclera is so large that its correction requires the use of free skin grafts as in repairing an ectropion. A. Preoperative view. B-C. Evidence of loss of cutaneous tissue. D. Free skin graft to close the raw area. E. Brown's dressing in place. F. Free graft integrated.

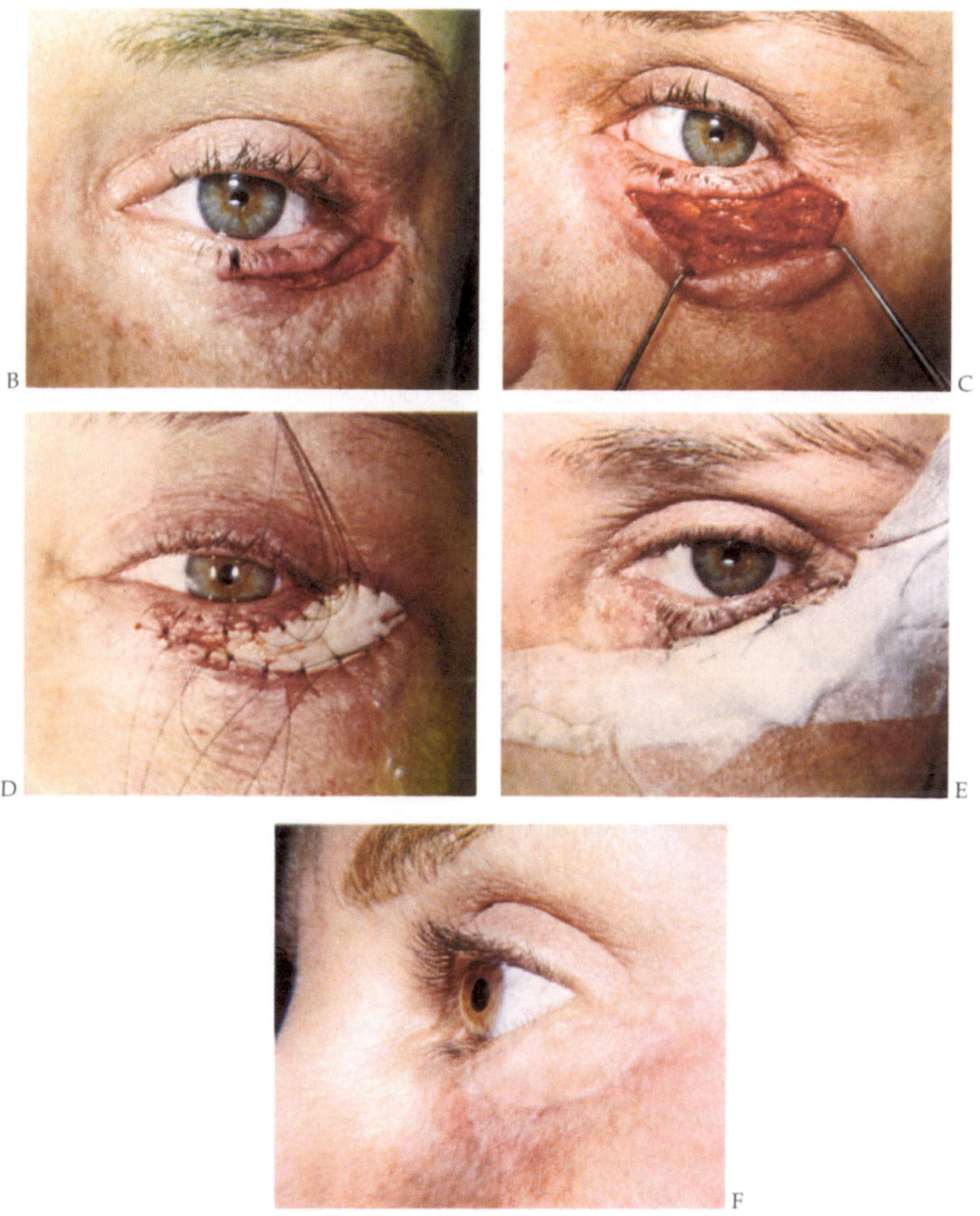

FIGURE 2.17

Additional Reading

ASTON SJ: Orbicularis oculi muscle flaps: A technique to reduce crow's feet and lateral canthal skin folds. *Plast Reconstr Surg,* 1980; 65:206.

BEYER CK, SMITH B et al: Ophthalmological aspects of blepharoplasty. *Eye Ear Nose Throat Mon* 1970; 49:242.

DHOOGHE P: Aesthetic blepharoplasty, ectropion and incipient ectropion. *Acta Chir Belg* 1978; 77:127.

EDGERTON MT: Causes and prevention of lower lid ectropion following blepharoplasty. *Plast Reconstr Surg* 1972; 49:367.

FOERSTER DW: A new method for tightening the orbicularis oculi muscles during blepharoplasty. *Aesthet Plast Surg* 1979; 3:265.

FOSATTI GH: Treatment of lower lid hipotonicity (a new procedure). *Rev Cir Plast Urug* 1967; 1:21. (in Spanish)

FRISHBERG IA: The technique of excision of surplus skin in eyelid of the ageing face. *Acta Chir Plast* 1976; 18,2:75.

KUHNT H and SZYMANOWSKY J: In Plastic and Reconstructive Surgery (p. 516–517) Padgett EC and Stephenson KL (ed) Springfield, Illinois, Charles C. Thomas, 1948.

LOEB R: Scleral Show. *Aesth Plast Surg* 1988; 12:165-170.

MACKINNON SE, FIELDING JC et al: The incidence and degree of scleral show in the normal population. *Plast Reconstr Surg* 1987; 80:15.

REES TD DUPUIS C: Cosmetic blepharoplasty in the older age group. *Ophthalmic Surg* 1970; 1:30.

SHORE JW: Changes in lower eyelid resting position, movement and tone with age. *Am J Ophthalmol* 1985; 99:415.

SMITH B, LISMAN RD: Cosmetic correction of Eyelid deformities associated with exophthalmos. *Clin Plast Surg* 1981; 8:777.

STASIOR OG: Complications of ophthalmic plastic and reconstructive surgery. *Trans Am Acad Ophthalmol Otolaryngol* 1976; 81:550.

TENZEL RR: Complications of Blepharoplasty. *Clin Plast Surg* 1981; 8:797.

3

Bulges of the Skin, Fat, Muscle, and Bone Tissue

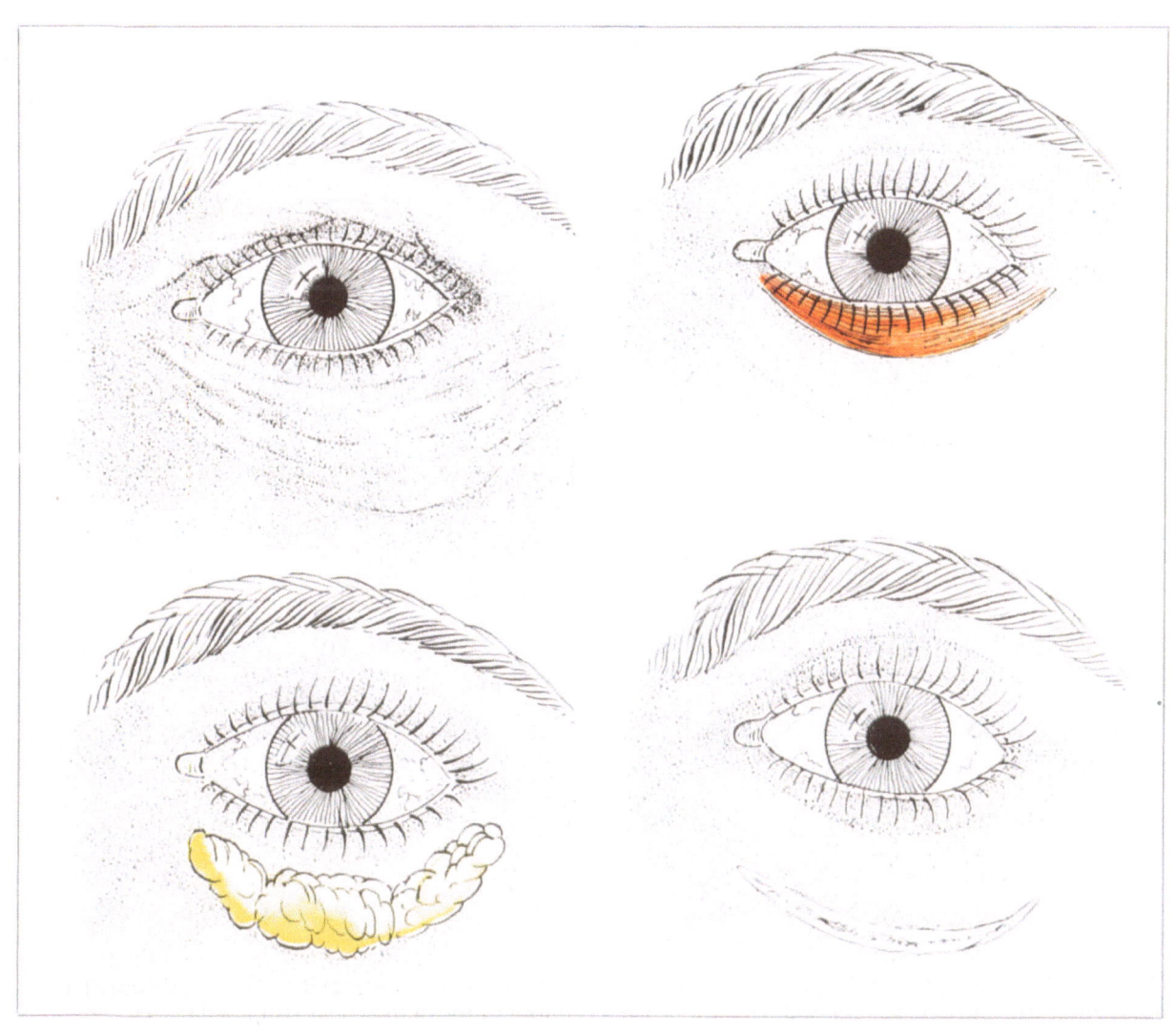

Introduction

Bulges in the eyelids, better known as baggy eyelids, can give a look of tiredness and/or aging to the face. They are very common occurrences and can exist at almost any age.

The bulges most commonly found are those caused by hypertrophy of the fat pockets. But there are also other types of bulges in the eyelids: those caused by excess of skin, of muscle, and of bony tissues (Fig. 3.1).

Each of these bulges has its own characteris-

tics, and each must be handled in its own specific manner. But all the treatments involve the adequate reduction of whatever excess volume is found. The diagnoses that differentiate between these various types of bulges should be quite precise: improper techniques subsequent to bad diagnoses can result in iatrogenesis. A complete understanding of the subject and of the therapeutic indications is essential. The following classification is proposed:

1. Skin bulges (looseness)
2. Fat bulges

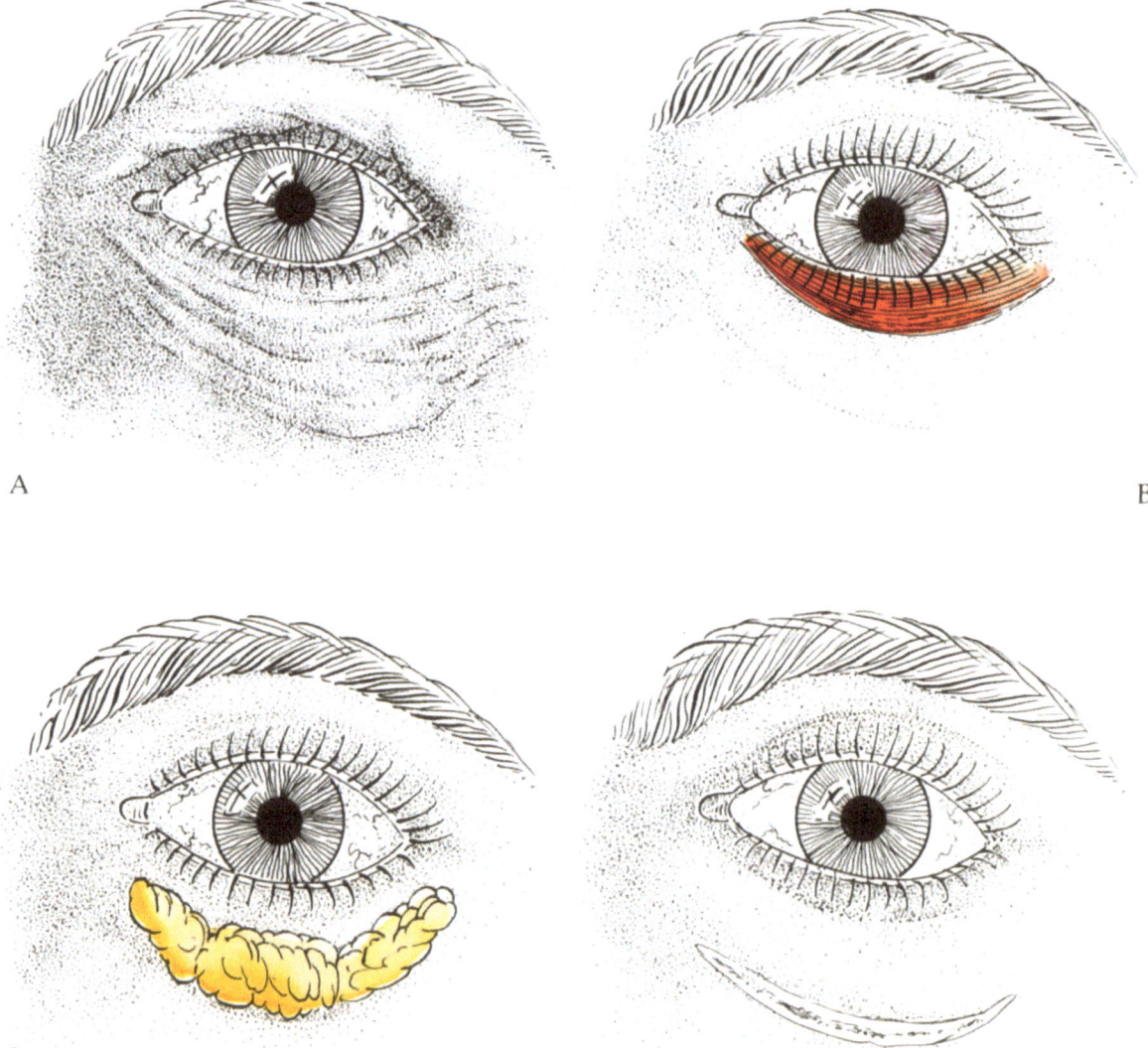

A

B

C

D

FIGURE 3.1 The four types of bulges: *A*. Cutaneous, occupying the surface of the lid. *B*. Muscular, localized in the pretarsal portion. *C*. Adipose, in the septal portion. *D*. Bony, at the level of the medial and central thirds of the lower palpebral border.

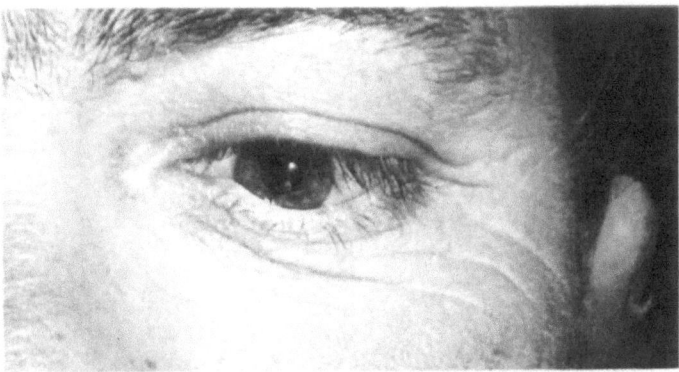

FIGURE 3.2. Typical case of loose skin.

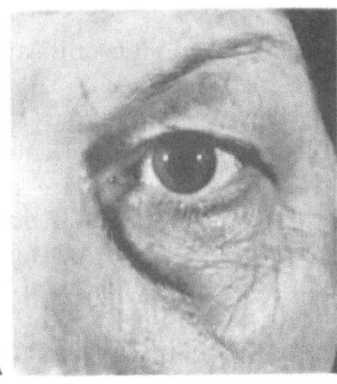
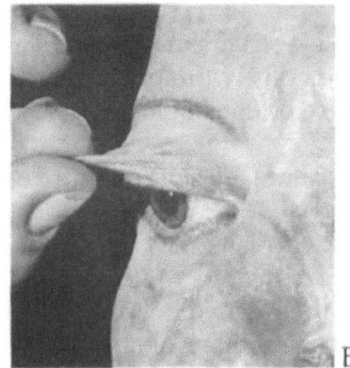

A   B

FIGURE 3.3. Skin looseness in both the upper and lower lids. *A.* Gravity has formed festoons. Those of the upper lids have formed "curtains" in front of the ocular globe. Those of the lower lid are not only in the tarsal but also in the septal portion. *B.* The palpebral

skin is pinched between the thumb and forefinger and pulled forward. One can thus evaluate the excess skin and test its tension and the slackness of the orbicularis oculi muscle.

3. Muscular bulges
4. Bony bulges

Two or three of these bulges can be found simultaneously in the same individual. When this happens, they all should be treated in one surgical procedure. However, it is also possible to find only one of the above types of bulges in a patient, for instance, the fat bulges in a young patient who does not yet show skin looseness. In this case, after making the diagnosis, the problem is resolved by the removal of the excess fat alone.

Care should be paid to the influence that the resection of one type of bulge can have on another type. For example, an exaggerated fat resection can cause the appearance of what was previously only an incipient muscular bulge.

Skin Bulges (Looseness)

General Considerations

Looseness of the skin of the eyelids can sometimes be great enough that it appears as bulges. This slackening of the skin (Fig. 3.2) can also include part of the orbicularis oculi muscle and may be located in both tarsal and septal portions of the lid. Sometimes the slackening is great enough to be confused with underlying fat or muscle hypertrophy. Skin looseness can range from light undulations to large cutaneous waves or festoons (Furnas, 1978) (Fig. 3.3A).

Bulges caused by loose skin can easily be grasped between the thumb and the forefinger and pulled forward without causing ectropion,

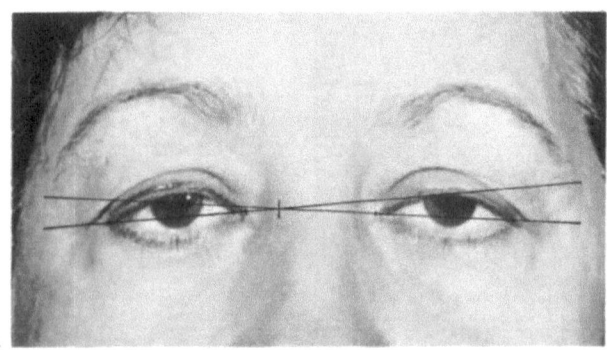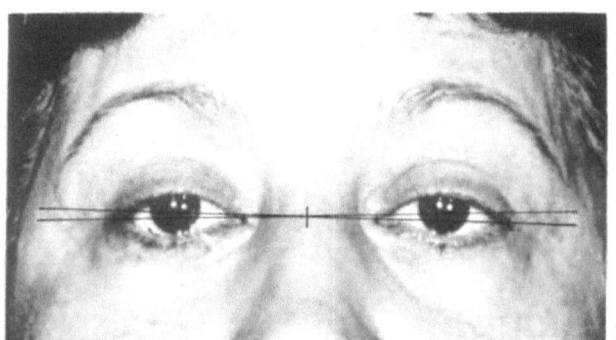

A   B

FIGURE 3.4. Patient approximately 50 years old presenting with blepharochalasis. *A.* Preoperative view. *B.* Postoperative view after resection of excess palpebral tissue.

indicating that there is a true skin excess (Fig. 3.3B). Fat and muscle bulges cannot be treated in this manner because of their tight fixation to the subjacent tissues.

Wrinkling is the most notable consequence of skin looseness of the eyelid. At times the wrinkles can be deep enough to cause an appreciable fold across the lid. Correction is routine, being one of the first procedures that young plastic surgeons perform (Gonzales-Ulloa and Stevens, 1967). Both the beginning and the experienced plastic surgeon handle and treat excess palpebral skin in their daily practice. Before learning the details of fat and muscular resections, and certainly before placing fat grafts into the lids, the neophyte learns how to correct looseness and wrinkles. The widespread use of these procedures is the reason for the detailed study here.

Etiology

The amount of looseness of the skin of the eyelids is a developmental phenomenon and varies with the patient's heredity and way of living. It begins with tiny, almost imperceptible wrinkles that are accentuated with age, sometimes becoming skin folds or true bulges.

Looseness of the upper eyelids is called "blepharochalasis" by many (Panneton, 1936), and has been used to describe various degrees of looseness. The word "blepharochalasis" comes from the Greek, meaning "relaxation of the

eyelids,"* and it is quite appropriate and widely accepted (Fig. 3.4).

Individuals suffer different degrees of blepharochalasis, depending on the quality of their skin. Some can expose themselves regularly to the sun without suffering consequences, while others, even youngsters, may have early wrinkles with little exposure (Rees, 1980). One thing is certain: Over the long term, skin abuse from the action of solar rays produces cutaneous scleroses and damages the skin's elasticity and appearance. In addition, excessive exposure results in exaggerated contractions and relaxations of the eyelid muscles, making the skin act like an accordion and contributing to the formation of those lateral extensions called "crow's-feet."

Hypermotility of the facial musculature can also be harmful, as in the case of persons with very expressive faces or of nearsighted persons who contract the orbicularis oculi muscle tightly to improve their vision (Furnas, 1981).

In some individuals, palpebral wrinkles are less common because the greater development of the zygomatic and malar areas causes a nota-

---

* We should emphasize, however, that in reality, true blepharochalasis is rare and of obscure etiology. It is characterized by a group of factors: loss of the normal elasticity of the upper eyelids, causing ptosis; extreme looseness of the septum orbitale; and herniation of the fat pockets, which become integrated with the ptotic tissue. Also associated is edema and telangiectasia.

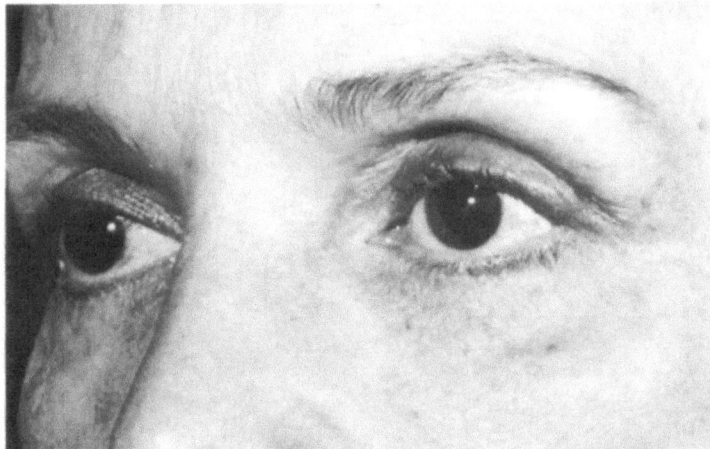

FIGURE 3.5. Patient approximately 50 years old with well-developed zygomatic and malar bone structure, making palpebral looseness less noticeable.

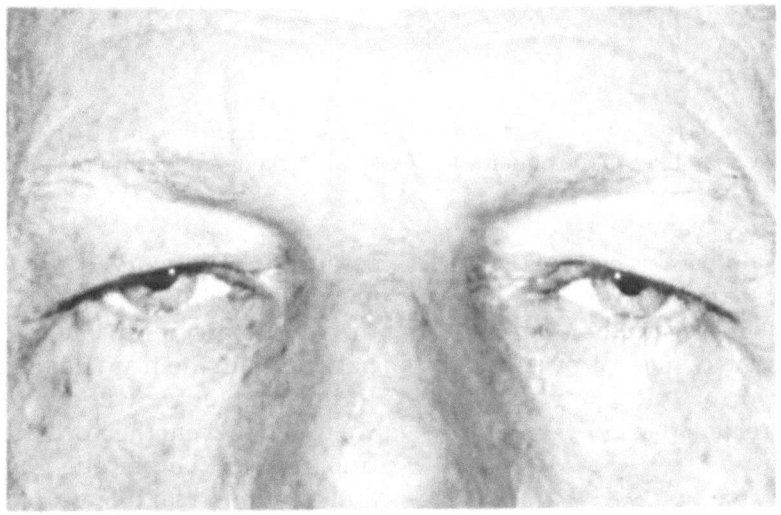

FIGURE 3.6. Palpebral pseudoptosis. In these cases the looseness of the upper lids can even reach the iris, covering the visual field and interfering with vision.

ble distension of the tissue of this region (Fig. 3.5). Other individuals do not have this enhanced bone structure, and the skin of the eyelids tends to wrinkle more rapidly because of lack of sufficient support.

Because of the opening and closing of the palpebral rim by the action of the levator and orbicularis oculi muscles, there are vertical movements in the upper lids that contribute greatly to the looseness of the septal portion (Gordon, 1951). In the lower lids, these vertical movements are accompanied by oblique motions that move the tissues in a medial direc-

tion. During exaggerated contractions, these oblique movements can reach intensities equivalent to the vertical contractions, thus accounting for the oblique slant of the wrinkles of the lower lids. The contractions of the orbicularis oculi muscle have great influence on the etiology of the looseness of the skin of the lids because of the intimate connections of the muscle with the palpebral skin.

In extreme cases the excess skin in the upper eyelids can cover the pretarsal area, even hiding the lashes. This can reduce the visual field, interfering with ocular function (Kahn, 1934). In

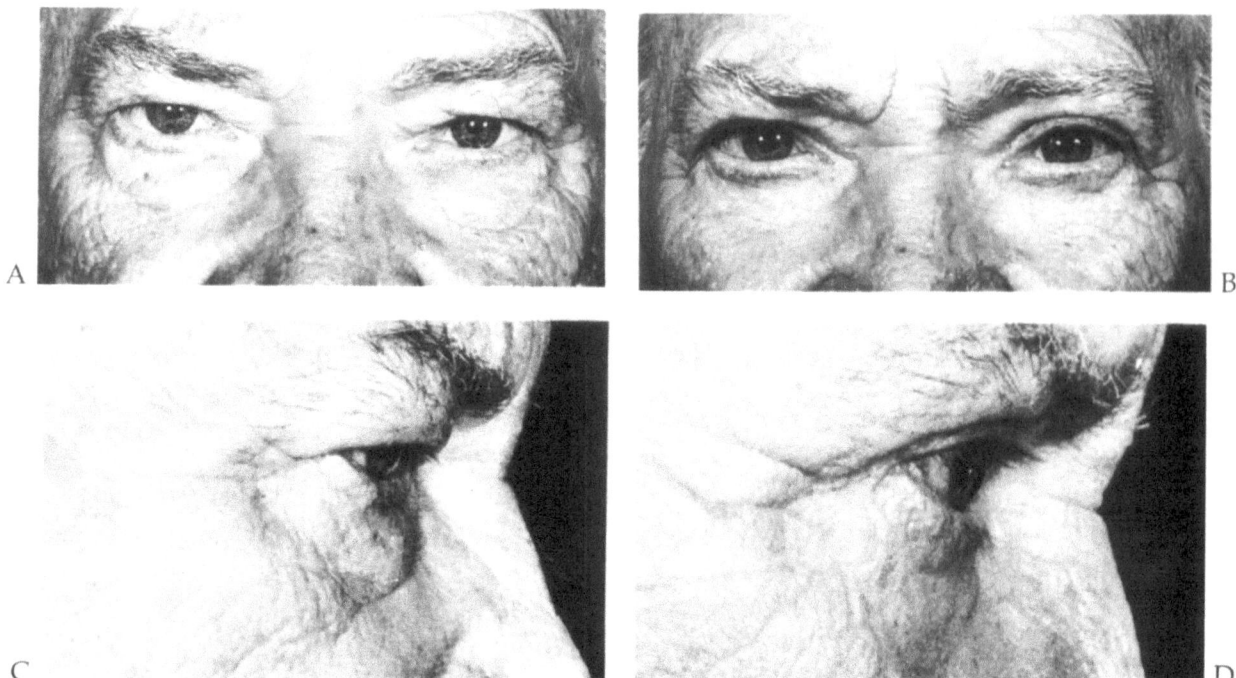

FIGURE 3.7. Blepharochalasis (palpebral pseudoptosis). These cases have benefitted greatly by an adequate tissue resection. *A-B*. Preoperative and postoperative views. *C-D*. Preoperative and postoperative views.

these cases a pseudoptosis[+] is created (Fig. 3.6). A patient with this condition, in order to see properly, must either elevate the eyebrows by contracting the frontal muscle, or throw his head back. A resection of the excess tissue generally resolves this problem (Fig. 3.7).

Treatment

Most cases of looseness of the eyelids can be corrected in the eyelids themselves, using variable incisions followed by appropriate underminings and resections. In this manner, wrinkles can be corrected and the depth of important folds, such as the upper palpebral and nasojugal, can be reduced (Converse, 1964).

Although these procedures may be well standardized, errors of calculation can occur in the

resections. The worst consequences are scleral show and ectropion. In our practice we have managed largely to avoid these, although patients with them are frequently referred to us. In this chapter we will demonstrate the details we use to prevent their occurrence. These procedures should be preceded by careful planning and cautious marking to reduce any possible margin of error.

In some cases, in order to eliminate palpebral looseness completely, it is necessary to perform such extrapalpebral procedures as peelings and brow liftings (Baker, 1962). These are discussed in Chapter 5.

Preoperative Care and Planning

Although the patients preoperative examination and test findings may be normal, with a good prognosis, the possibility of complications during a blepharoplasty cannot be discarded, and many precautions are necessary before the surgery begins.

All routine surgery is planned with great care. Important details are noted in the patient's file,

---

[+] Pseudoptosis should not be confused with true ptosis, in which the palpebral border droops because of paralysis of cranial nerve III. We will not deal with this subject here, as it has been studied extensively by others.

along with preoperative photographs and diagrams. This document should be present in the operating room and easily available during surgery.

The success of the blepharoplasty will depend on careful patient examination, an analysis of his/her medical history, and a thorough planning of every procedure.

Anesthesia

Regardless of the patient's preference for local or general anesthesia, the surgeon must decide the type most suited to the individual case, based on the patient's physical and mental state. We generally find local anesthesia with sedation (preferably with an anesthetist) to be adequate, even for cases of hypertrophic fat pockets that require deep dissection. The type of anesthesia, however, should be adequate for the particular case. For instance, for skin resections only, we just use local anesthesia.

Premedication

We ask the patient to take 10 mg of diazepam nightly for two days before the operation. About an hour before surgery, an appropriate intramuscular injection of meperidine, atropine, and an antipyretic is given.

Sedation

Sedation is always a complement to the local anesthesia given by the surgeon. The patient comes to the operating room having already received his preanesthesia medication. Serum is transfused intravenously. There is continuous ECG monitoring and blood pressure it taken frequently. The anesthetist administers a dilute amnestic tranquilizer, (medayepam), and a morphinetype analgesic, (fentanyl, meperidine, or innovar), intravenously in small controlled doses.

At times, small intravenous doses of anesthetic are administered when giving local anesthesia by infiltration. The anesthetist should be careful not to depress respiration. Swallowing of the tongue can be avoided by the use of a pharyngeal cannula or, better yet, by traction on a transfixed suture in the tip of the tongue.

Sedation should always be such that the patient remains calm and can respond to requests to open or close the eyes, to breathe deeply, or to complain of pain when further anesthesia becomes necessary. The progress of the sedation should be planned so that at the end of the surgery the patient is able to care for him/herself.

Local Anesthesia

We initiate local anesthesia with an insulin needle, followed by a larger gauge. We use 1% or 2% Xylocaine, diluted in accordance with the patient's preoperative cardiovascular evaluation. In patients with a history of high blood pressure, we use adrenaline very conservatively, or avoid it completely. We also use local anesthesia when the patient is under general anesthesia, and intubation if the anesthetist finds it advisable.

We believe that local anesthesia is ideal for a blepharoplasty because it facilites the detection of possible future occurrences of scleral show or ectropion: The patient can be asked to raise his/her head so that gravity will exert its pull on the lids, and then asked to open and close the lids. If sedation is deeper than usual, or if general anesthesia is being used, the surgeon, or another member of the operating team, can raise the patient's head.

In highly emotional patients with a history of variable blood pressure, we use local anesthesia with stronger sedation, controlled by the anesthetist.

General Anesthesia

For those patients with a record of variable blood pressure, as well as for those with a background of tachycardia or arrhythmia, we request that an anesthetist be present, and we use general anesthesia with the patient intubated.

The preparation for general anesthesia is the same as that for a local: ECG monitorization, frequent blood pressue readings and the injection of an amnestic and a hypnotic, (midazolam, medoyepam, etc) and of an analgesic (fentanyl).

We use an intravenous anesthetic (thiopental sodium, hypnomidate, or midazolam), followed by curarization with succinylcholine. After manual respiration with a mask and oxygen, a dis-

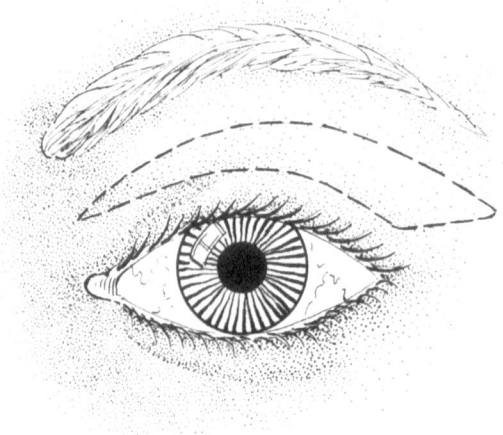

FIGURE 3.8. Preoperative markings for incisions in the preseptal portion.

posable balloon catheter is placed in the trachea and mechanical breathing is initiated. Anesthesia is maintained with oxygen, nitrogen protoxide, and an inhalant (halothane, enflurane, etc). Curarization is maintained with a (depolarizing) agent, such as pancuronium or alcuronium.

After surgery atropine, neostigmine, and, at times, an antimorphinic (naloxone), is given, and the patient is taken to the recovery room for careful observation.

Markings

Using an indelible pen or pencil, the markings are placed exactly where the incisions will be made. They should enclose the surface to be resected within the limits of the preseptal portion, since the resulting scar must coincide with the supratarsal fold (Fig. 3.8).

In the lower lid the markings are placed only where the incisions will be made. The area to be resected is *not* marked, since this can only be determined after the undermining has been completed.

Surgical Steps

There are three principal surgical steps: incision, resection and suturing. In addition, in the lower lid only, undermining is performed.

Incisions

The incisions should result in scars that are undetectable or nearly so. The following principles should be followed: (1) Vary the level of the incision line, (2) avoid making the incision inside a principal sulcus (this is just for the lower lids), and (3) observe details at the extremities of the incision.

Vary the Level of the Incision. In the lower lids it is necessary to vary the distance that separates the incision line from the palpebral rim according to the requirements of each patient. We rarely use a rim incision (Fig. 3.9), since it favors scleral show and ectropion. We prefer to place it approximately 1.5 mm below the lash implantation, thus reducing the traction on the rim (Fig. 3.10).

When the looseness of the eyelids reaches as far as the cheek and malar regions (Fig. 3.11A), it is advisable to place the incision even lower (Converse, 1964), putting it between the lower palpebral and the nasojugal sulci (Figs. 3.11B and 3.12). This type of incision can, however, favor a postoperative swelling of the septal portion. Such a swelling absorbs very slowly, so the incision is rarely used. In these cases we prefer to use the technique of prolonging the incision laterally (See page 49).

Avoid Placing the Incisions Inside One of the Principal Sulci. When a scar matures, it contracts.

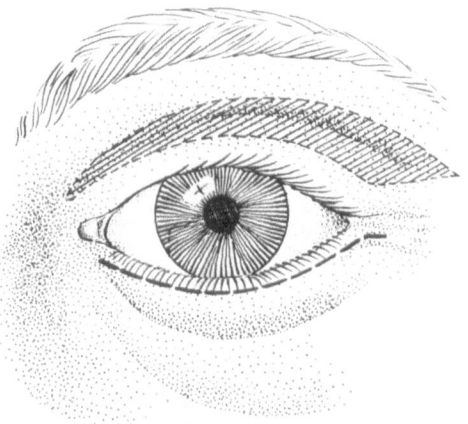

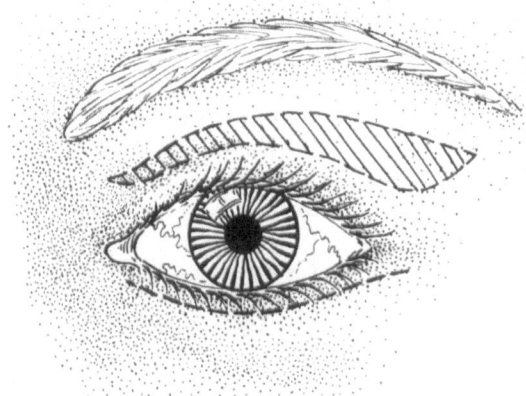

FIGURE 3.9. Rim incision in the lower lid. We rarely use this type of incision because there is a great risk of postoperative scleral show and/or ectropion.

FIGURE 3.10. Preferred incision in the lower lid. Because it is approximately 1.5 mm below the rim, the possibility of scleral show and/or ectropion is reduced.

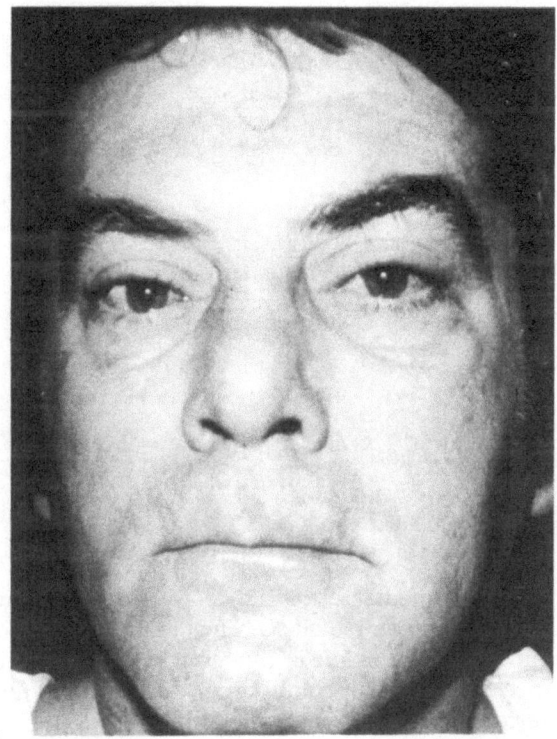

A

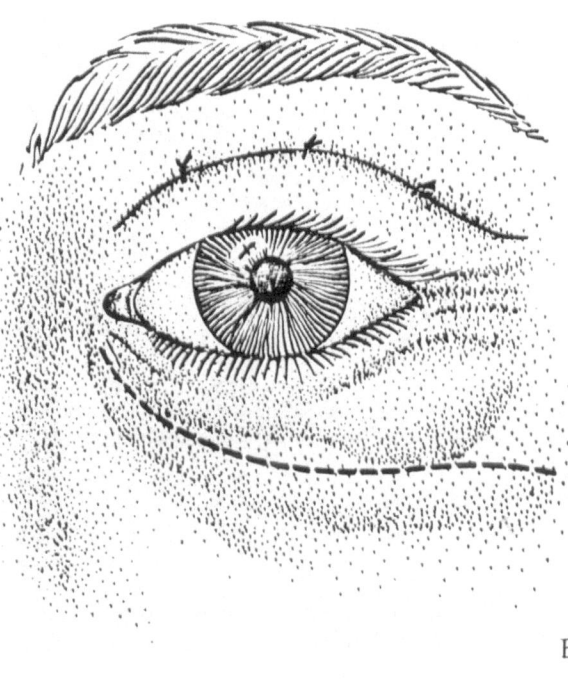

B

FIGURE 3.11. The low incision. *A.* In some patients the looseness of the lower palpebral skin can reach as far as the cheek and malar areas. In these cases we use a low incision. If this is deemed inadvisable because of the possibility of marked postoperative swelling we use the prolonged incision shown in Fig. 3.32 *B.* The low incision is placed below the lower palpebral sulcus in a line parallel to one of the fine wrinkles of the area. This incision is rarely used.

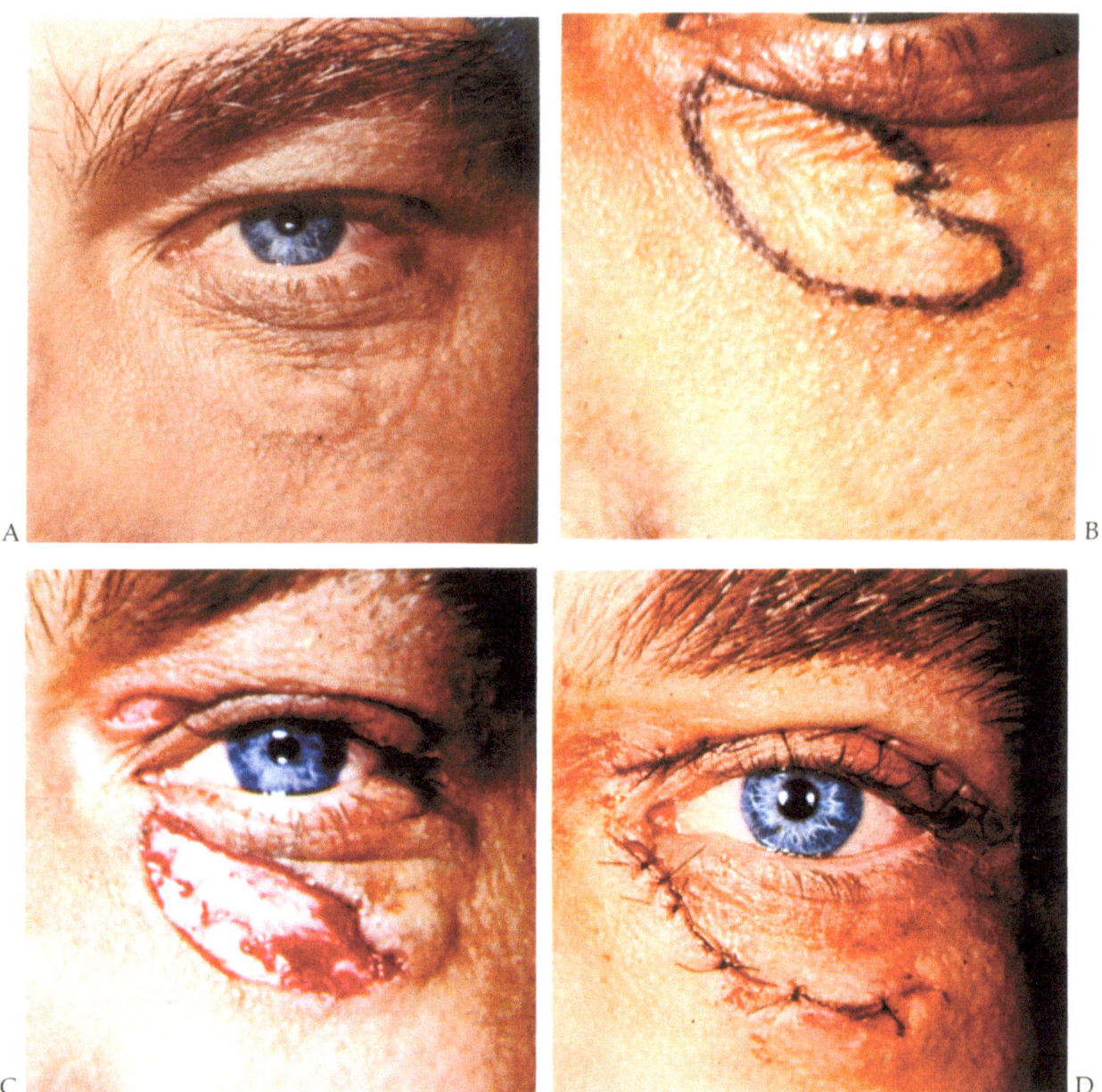

FIGURE 3.12. The low incision. A contribution to the standardization of skin resection. This case of extensive resection of a xanthelasma served to convince us that the use of a wide preseptal skin resection using a low incision would not result in scleral show or ectropion. *A.* Xanthelasma occupying all of the central and medial thirds of the lower lid. *B.* Closeup. *C.* Resection completed. *D.* Final suturing. The tension on the suture line is great, but because of its distance from the palpebral border, there is little force exerted there. There is no scleral show.

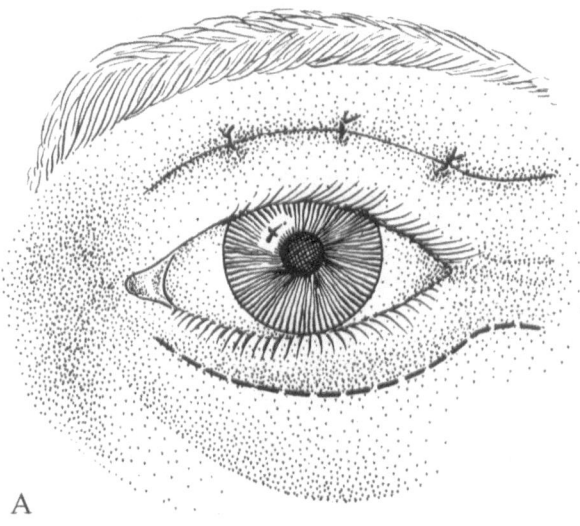

A   B

FIGURE 3.13. In the lower lids, incisions that coincide with the principal sulci should be avoided. *A.* Erroneous incision coinciding with the lower palpebral sulcus. *B.* Erroneous incision coinciding with the nasojugal sulcus.

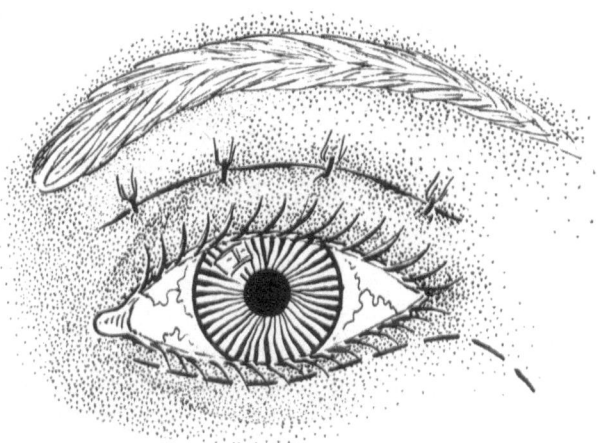

FIGURE 3.14. A downward-pointing incision in the lateral portion of the lower lid, giving a sad expression to the eye. *We do not recommend this type of incision.*

Such a contraction at the bottom of a sulcus will therefore tend to deepen it (Fig. 3.13). To avoid accentuating these, we prefer to place the incisions parallel to, either above or below, any sulcus.

Observe Details at the Extremities of the Incisions. The most important of these details are:

1. Do not allow the medial and lateral extremities of the incisions to extend downward too much. The scars that result from a downward pointing incision can confer a look of sadness on the face. There is considerable disagreement among authors as to the direction of the lateral extension of the incision in the lower eyelid. Some feel that to avoid "dog ears," it should point sharply down, in a malar direction (Fig. 3.14). *We are not in agreement with this.*

We manage to avoid the "ears" by extending the lateral excision parallel to the long axis of the rim of the palpebra, but not heading caudally at the lateral end (Fig. 3.17). In the medial portion, a downward slant also is con-

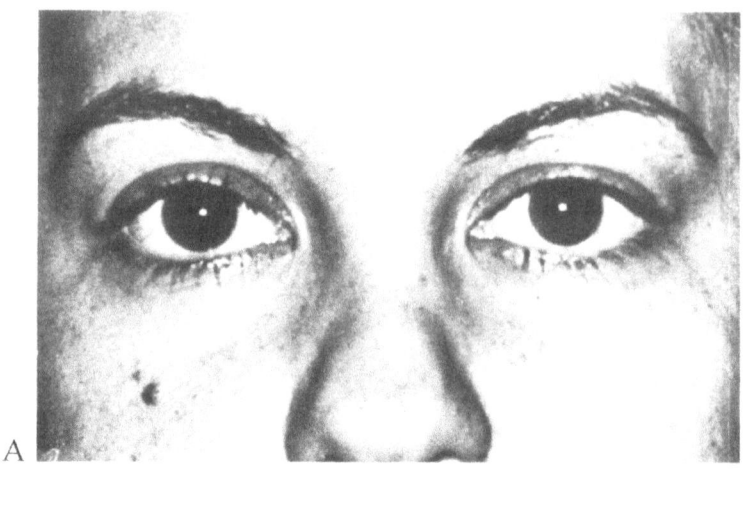

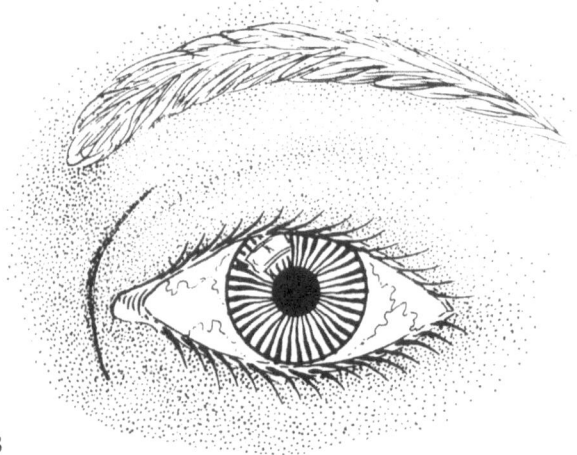

FIGURE 3.15. *A.* Patient presenting with epicanthus. *B.* Diagram showing a slight epicanthus connecting the upper and lower lids. Care should be taken during a blepharoplasty not to exacerbate this.

traindicated, particularly when there is a preoperative tendency to epicanthal fold, since the resulting scar can exacerbate this fold (Fig. 3.15). For this reason, the incision should have its mesial extremity directed upward, so as not to coincide with the fold (Fig. 3.16).

2. Separate the extremities of the upper and lower incisions from each other. The lateral portions of the upper and lower incisions should be a minimum of 1 cm apart (Fig. 3.17) to avoid cicatricial contractures near the lateral angle of the eye.

3. Elongate the incisions laterally. When correcting accentuated "crow's-feet," the incisions should be prolonged laterally to permit ample resection of the tissues there as well as in the malar and zygomatic areas (Fig. 3.18).

Undermining

These are the techniques by which the surgeon liberates the palpebral tissue from its subjacent planes to permit easy mobilization.

Upper Eyelid. There is no need for undermining in the upper eyelid because the skin can easily be separated from the plane below it.

Lower Eyelid. Either subcutaneous or myocutaneous undermining is used (Rees, 1981), but the former is rare because it can cause major scleral show or ectropion. Skin-muscle undermining produces flaps that contain all or part of the thickness of the orbicularis oculi muscle (Beare,

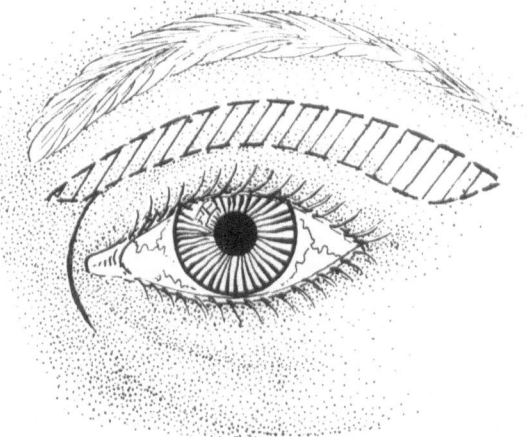

FIGURE 3.16. In the upper lid, the incision above the mesial angle of the eye should have an upward trend in order not to coincide with the epicanthal fold.

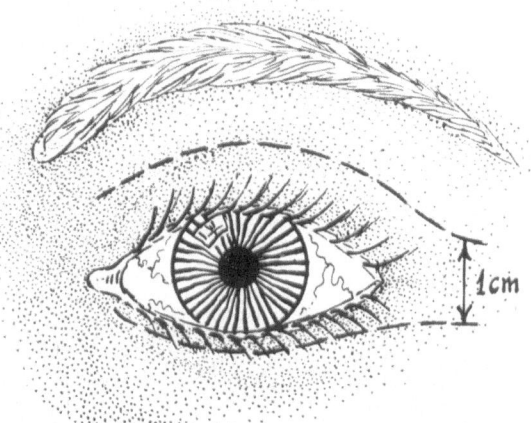

FIGURE 3.17. Recommended distance between the lateral extremities of the incisions in the upper and lower lids. This will help to prevent contractures.

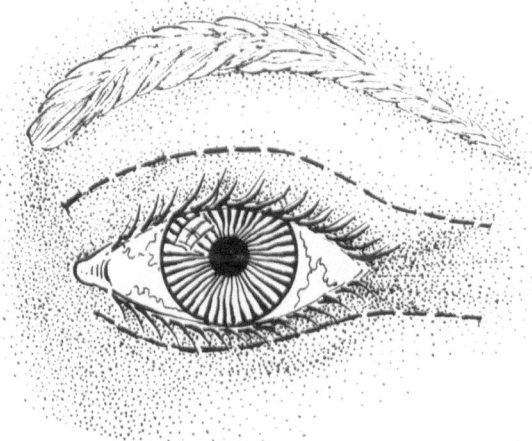

FIGURE 3.18. The dotted lines show the lateral extention of the incision lines used in the correction of "crow's-feet."

1967), and is the preferred procedure. If the undermining is adequately done, it should not reduce the tonus of the orbicular muscle of the eye. When the looseness of the lower lid is only in the pretarsal region, undermining is necessary only in that part; one does not have to undermine the preseptal portion (Fig. 3.19).

The bundles of the orbicularis oculi muscle are separated, and about one third of the muscle is included in the flap. In other cases the entire thickness of the orbicularis oculi muscle can be included in the flap (Figs. 3.21 and 3.22).

When the looseness is also in the preseptal portion, or when it is necessary to treat the fat pockets there as well, the skin-muscle undermining must be extended in front of the septum orbitale in the septal portion of the lid. When the looseness reaches as far as the cheek, undermining may also be done at this level (Fig. 3.20). Generally, skin-muscle undermining varies as a function of the degree of wrinkling and/or looseness. Please refer to page 42 for further discussion.

Resections

Resections should always begin first in the upper lids and *never in the lower*. If this order is reversed, serious problems can arise, because

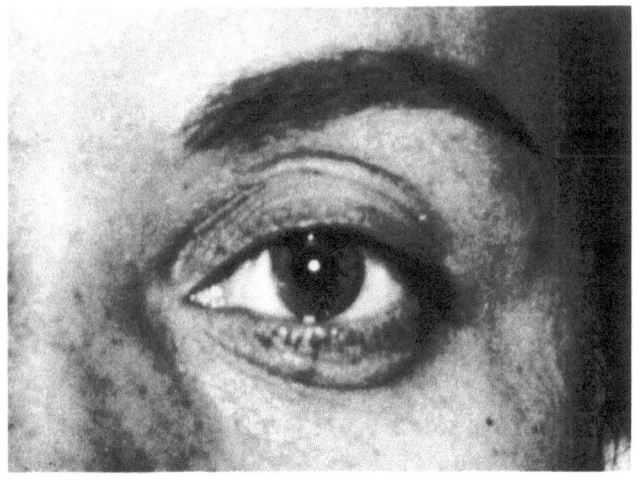
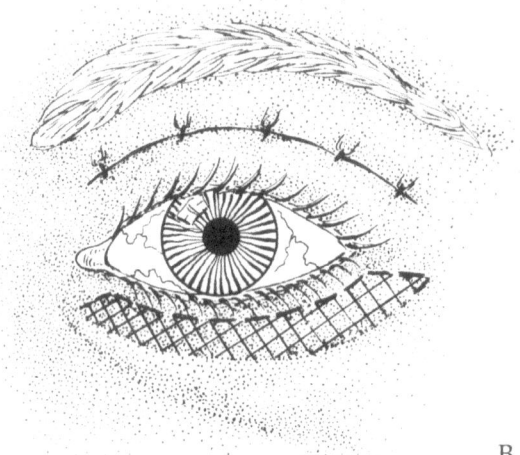

A   B

FIGURE 3.19. Pretarsal undermining used when the looseness is localized only in that portion. *A.* Clinical case. *B.* Drawing of the area to be undermined.

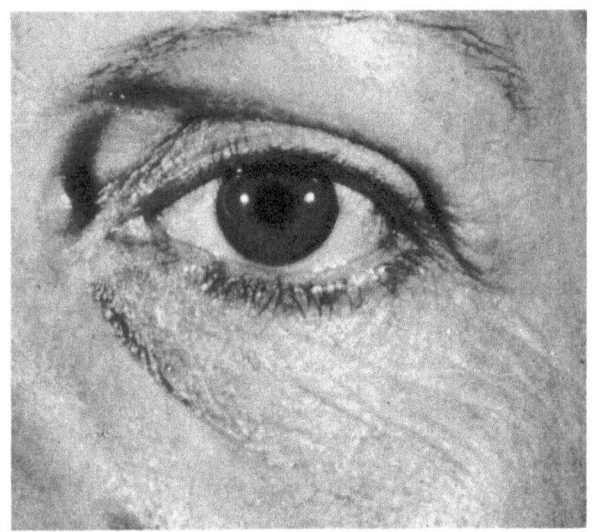
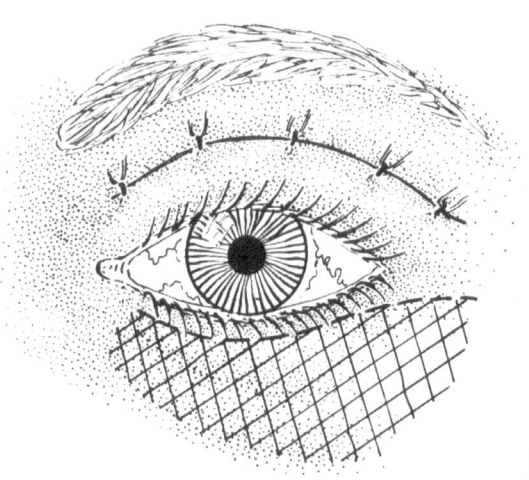

A   B

FIGURE 3.20. Pretarsal and preseptal skin-muscle undermining is used when the looseness is in these regions as well as in the malar and zygomatic areas.

A. Clinical case. *B.* Diagram of the area to be undermined.

during healing the pull coming from below is added to the pull of gravity, and these together can cause contractures at the lateral angle of the eye, in addition to scleral show and/or ectropions (see Chapter 5 "Complications").

The relationship between looseness in the upper and lower lids is very significant. It is accentuated by the fact that at the lateral angle of the eye, the skin of both lids slides easily over the underlying periosteum. The tension generated by resections and suturing in the upper lid brings about an elevation of the lateral angle of

the eye, reducing or even eliminating the looseness in the lateral third of the lower eyelid.

It is during resection that great care must be taken to retain the anatomical and functional integrity of the lids, as this is where errors bring about most of the scleral show and/or ectropion problems. The patients are generally operated in a supine position. In this position the eyelids are dislocated ventro-dorsally. It is thus convenient to elevate the head to a vertical position, a maneuver that must be made more than once during the operation. This maneuver is helpful in

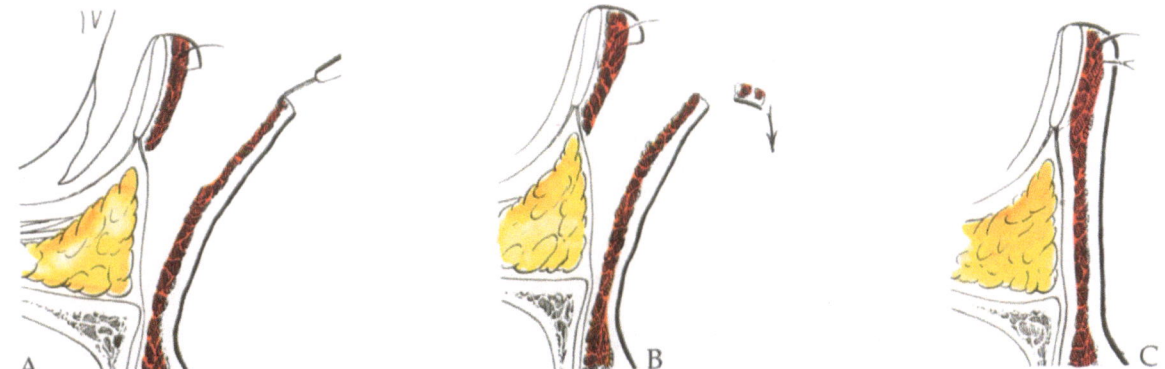

FIGURE 3.21. *A.* The incision is made 1.5 mm below the ciliary rim and the flap is undermined, leaving about one third of the thickness of the orbicular muscle on the pretarsal portion. *B.* The flap is shortened by adequate skin-muscle resection. *C.* The flap is replaced, with adequate muscular tissue remaining.

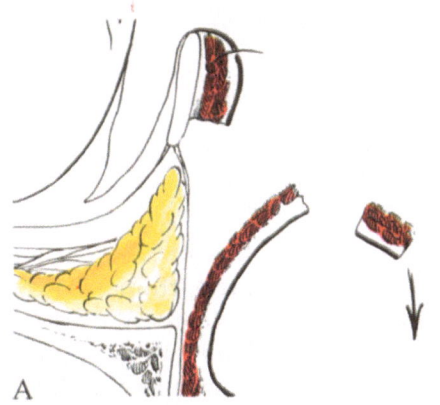

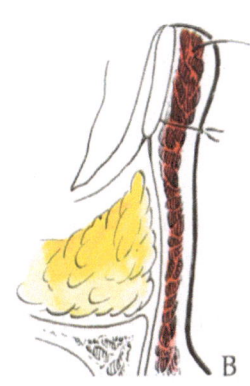

FIGURE 3.22. *A.* Here the incision is made 2 to 3 mm below the ciliary margin. In this way, sufficient orbicular muscle remains in the tarsal portion to maintain good tonus. *B.* The flap is replaced with adequate muscular tissue remaining.

observing any existing scleral show or ectropion.

To help prevent scleral show, two precautions relative to the resection of the orbicular muscle should be noted:

1. When using the subciliary incision, we recommend that no more than one third of the thickness of the orbicular muscle be resected in the tarsal portion. Enough of the muscle should be left to ensure normal contractive capacity and adequate support of the palpebral rim (Fig. 3.21).

2. An alternative to the above is to make the incision 2 to 3 mm below the ciliary margin, and then to resect the entire thickness of the orbicular muscle as far as the tarsal cartilage. The remaining muscle volume in the tarsal region will be enough to maintain the tonus of the lid (Fig. 3.22).

It should be emphasized that it is better to leave a postoperative excess of skin, causing an earlier reappearance of the wrinkles, than to remove too much and thus generate a scleral show or ectropion. Patients know that their wrinkles are going to return sooner or later and easily accept them. The same cannot be said of a scleral show or an ectropion; the patient's reation to these is total dissatisfaction.

Suturing

We do not normally suture either the orbital fascia or the orbicularis oculi muscle. Suturing is done only in the skin, using 6-0 nylon discontin-

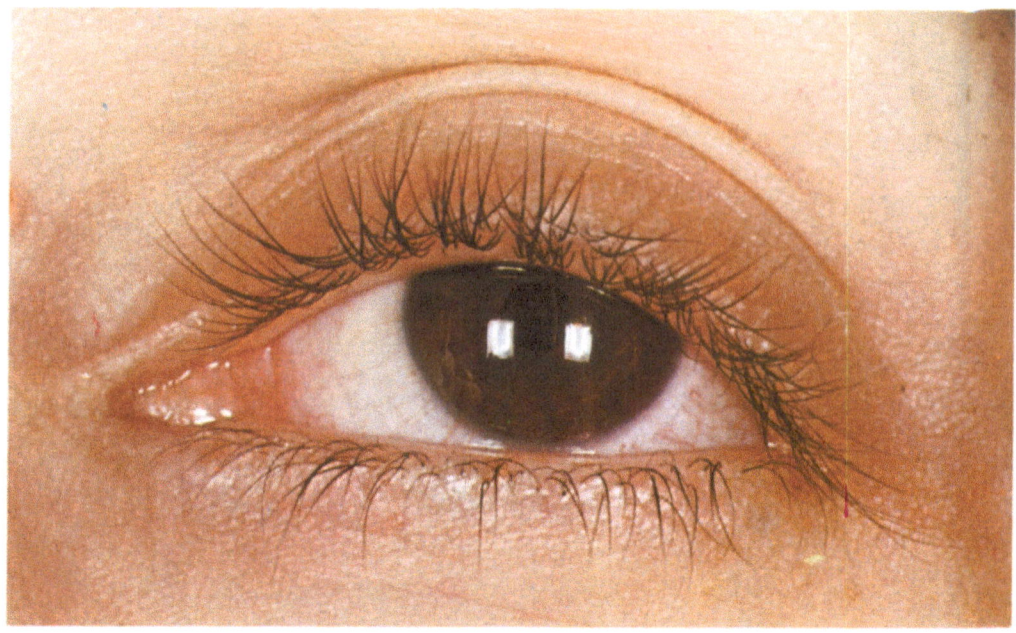

FIGURE 3.23. First-degree wrinkles. The looseness is located almost exclusively along the line of the upper palpebral sulcus.

ous stitches. These are removed 48 hours after surgery. Continuous suture can also be used.

Classification of the Wrinkles of the Eyelid

For the purposes of improving the understanding and planning of the correction of tissue looseness, we classify eyelid wrinkles into grades 1, 2, and 3, according to age level and the progressive wrinkling.

Independent of individual variations, generally we find first-degree wrinkles in patients in their second decade of life; second-degree wrinkles in the third and fourth decades, and third degree in the decades that follow. For each of these degrees we have a specific type of surgical orientation.

In all three degrees of wrinkling, the incisions, undermining, and suturing are done similarly, as described above. The resections, however, differ according to the degree of wrinkling involved. The reason for this is described above, but we repeat it here for emphasis: *since the resection of a substantial portion of tissue from the lateral third of the upper eyelid increases the tension on the tissue in the lateral third of the lower eyelid, thereby reducing its flaccidity, there is often no need for resection of the lower lid.*

The result of this increase in tension varies and is directly proportional to the degree of wrinkling: in first-degree wrinkling there is no looseness in the lateral third of the lower eyelid; in second-degree wrinkling, the looseness is small and can often be corrected by the tension produced by the resection and suturing of the upper eyelid; in third-degree wrinkling, the excess tissue is exaggerated in the lateral third of the lower eyelid, and the resection and suturing of the upper eyelid does not completely correct the looseness. Thus, only in cases of third-degree wrinkling is it necessary to ressect additional tissue from the lateral third of the lower lid.

First-Degree Wrinkles

The first degree represents the least serious type of looseness. It is localized in the upper eyelid and, at times, causes small wrinkles close to the lateral angle of the eye. Looseness in the lower lids is not seen (Fig. 3.23). Resections are done only in the upper eyelids.

Repair Technique. The surface to be resected, including its precise angles, is marked, outlining a cutaneous segment in the form of a crescent (Fig. 3.24A). The amount to be resected depends

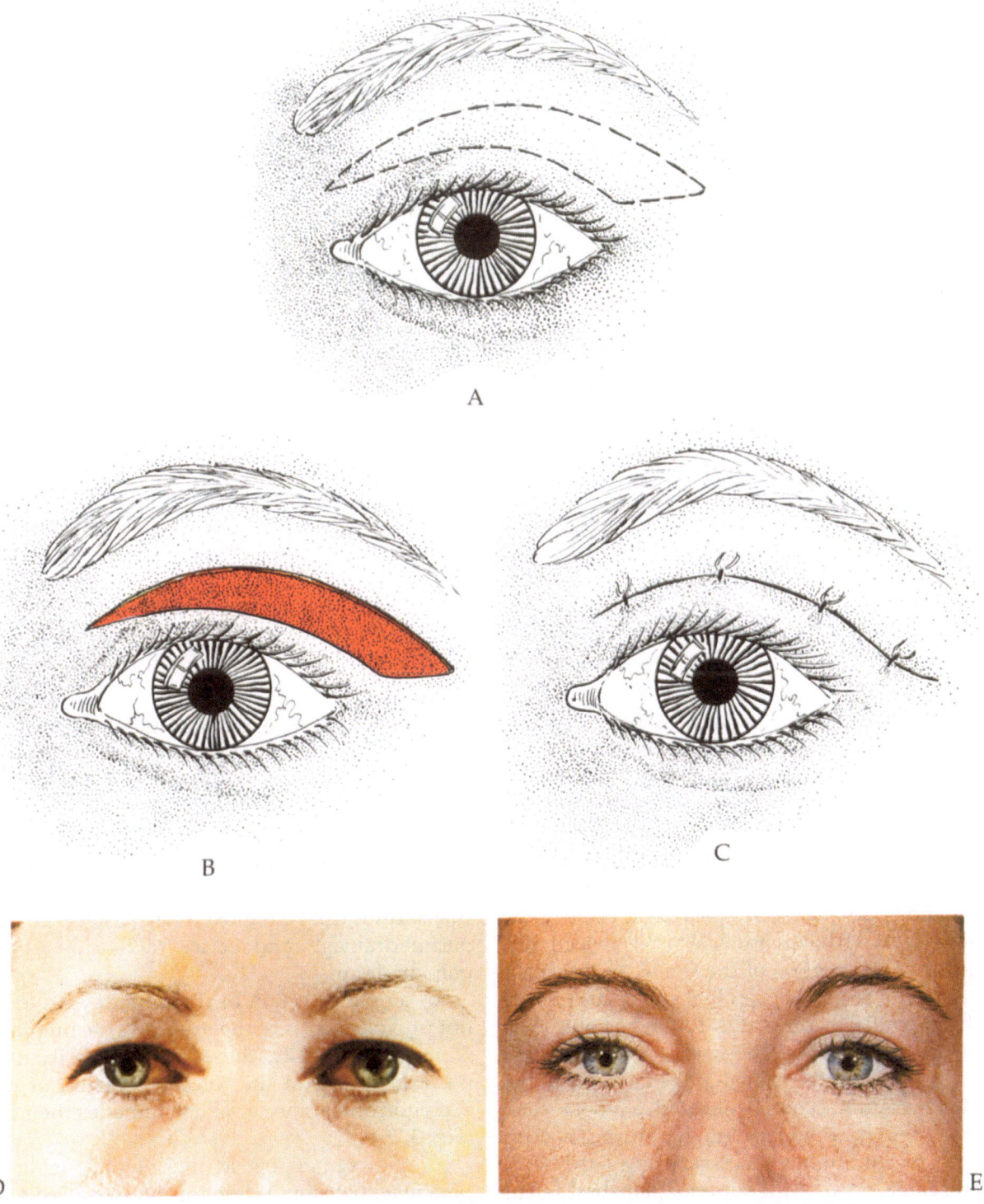

A

B

C

D

E

FIGURE 3.24. Tissue resection for first-degree wrinkl-ing. *A.* Markings. The resection should be about 1.5 cm at its widest part over the lateral angle of the eye.

B. Tissue resection accomplished. *C.* Suturing. *D, E.* Pre- and postoperative views.

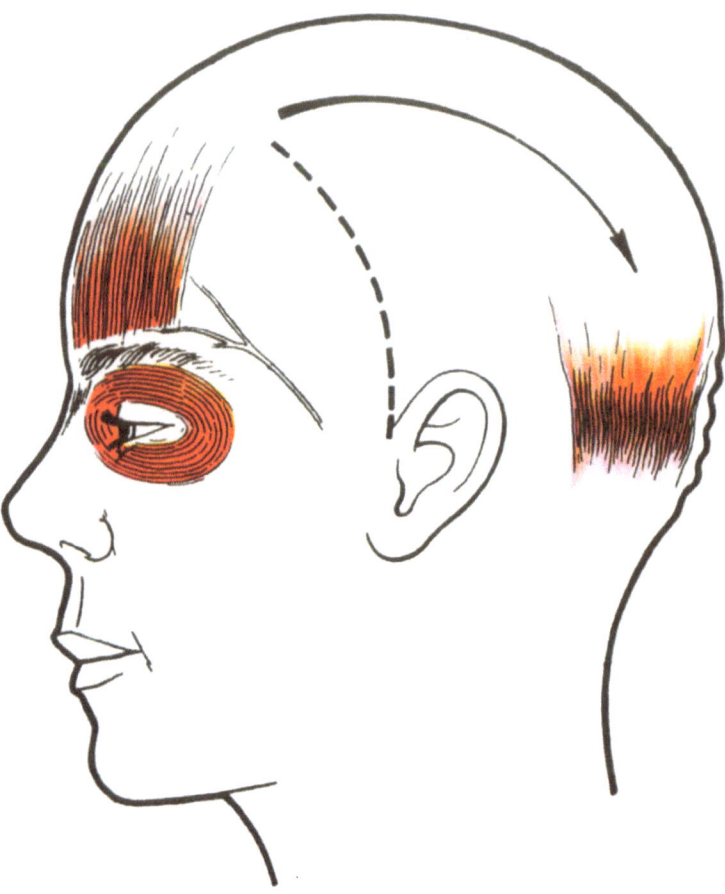

FIGURE 3.25. The eyebrows do not become ptotic after the resection of tissue from the upper lid because of the strong tension of the occipito-frontalis muscle. (From: Loeb R: Surgical procedure to avoid paralysis of the occipital belly of the occipito-frontalis muscle in rhytidoplasty. Reprinted from Excerpta Medica Foundation – Trans Fourth Int Cong Plastic Reconstr Surg. Rome, October 1967, pp 1116–1119).

on the aesthetic judgement of the surgeon. The widest part of the resection is approximately 1.5 cm and is situated above the lateral angle of the eye (Fig. 3.24B). Anatomically, this resection is in the septal portion of the eyelid, in the space below the superior palpebral sulcus and above the orbital portion of the lid and about 1 cm below the eyebrow. The width of the resection increases from the mesial to the lateral portion. Hemostasis is accomplished with a bipolar cautery. There is no undermining. Suturing is done with discontinuous stitches, using 6-0 Nylon, and coincides with the superior palpebral sulcus (Fig. 3.24C). The tissue lateral to the lateral angle of the eye is stretched by the suturing, and therefore any looseness at this level is corrected. This suturing also raises the level of the lateral angle of the eye (Fig. 3.24D).

We prefer discontinuous sutures because if there is any hematoma or scleral show, one or two sutures can be removed where necessary to permit drainage or to reduce the tension on the palpebral rim.

An ample resection of the upper eyelid does not provoke ptosis of the eyebrows, as might be supposed. Actually, the eyebrows are fixed in position owing to the force of traction of the occipitofrontal muscle, which impedes their fall (Fig. 3.25).

In the upper eyelid we avoid using a periciliary incision. When this type of incision is used, the excess tissue is taken from the pretarsal portion and *not from the preseptal portion as it should*. After suturing, the superior palpebral sulcus is too low (Fig. 3.26), being wrongly placed in the tarsal portion, whose width has

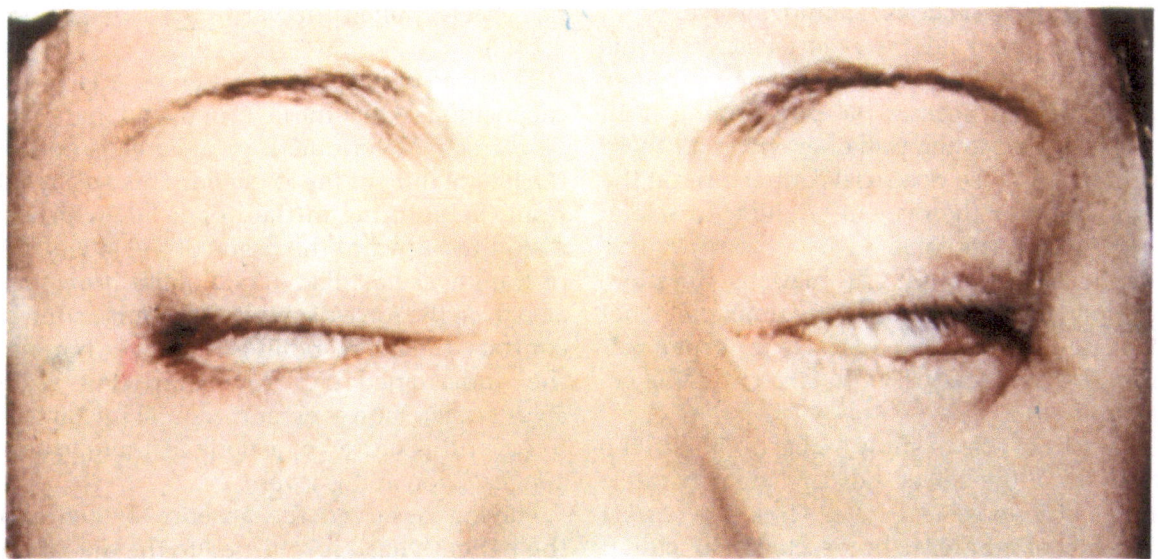

FIGURE 3.26. Erroneous resection of tissue from the pretarsal instead of the preseptal portion of the upper lid. As a consequence, the resulting scar is situated next to the palpebral rim, reducing the natural height of the pretarsal portion of the eyelid. The preseptal portion is excessively increased in the vertical dimension, and the looseness of the preseptal portion persists. These resections in the pretarsal portion of the upper eyelid can, among other things, cause scleral show, as in this patient.

been overly reduced. The worst problem in these cases is that an excess looseness remains in the septal portion, which was not resected when it should have been. There often is scleral show in these cases (Fig. 3.26).

Second-Degree Wrinkles

These are the most frequent cases, with the patients usually in their third or fourth decade of life (Fig. 3.27).

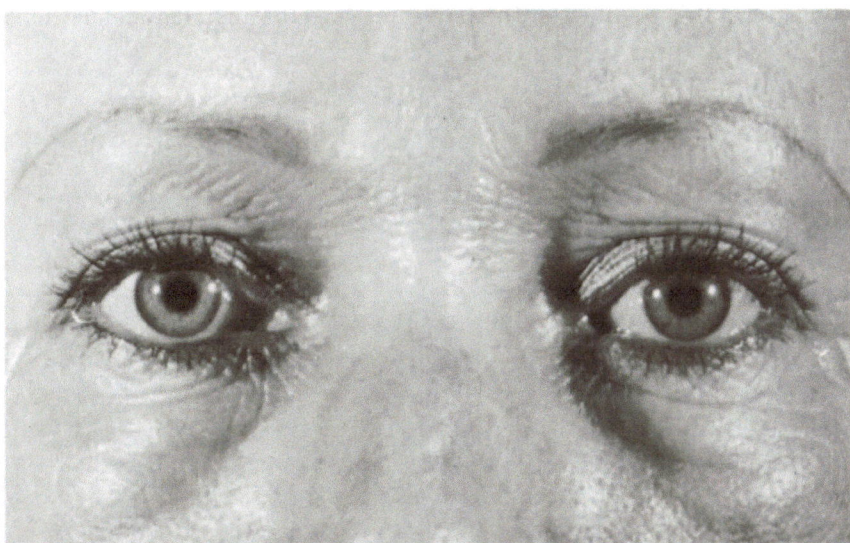

FIGURE 3.27. Second-degree wrinkles. Looseness in the upper eyelids along their entire length and in the lower lids in the medial and intermedial thirds. There is little in the lateral third of the lower lid.

To repeat: Resections should always begin first in the upper lids *never in the lower.* If this order is reversed, serious problems can arise because during healing the pull coming from below is added to the pull of gravity, and these together can cause cicatricial contractures at the lateral angle of the eye, in addition to scleral show and/or ectropions.

In the upper eyelids the marking, incision, resection, and suturing are done similarly to that of first-degree wrinkles, that is, in the septal portion and with a greater width taken from the lateral third.

The risks of scleral show and ectropion in the lateral third the lower lids are great because there is little looseness here. Thus, the correct evaluation of the area to be resected is difficult. It is excessive tissue resection in this area that causes scleral show and ectropion to occur. Special care should be taken about what is resected, as demonstrated in the technique that follows.

Repair Technique. Surgery is initiated with markings on the upper and lower lids (Fig. 3.28A). Resections are made and sutures placed in the upper lids similarly to that done in cases of first-degree wrinkles. An incision is made in the lower lid, followed by skin-muscle undermining (Fig. 3.28B). The amount of tissue to be resected is then evaluated, and in accordance with this, two complementary incisions a few milimeters in length are made in the skin flap. Two temporary sutures are placed at this point, after the flap

has been pulled upward and inward (Fig. 3.28C).

The head of the patient is then raised to a vertical position so that the level of the lid margin can be correctly determined. A raw area is noted in the lateral third of the lower lid. This area results from the suturing in the upper lid, which has dislocated upward the tissue of the lateral third of the lower lid, (Fig. 3.28D, *upper arrow*), and also from the force of gravity, which is acting in a contrary direction, pulling the lower border of the undermined flap downward (Fig. 3.28D, *lower arrow*). However, sufficient skin still exists to cover this raw area, as long as there is no tissue resection at this level.*

Having observed the absence of ectropion, the patient's head is returned to the dorsal position. The excess skin is then resected from the medial and central thirds of the lower lid (Fig. 3.28E). The final sutures are placed (Fig. 3.28F). Two clinical cases of second-degree wrinkles are presented in Figures 3.29 and 3.30.

---

* Considering that no tissue is resected from the lateral third of the lower lid, it would appear unnecessary to carry the incision beyond the lateral angle of the eye, as shown in Fig. 3.28E. However, sometimes such a lateral extension may be useful, as it facilitates the freeing of the flap, which is pulled medially. Also, at times the fatty tissue of the lateral pocket or the superficial layers of the orbicularis oculi muscle is resected through this lateral extension.

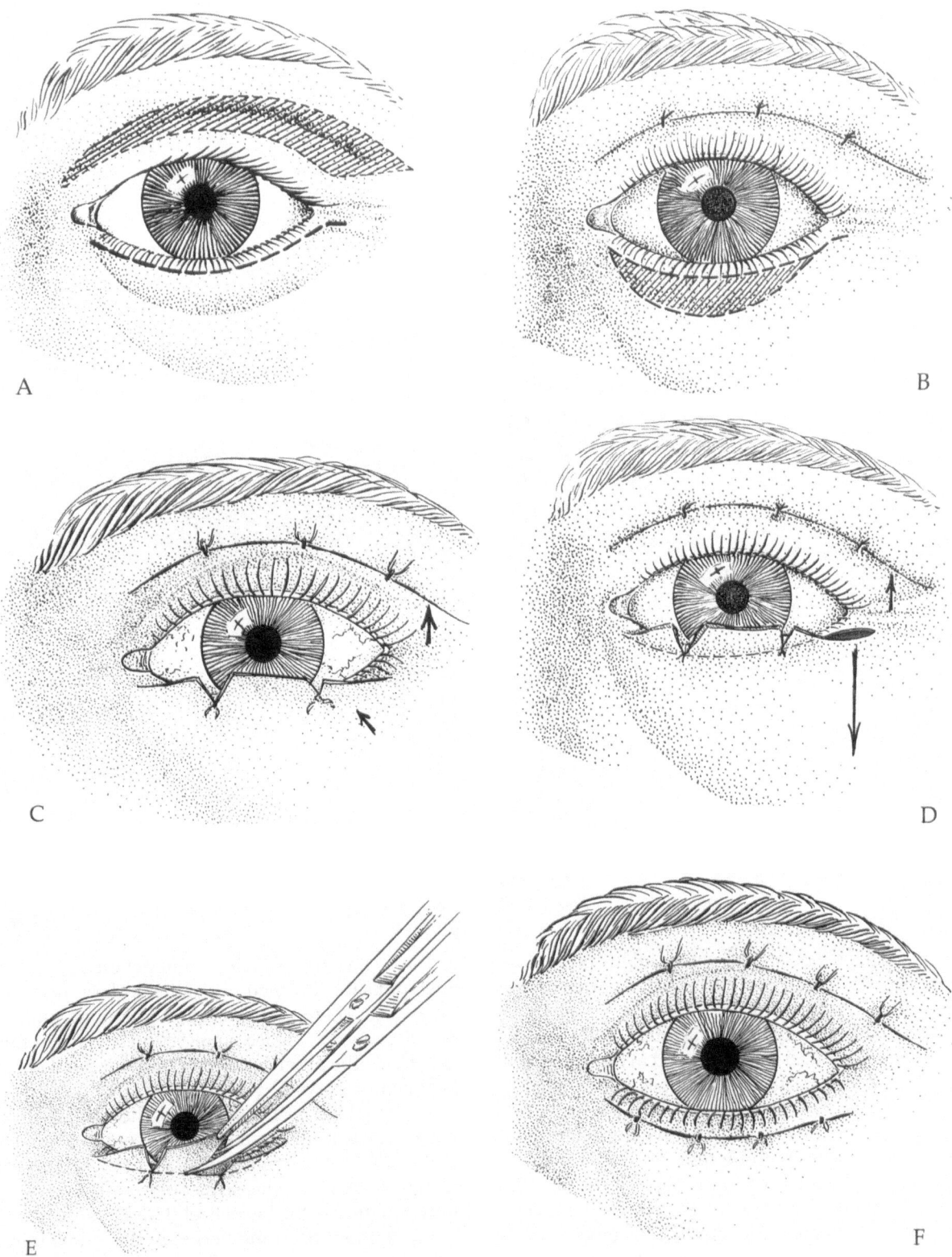

FIGURE 3.28. Tissue resection for second-degree wrinkles. Diagrams of the surgical steps are described on page 46. (From Loeb R: Esthetic blepharoplasties based on the degree of wrinkling. *Plast Rec Surg* 1971; 47:33).

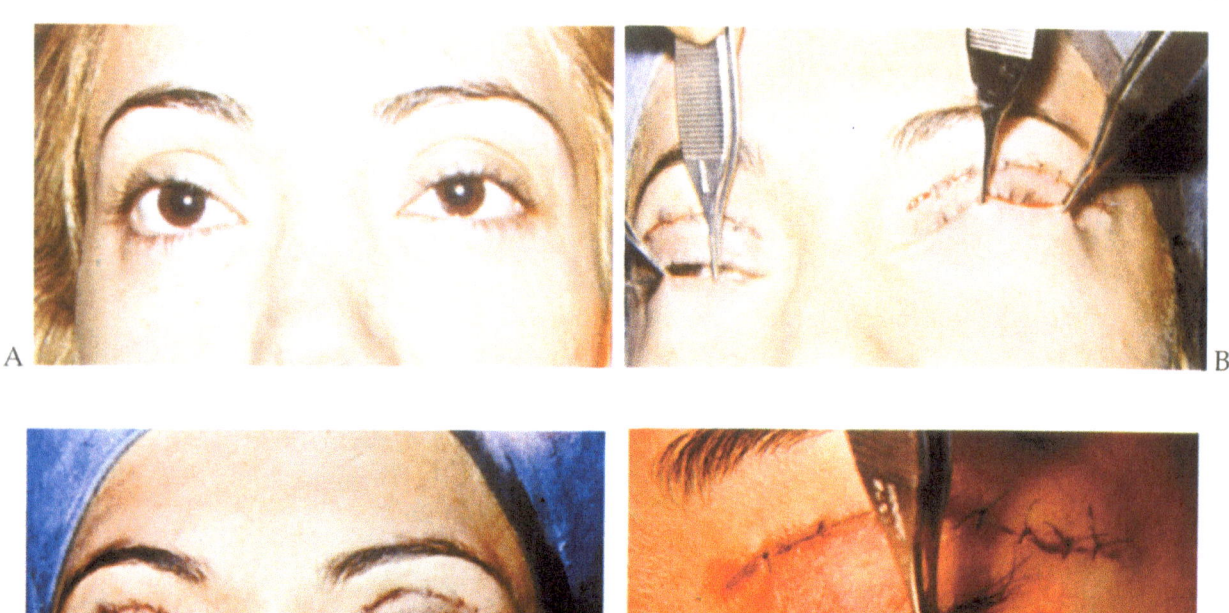

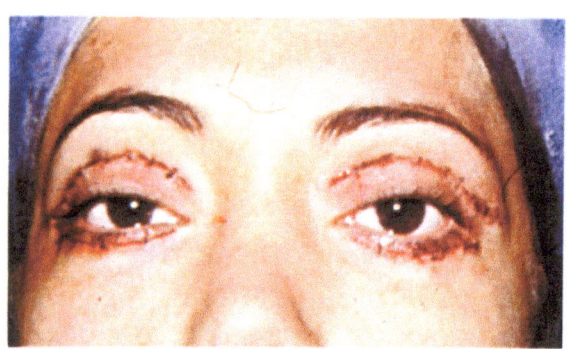

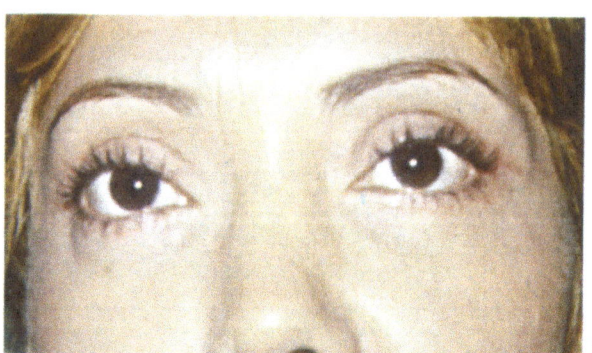

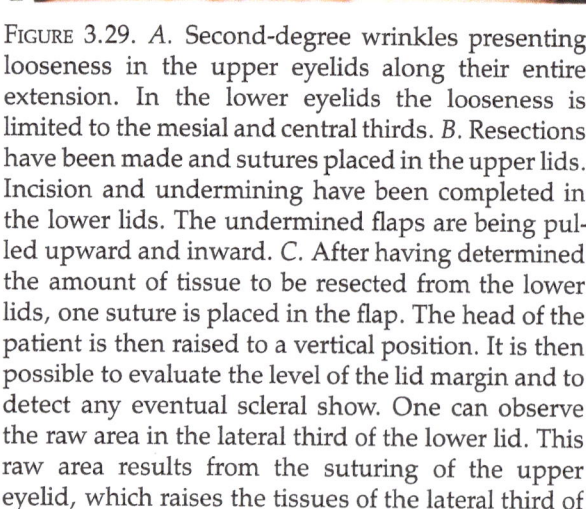

FIGURE 3.29. *A.* Second-degree wrinkles presenting looseness in the upper eyelids along their entire extension. In the lower eyelids the looseness is limited to the mesial and central thirds. *B.* Resections have been made and sutures placed in the upper lids. Incision and undermining have been completed in the lower lids. The undermined flaps are being pulled upward and inward. *C.* After having determined the amount of tissue to be resected from the lower lids, one suture is placed in the flap. The head of the patient is then raised to a vertical position. It is then possible to evaluate the level of the lid margin and to detect any eventual scleral show. One can observe the raw area in the lateral third of the lower lid. This raw area results from the suturing of the upper eyelid, which raises the tissues of the lateral third of the lower lid, and also from the action of gravity, which pulls the lower border of the undermined flap downward. There is, however, still enough skin to cover the raw area, since no resection is made at this level. Once the absence of ectropion or scleral show has been observed, the head of the patient is returned to the dorsal position. *D.* The excess skin is then resected from the mesial and central thirds of the lower lid. Care should be taken in these cases of second- degree wrinkles so as not to resect tissue in the lateral third of the lower eyelid. *E.* The sutures are placed (without resecting tissue) in the lateral third. *F.* Post-operative results 60 days after surgery. (From Loeb R: Esthetic blepharoplasties based on the degree of wrinkling. *Plast Reconstr Surg* 1971; 47:33).

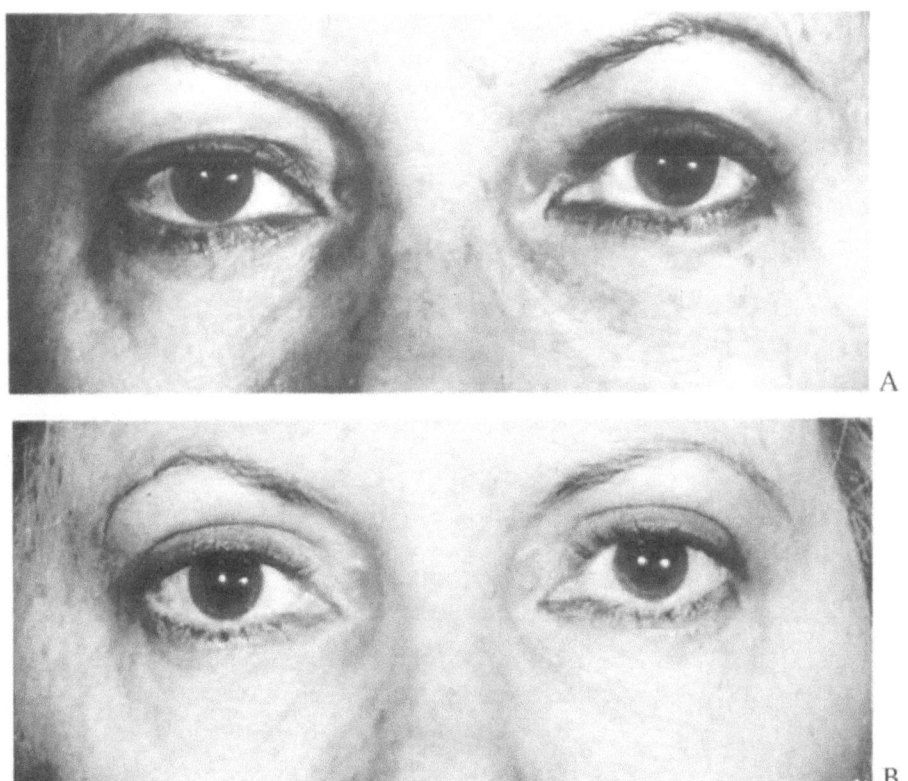

FIGURE 3.30. Second-degree wrinkles. *A*. Preoperative view showing looseness and fat pockets in the upper and lower lids. *B*. Postoperative view after resection of skin, muscle, and fat tissues.

Third-Degree Wrinkles

This degree of wrinkling generally occurs in patients in their fifth or greater decade of life. In these cases there is a great excess of tissue in both the upper and the lower eyelids, chiefly in the lateral third. Because of this excess tissue, the risks of scleral show and ectropions are less, and tissue can be resected from the lateral third of the lower lids.

Repair Technique. The resections in the upper eyelids are done in a manner similar to that already described for the correction of first-degree wrinkles. In these cases of third-degree wrinkles, the tension achieved by the resection and suturing in the upper lid is not sufficient to correct completely the looseness of the lateral third of the lower lid (Fig. 3.31). Thus, tissue resection is also required there, in addition to that done in the mesial and central thirds (Fig. 3.31 C). Suturing is completed (Fig. 3.31 D).

Correction of "Crow's-Feet" and Low Palpebral Looseness Using Tissue Resections Extended Laterally

In these cases, the upper and lower incisions are prolonged laterally (Fig. 3.32 and 3.33). This is followed by a wide skin-muscle undermining and resection of the region situated laterally to the lateral angle of the eye. In this way, the risk of ectropion is reduced because the tension at this level does not act over the lateral third of the lower eyelid; rather only on the soft tissues of the zygomatic region, situated laterally to the lateral angle of the eye. The resultant scars are inconspicuous because they follow the natural lines of the region. This technique is useful in those cases where peeling is contraindicated because of a tendency toward over-pigmentation. It is also a satisfactory substitute for the technique of using division and suspension of the orbicularis oculi muscle in the periorbital region.

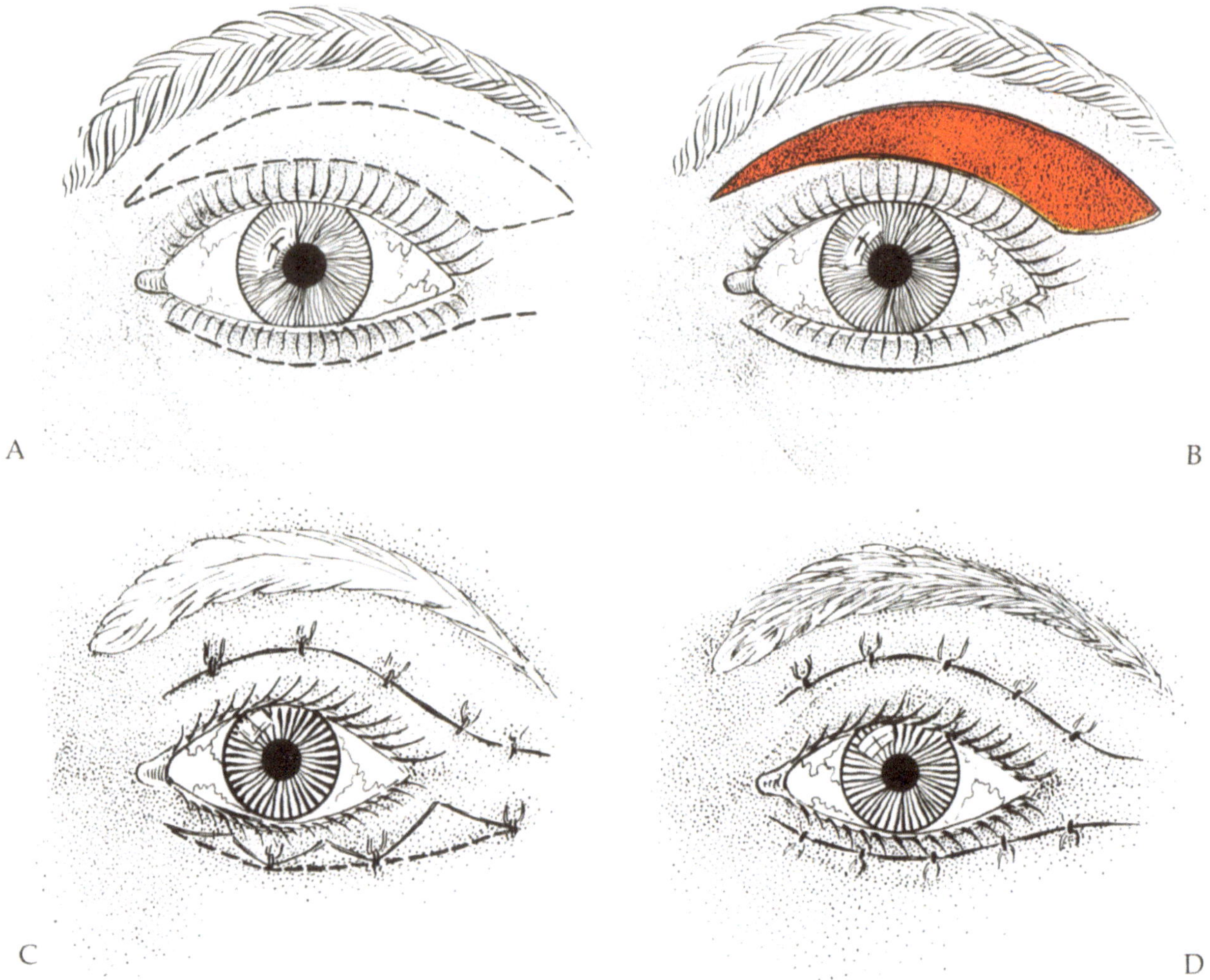

A

B

C

D

FIGURE 3.31. Operation for third-degree wrinkles. In these cases resection is also done from the lateral third of the lower eyelid. *A.* Marking. *B.* Upper lid resection and lower lid incision. *C.* Resection from the lateral third of the lower lid. *D.* Incisions sutured.

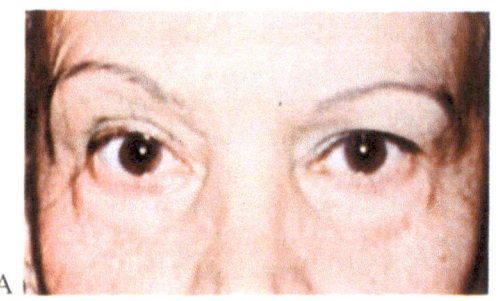

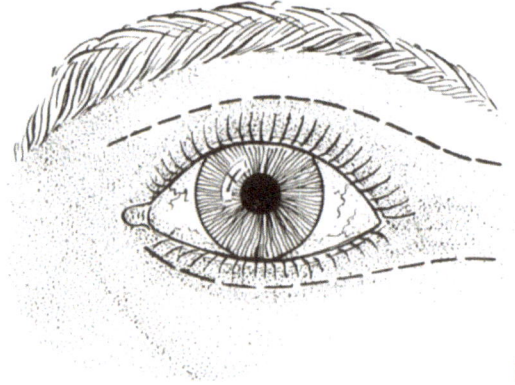

FIGURE 3.32. *A.* Preoperative view showing skin looseness and hypertrophic fat pockets of the upper and lower lids. The "crow's-feet" are very marked. *B.* Lateral prolongations for the incisions in the upper and lower eyelids. *C.* Following the markings, the lateral extensions of the cutaneous incisions should be prolonged. *D.* Prolongation of the incision and wide undermining, permitting the exposure of the orbital septum and the orbicularis oculi muscle. *E.* Flap undermined and raised. *F.* Complementary incision

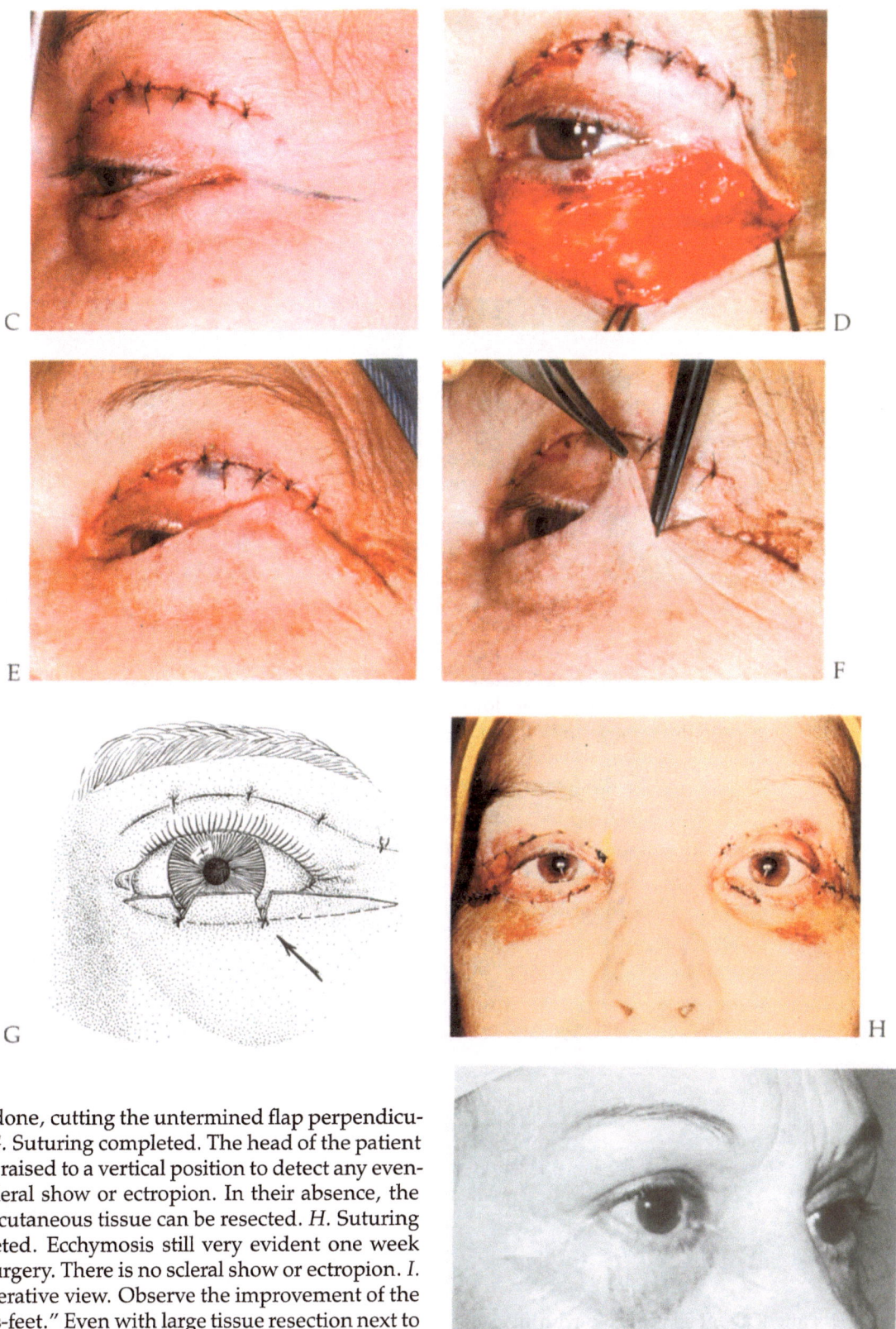

being done, cutting the untermined flap perpendicularly. *G.* Suturing completed. The head of the patient is now raised to a vertical position to detect any eventual scleral show or ectropion. In their absence, the excess cutaneous tissue can be resected. *H.* Suturing completed. Ecchymosis still very evident one week after surgery. There is no scleral show or ectropion. *I.* Postoperative view. Observe the improvement of the "crow's-feet." Even with large tissue resection next to the lateral angle of the eye, scleral show and ectropion were avoided.

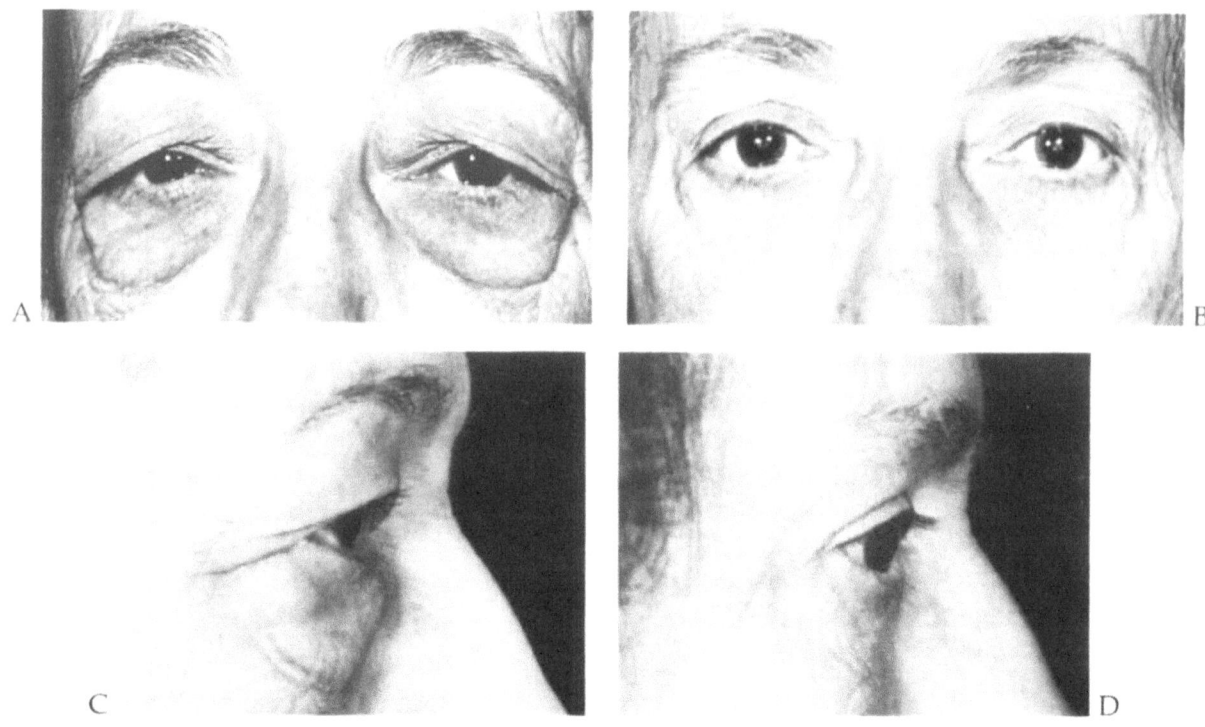

FIGURE 3.33. Correction of looseness and fat pockets using a prolonged lateral incision. The tissue looseness of the upper lids is so great as to form "curtains" that partially cover the visual field. In the lower eyelids the looseness is in the mesial, central, and lateral thirds. In addition, there are extensive fat pockets, which form bulges that add to the looseness of the tissue. A, B. Frontal views, pre- and postoperative. C, D. Profile views, pre- and postoperative

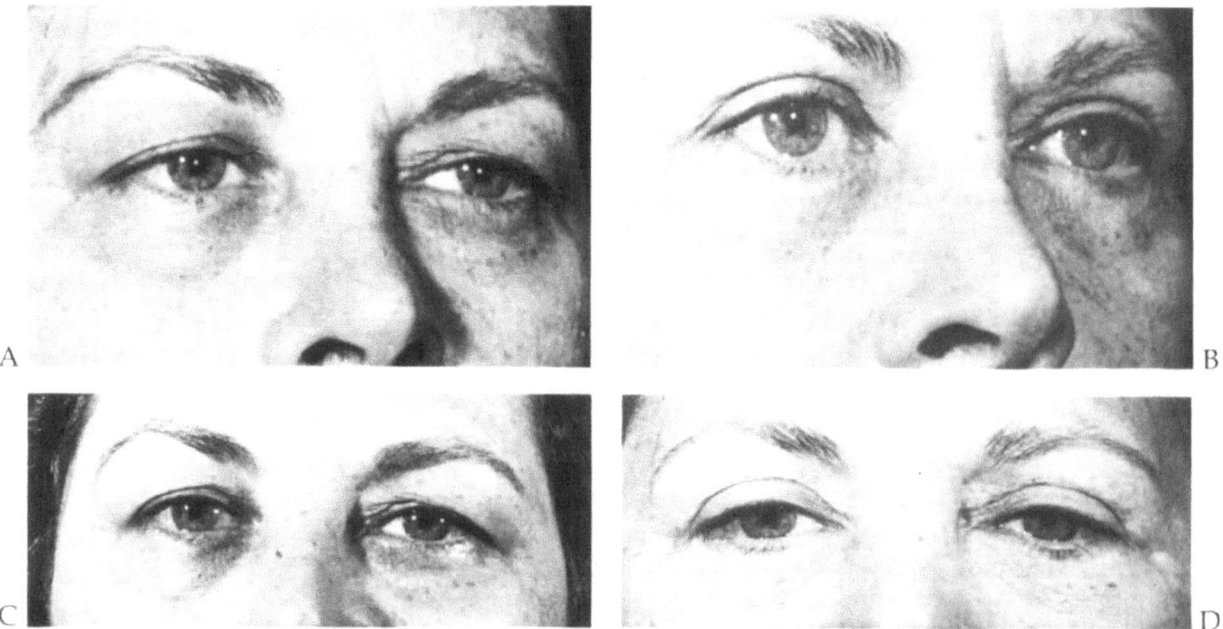

FIGURE 3.34. Patient about 50 years old with an exaggerated excess of skin of the upper eyelids (blepharochalasis), principally on the left side. She also has fat pockets and looseness in the lower eyelids. These defects give her an "austere" air that does not correspond to her personality. Correction was done by means of the techniques described in Figure 3.28. Fat resections in both upper and lower lids. A, C. Preoperative views. B, D. Postoperative views.

Two Examples of the Treatment of Third Degree Wrinkles in the Septal and Malar Regions Through a Low Elongated Incision Are Shown in Figs. 3.35 and 3.36.

FIGURE 3.35. *A.* Patient needing improvement in palpebral appearance for artistic-professional reasons. There are fat pockets and looseness in both upper and lower lids. In the lower lids the looseness also occupies the lower portion of the lid, invading the upper part of the cheek region. *B.* Upper eyelids completed. In the lower eyelids we use a low and prolonged incision and do wide undermining. *C.* The flap was sectioned to estimate the tissue resection to be made. Sutures already done. *D.* Postoperative appearance after 2 days, showing absence of scleral show and ectropion. *E.* Postoperative results after 3 months. In this case there was not the heavy postoperative edema that often occurs with this type of low incision. With the disappearance of the slight edema, one can see a reduction in any tendency toward scleral show.

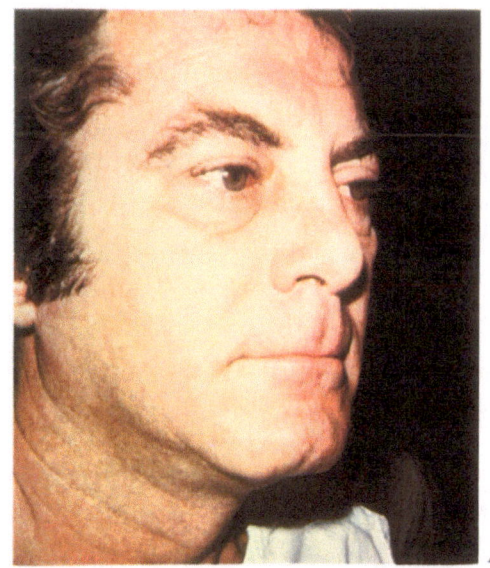

A

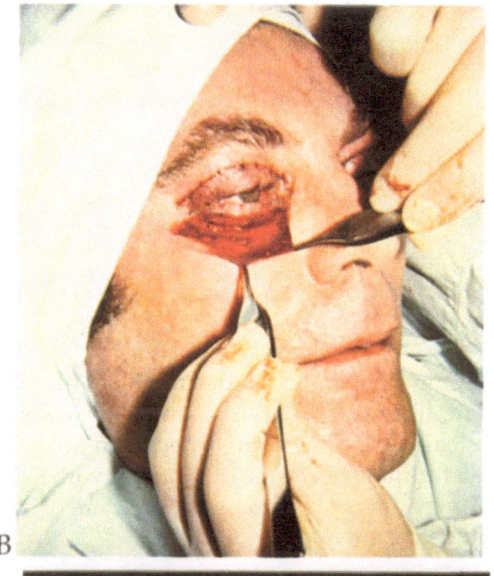

B

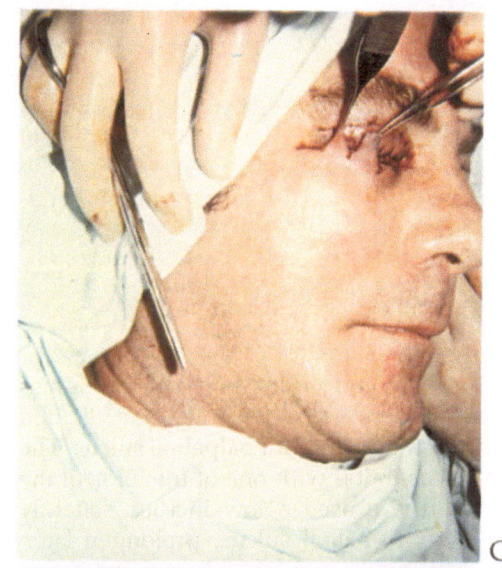

C

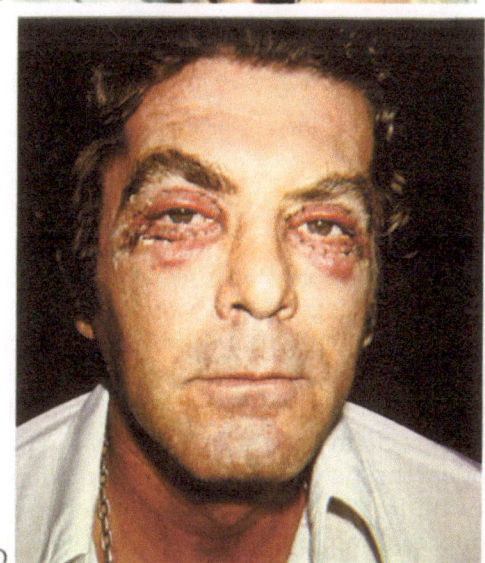

D

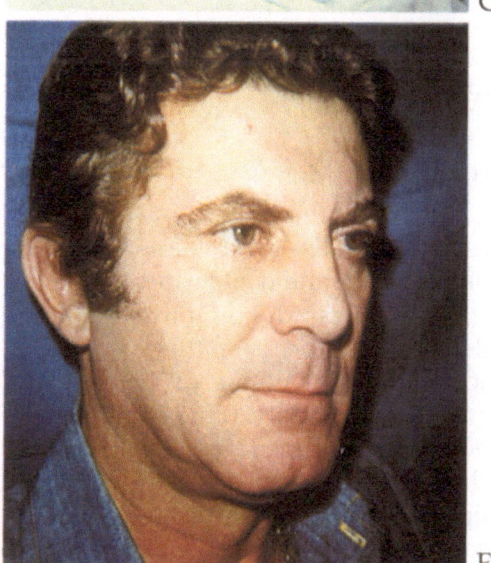

E

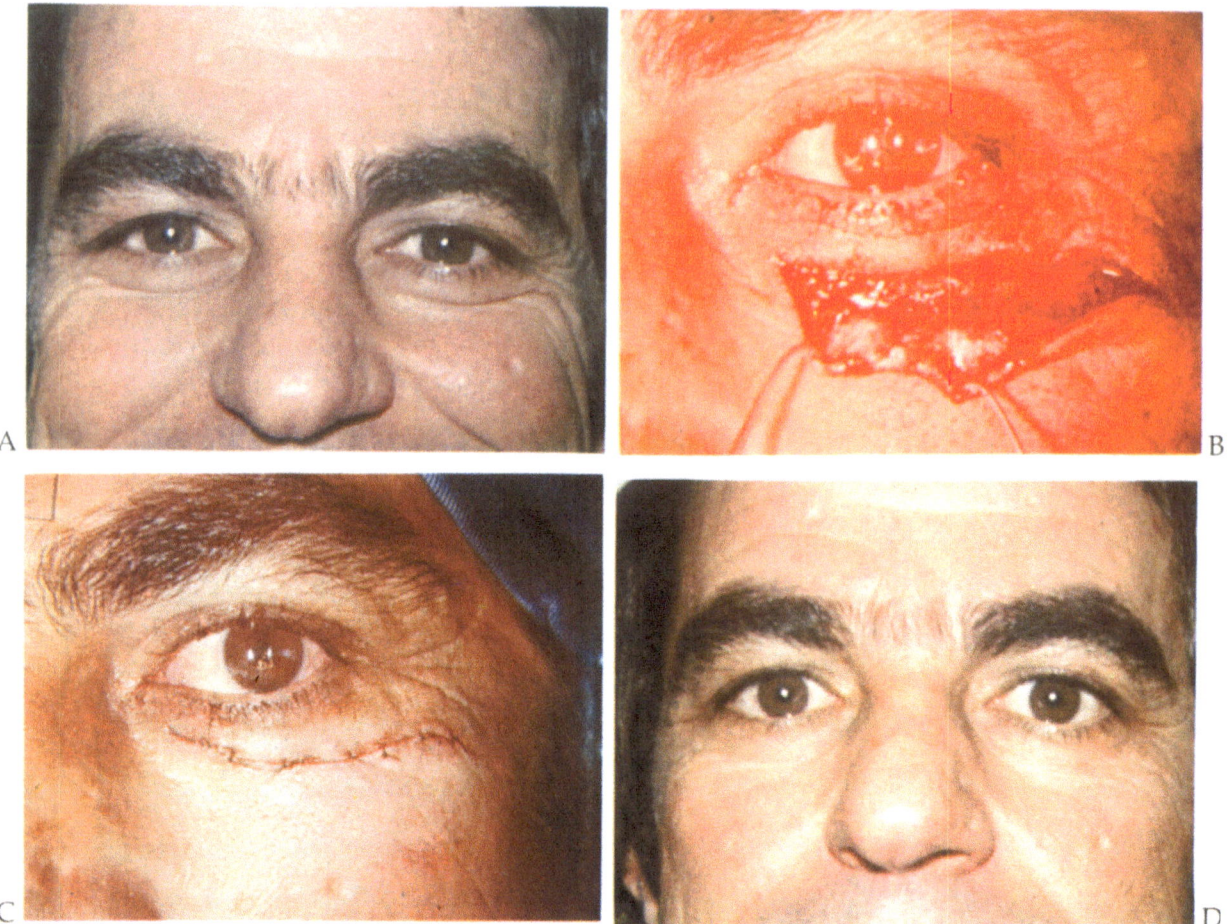

FIGURE 3.36. *A.* Exaggerated looseness of the tissues of the tarsal portion of the lower eyelids, limited inferiorly by a retracted inferior palpebral sulcus. The end of the sulcus unites with one of the folds of the "crow's-feet." *B.* We used a low incision, slightly above the lower palpebral sulcus, prolonged later-ally, and did a wide undermining of the skin-muscle flap, liberating the retraction of the lower palpebral sulcus. *C.* Excess tissue resected in accordance with the technique on page 51. Sutured with 6-0 nylon. *D.* Three months postoperative. There was no postoperative edema.

Fat Bulges

General Considerations

Fat bulges constitute the most voluminous projections of the eyelids and usually develop in the septal region, at times extending into the tarsal and cheek regions. On occasion they are marked by an increase in the volume of fat compartments of the orbital cavity (Hugo and Stone, 1974). Because of the way the light hits the bulges, the skin superficial to them normally appears lighter in color than the surrounding tissue and contrasts markedly with the darkness of the neighboring sulci and depressions (Fig. 3.37).

Etiology

The etiology of these exaggerated bulges has been discussed extensively. Castanares, (1964), is of the opinion that they occur on account of a herniation at the level of the orbital septum because of the internal pressure of the fat tissue. Others claim it is a simple increase in the volume of fat tissue, without any herniation (Bames, 1958). It is to be noted that these hypertrophied pockets are generally situated below the septal

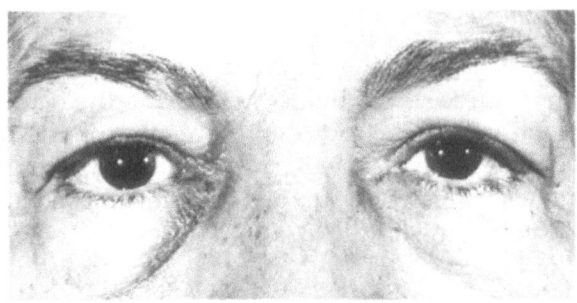 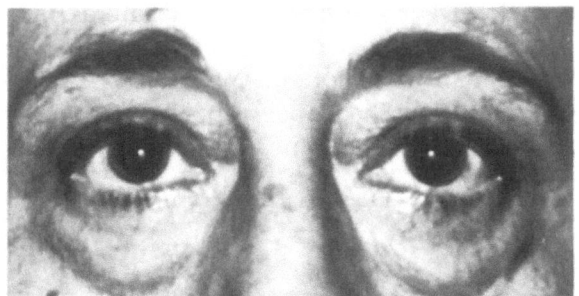

FIGURE 3.37. Because of their prominence, fat bulges receive more light and thus appear lighter than the surrounding areas.

portion of the orbicularis oculi muscle, whose thickness there is homogeneous. Actually, there is no herniation, because no herniary opening exists, although it has been described by some authors.

The thickness of the orbital septum varies from person to person and also within the same individual. When the septum is thin along its entire length, the fat pockets can be seen along the entire surface of the preseptal portion of the eyelids. When the orbital septum is thinner only in a portion of the eyelid, it is here that a fat bulge occurs.

Palpebral bulges that accompany thyroid or renal pathologies have an appearance similar to that typical of hypertrophied fat pockets, but the two should not be confused. The patient's history certainly will indicate the different causes.

Hypertrophied fat pockets often cause psychological and emotional problems, and the subjects are frequently the target of negative comments: "She leads a dissolute life and sleeps badly," "he is drinking a lot," etc. In reality, the problem could be entirely different: a person with an exemplary life can also have exaggerated fat pockets. It is true that senility, worries, precarious health, genetic factors, excess alcohol, too much night life, all these and others, together or separately, can contribute to the tired look caused by fat pockets.

Exaggerated growth of the orbital fat tissue puts pressure on the orbital septum, and frequently persons with enlarged fat pockets complain of a sensation of discomfort. According to them, this discomfort is relieved with the reduction of the hypertrophied fat tissue. This is one of the various reasons that bring patients to seek surgery for the correction of their fat pockets.

Upper Eyelids

In the upper lids the fat pockets are seen in the mesial and central thirds of the preseptal por-

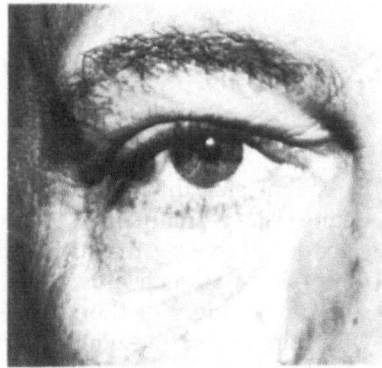 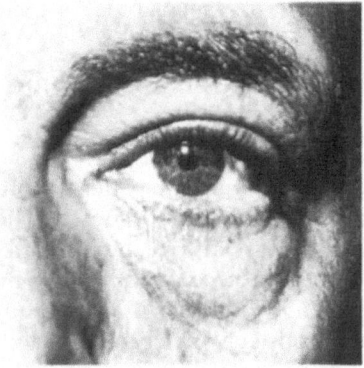

FIGURE 3.38. Hypertrophy of the fat in the upper eyelids, forming a pseudoptosis, principally on the right side. The palpebral border is lowered, reducing the visual field.

tion, (Rees, 1980), and rerely, in the lateral third (Owsley, 1980). In extreme cases, such a hypertrophy at the level of the mesial and central thirds can lower the palpebral border, creating a pseudoptosis that, at times, can reduce the visual field (Fig. 3.38).

Treatment

Before surgery, the surgeon should accentuate the volume of the bulge by pressing the ocular globe gently. This aids in the evaluation of the fat volume to be resected. The patient is appropriately sedated. The surgical techniques used are described in Figure 3.39.

Surgical Sequence for the Reduction of Fat Bulges in the Upper Eyelids (Fig. 3.39 A – K)

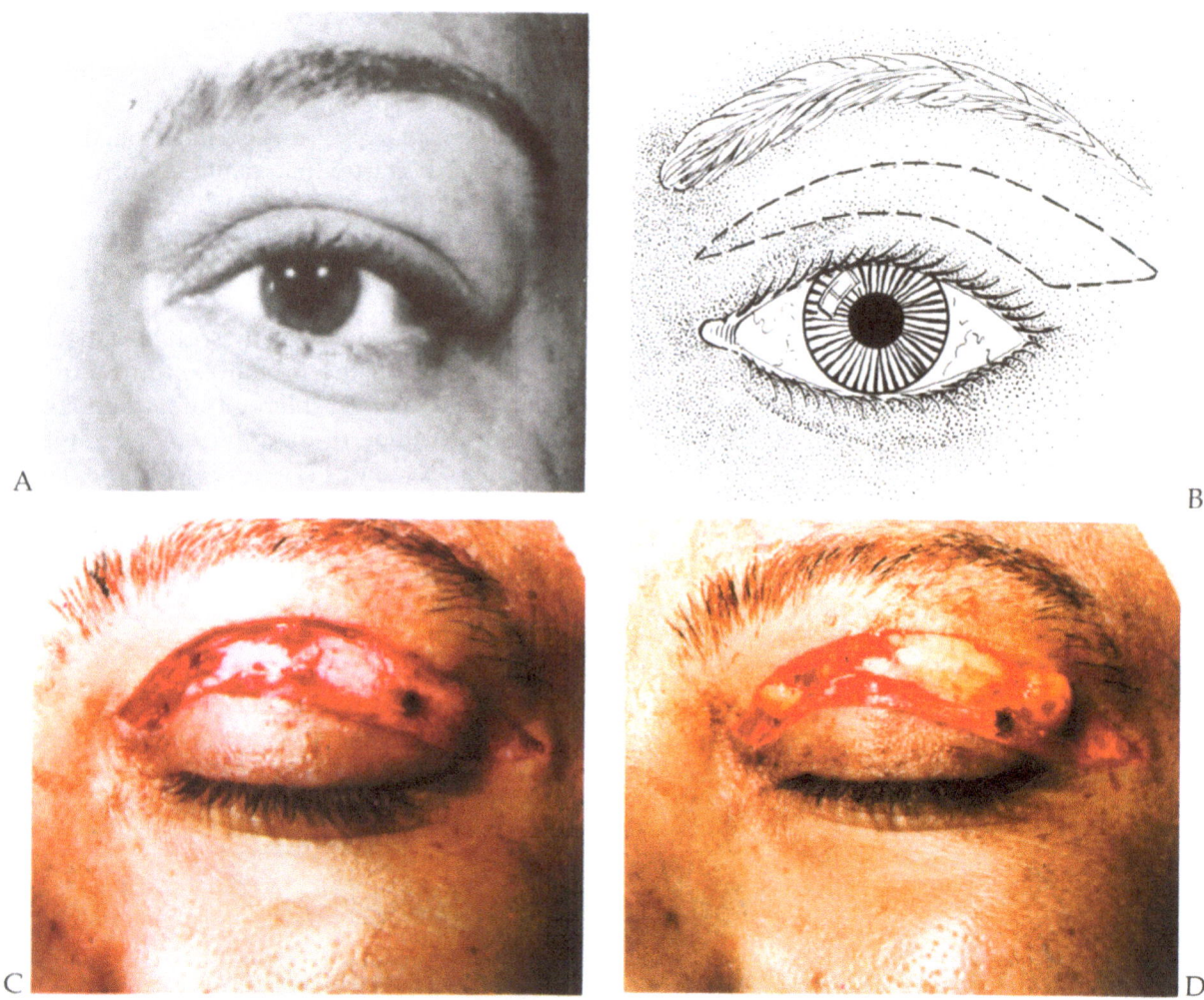

A   B

C   D

FIGURE 3.39. *A.* Preoperative view of patient. Both eyelids need reduction of fat and skin tissues. *B.* The skin of the upper eyelid is marked with indelible ink, indicating the area to be resected. Anesthesia is by local infiltration using 1 % Xylocaine, with or without adrenaline. *C.* The excess tissues have been resected. Observe the raw area in the septal portion beyond the lateral angle of the eye. The extremity of the resection in the mesial third is oriented upward. Careful hemostasis is maintained, preferably with bipolar electrocautery. *D.* After having divided the fibers of the orbicularis oculi muscle with fine-pointed scissors, the borders of the muscle were pulled aside with skin hooks, revealing the orbital septum, which was then sectioned. The fat of the central and medial fat pockets has herniated. Note the lateral extension.

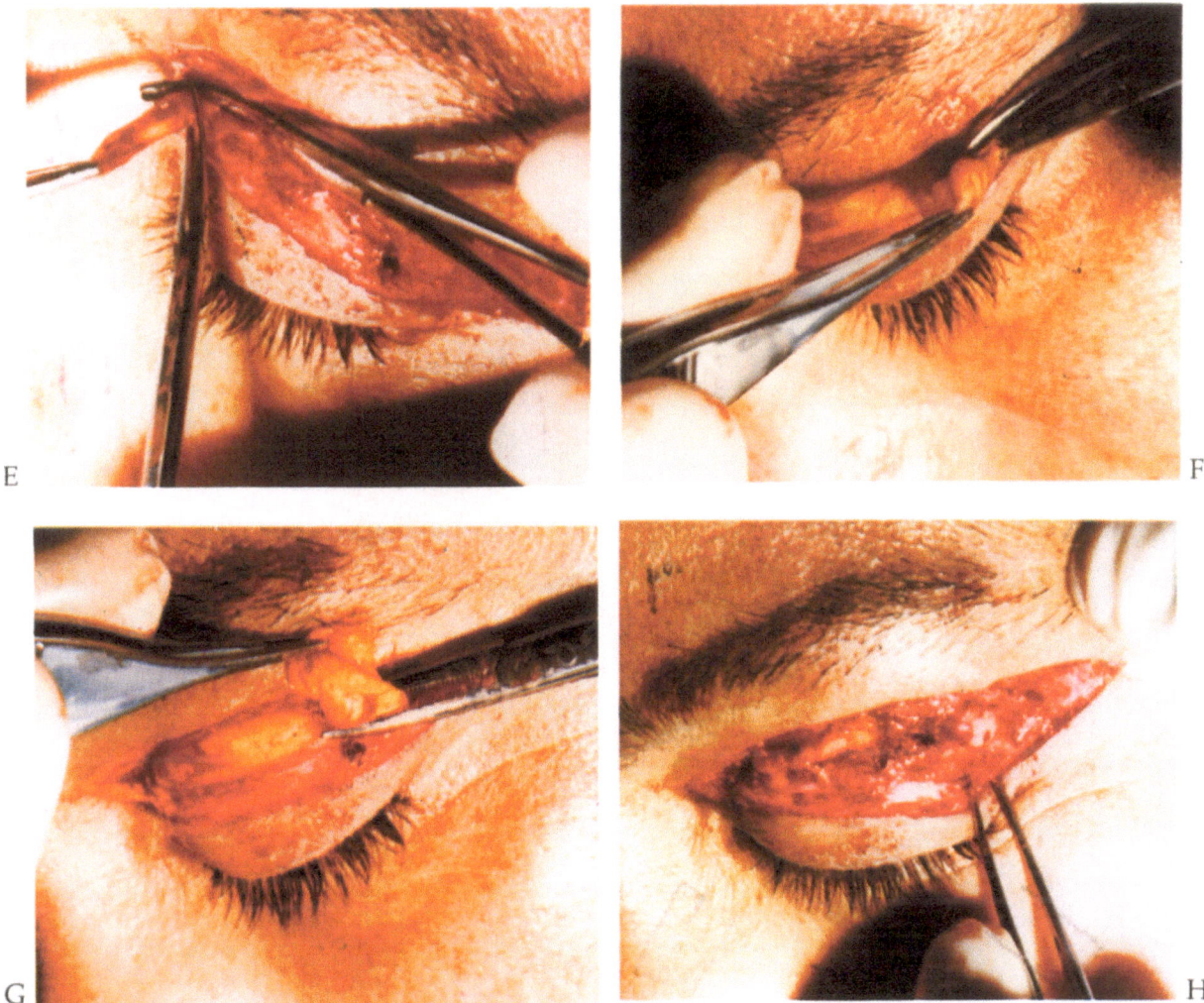

FIGURE 3.39. *E.* The excess fat has been resected from the central pocket. The excess in the mesial pocket is then assessed. To avoid hemorrhage, this excess is pinched with a curved hemostat and cauterized before being excised. These medial pockets are always difficult to access. They are characterized by being deep, fibrous, and well encapsulated, and they have fat whiter than the central pockets. *F.* The fibers of the lateral third of the orbicularis oculi muscle have been divided so as to reach the lateral extension of the central fat pocket. When the orbital fascia, which is deep at this level and difficult to reach, is sectioned, the fat herniates. The lateral extension is being tractioned and its excess evaluated and pinched with the hemostat. *G.* The excess fat is being excised from the lateral extension with curved scissors. Great care should be taken to avoid damage to the underlying lacrimal gland. *H.* Careful hemostasis is used. Note the lacrimal gland below the area from which the excess fat was resected.

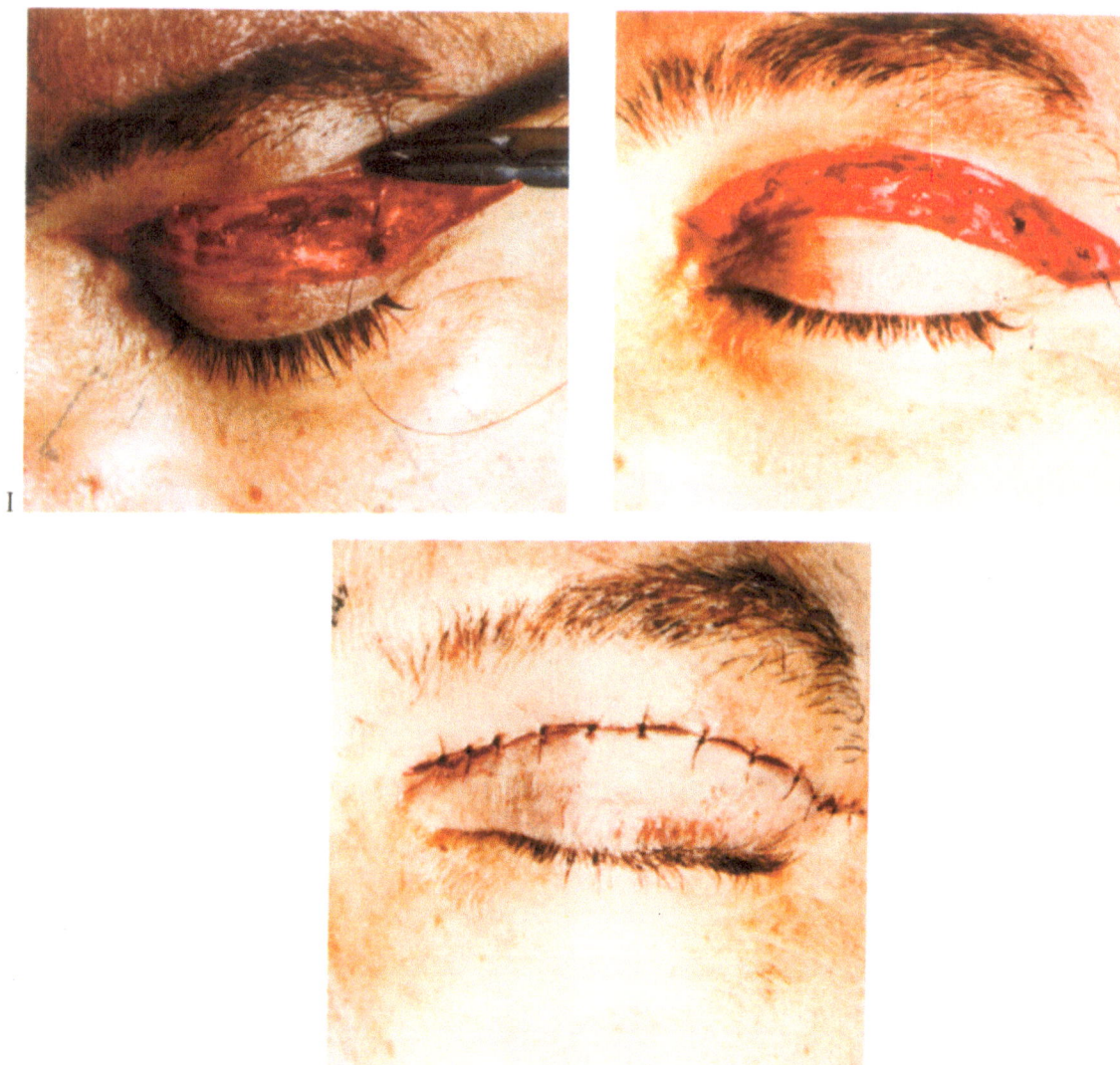

FIGURE 3.39. *I.* The orbicularis oculi muscle is sutured above the lacrimal gland, reconstructing the protective muscular wall. *J.* Muscular sutures completed.

K. Discontinous cutaneous suture of 6-0 nylon. Note that the suture line corresponds with the upper palpebral sulcus.

Lower Eyelids

The hypertrophied fat pockets of the lower eyelids are generally situated in the mesial and central thirds of the septal portion, between the nasojugal and the lower palpebral sulci. They may invade the tarsal portion of the eyelid. They are also found, but with less frequency, in the lateral third of the eyelid.

Treatment

Fat resections should be done conservatively to avoid the occurrence of depressions. One should always keep in mind that a flat lower eyelid is ideal, and everything should be done to enable this to be accomplished. Exaggerated resections from the medial pocket can deepen the nasojugal sulcus and are a factor in the formation of scleral show (technique in Fig. 3.40).

Surgical Sequence for the Reduction of Fat Pockets in the Lower Eyelids (Fig. 40A – H)

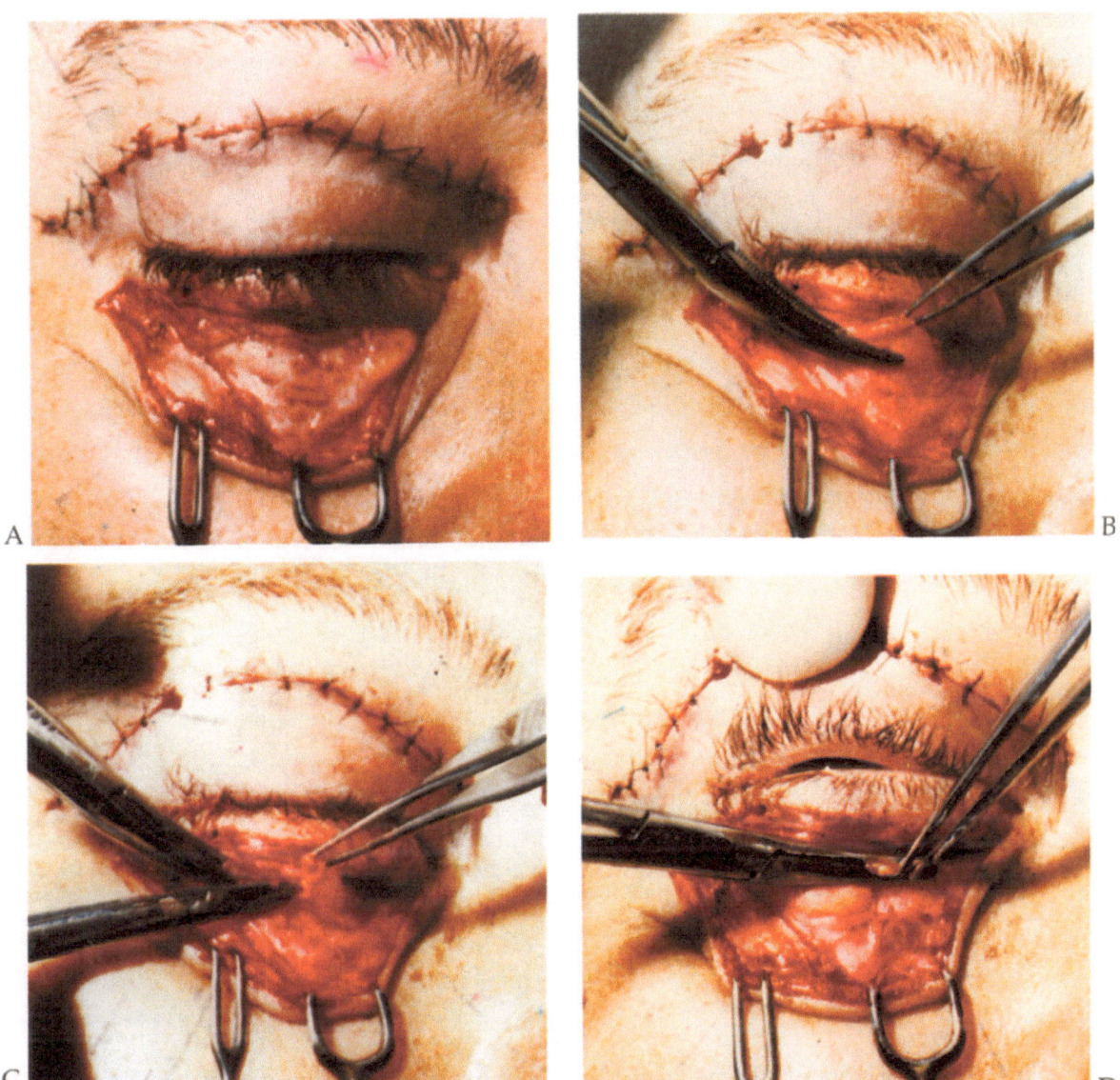

FIGURE 3.40. *A.* Incision and undermining of the skin muscle flap has been already performed. In the septal portion, the undermining is done over the orbital fascia, which has a typical "pearly" appearance. The fascia is sectioned above the mesial, central, and lateral pockets, and the fat of the three pockets herniates. The fat from the mesial pocket is white, while that from the other two pockets is yellow. *B.* The central pocket has been exteriorized. The excess fat is evaluated and pinched with a curved hemostat. *C.* The excess fat of the central pocket is sectioned with curved scissors. *D.* After removal of the excess fat, the area is coagulated with bipolar electrocautery.

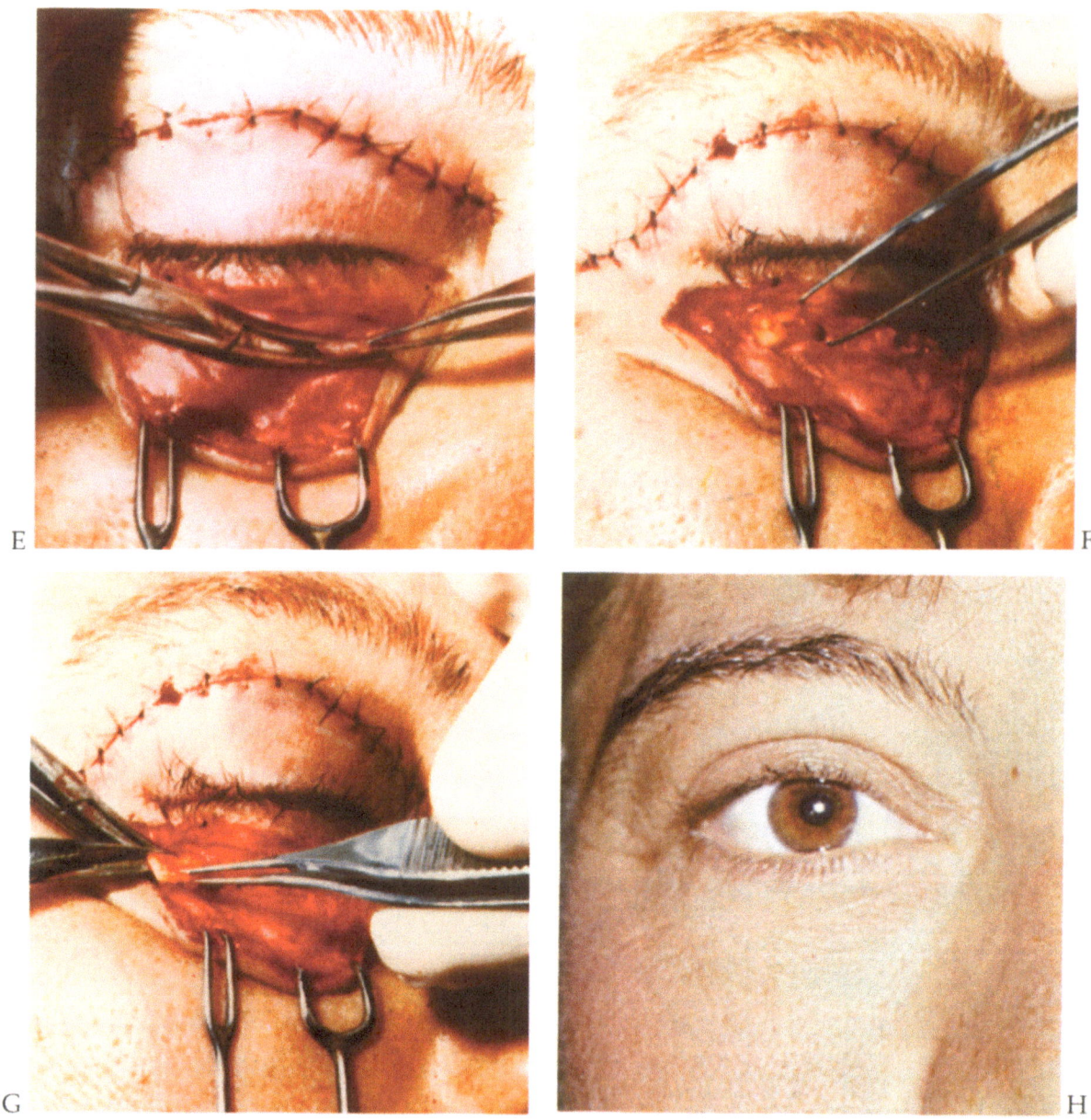

FIGURE 3.40. *E.* The same is done in the mesial pocket. *F.* The excess fat has been resected from the mesial and central pockets and cauterized. The forceps are ready to grasp the lateral fat. *G.* The lateral fat has been pinched with the curved hemostat, and the excess fat is sectioned with scissors. *H.* Postoperative view, 60 days after surgery.

Intraoperative and Postoperative Concerns

During surgery, the excised fat is kept at hand so that a little can be replaced as a free transplant if it becomes evident that too much was removed. However, these excessive reductions are not always evident immediately after surgery, or even in the later postoperative period, since edema can obscure them. With the disappearance of the edema, the lid becomes concave because the skin is pulled toward the back of the cavity (Rees, 1980). A depression becomes visible and the potential of scleral show is increased.

Examples of Reduction of Fat Pockets (Figs. 3.41–3.44)

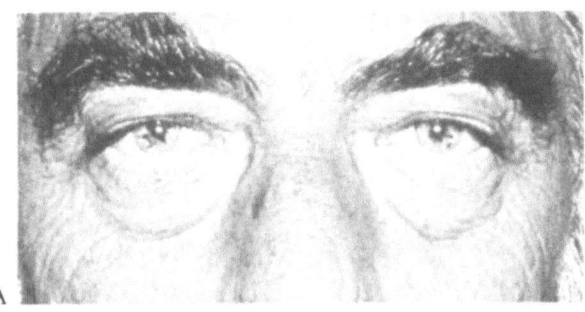

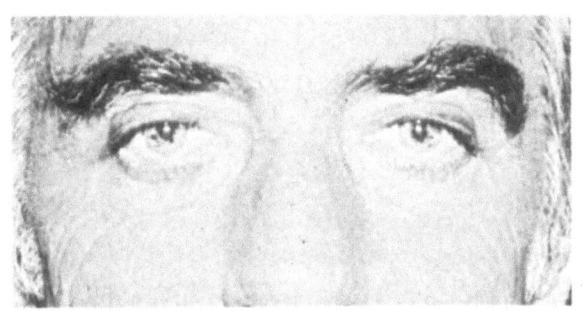

FIGURE 3.41. Hypertrophy of the fat pockets of the upper and lower lids associated with excessive skin looseness. *A.* Preoperative view. *B.* Postoperative view. (From Loeb R: Improvements in blepharop-

lasty: Creating a flat surface for the lower lid, in: *Transactions of the Seventh International Congress of Plastic and Reconstructive Surgery.* São Paulo, Sociedade Brasileira de Cirurgia Plástica, 1979, pp 390-393).

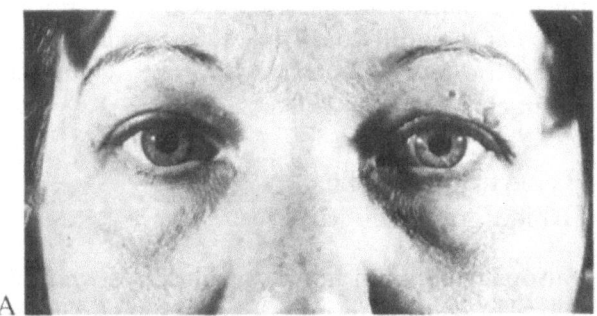

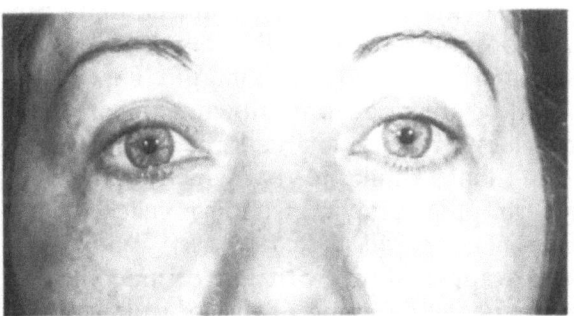

FIGURE 3.42. Patient of about 40 years of age presenting skin looseness and fat pockets in the upper and lower eyelids. Fat and skin-muscle resections were

done, including extirpation of a nevus in the lateral third of the left upper lid. *A.* Preoperative view. *B.* Postoperative view.

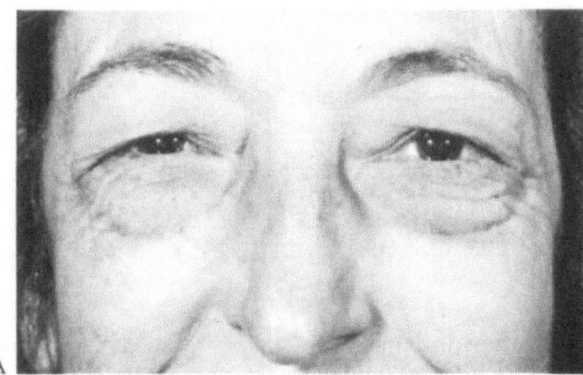

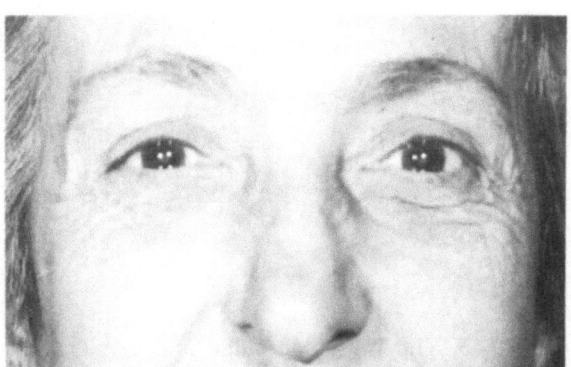

FIGURE 3.43. Fat pockets invading the cheek and malar regions. *A.* Preoperative view. *B.* Postoperative view.

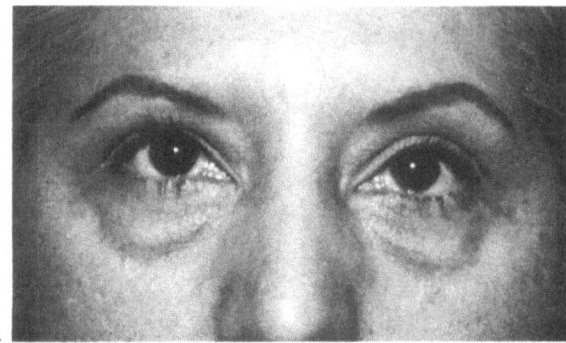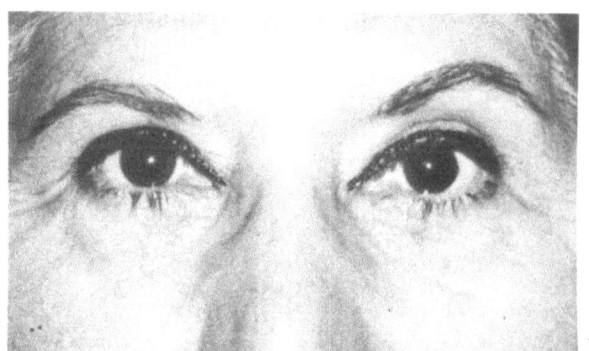

FIGURE 3.44. Fat pockets in the lower lid. *A.* Preoperative view. *B.* Postoperative view showing the flat surface obtained.

Muscular Bulges

General Considerations

Muscular bulges are caused by an increase in the volume of the orbicularis oculi muscle in the pretarsal portion of the lower lid, between the lower palpebral sulcus and the lid margin (Fig. 3.45).

If these bulges are present when the orbicular muscle is at rest (static situation), the patient has a tired look, similar to that which occurs with hypertrophied fat pockets. This is called: *"hypertrophy of the orbicularis oculi muscle."* When these bulges appear only with the contraction and consequent thickening of the orbicular muscle (the dynamic situation), a jovial expression appears, and the aesthetic effect is pleasing. This is called: *"transitory hypertrophy of the orbicularis oculi muscle."*

The faces of individuals with hypertrophy of the orbicularis oculi muscle can exhibit a sudden and paradoxical duplicity of expression: tired when the muscle is relaxed; happy when it is contracted.

Hypertrophy of the Orbicularis Oculi Muscle

Various factors can cause exaggerated lower palpebral bulges in this muscle while it is static (Fig.

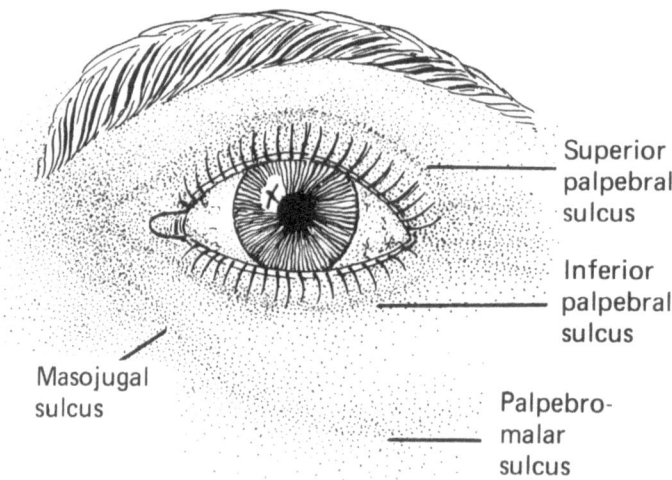

Superior palpebral sulcus

Inferior palpebral sulcus

Masojugal sulcus

Palpebromalar sulcus

FIGURE 3.45. The muscular bulge is caused by the hypertrophy of the orbicularis muscle and is situated in the tarsal portion of the lower eyelid, between the lid margin and the inferior palpebral sulcus. It should not be confused with skin, fat, or bony bulges.

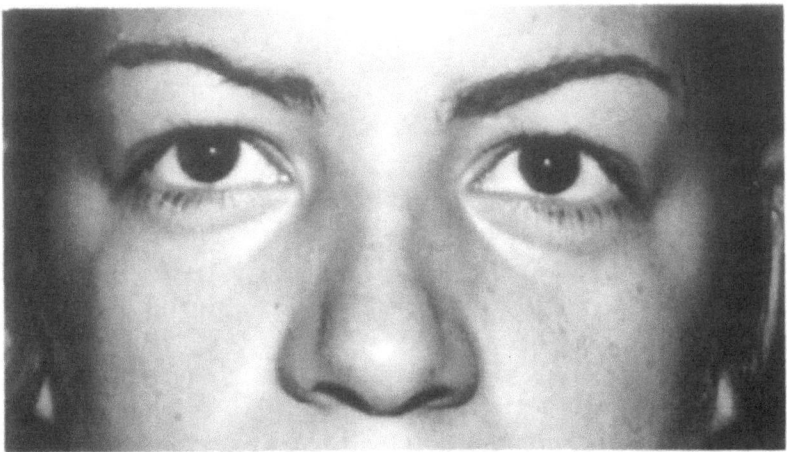

FIGURE 3.46. Hypertrophy of the orbicularis oculi muscle. A 30-year-old patient presenting with typical muscular hypertrophy in the tarsal portion of the lower lids, with the characteristic tired expression of the face. Note the bulging tarsal portion in relation to the septal portion. The orbicularis oculi muscle is static.

3.46). In the pretarsal portion of the upper eyelid, one does not see such hypertrophies, but at times there can be a small increase in the septal portion of this lid.

Classification of the Hypertrophies of the Orbicularis Oculi Muscle

The hypertrophies of the orbicularis oculi muscle can be developmental or iatrogenic.

Developmental

Frequently a muscular bulge is found in the pretarsal region of the lower lid in young people. While it is characteristic of infancy, it can also be found in adults. These bulges are often more evident when there is a depression of the septal region. If the muscular bulge is exaggerated when the muscle is static, it can have an appearance similar to a fat palpebral pouch, and the aesthetic effect is poor. In this circumstance, the excess muscle must be reduced surgically in the tarsal region. Sometimes a fat graft can be inserted below the orbicularis muscle in the septal region.

Iatrogenic

Bulges of an iatrogenic origin can occur as a consequence of undue resection of fat from the central and mesial pockets of the lower lid. Usually in these cases, hypertrophy of the tarsal portion of the orbicularis oculi muscle had already existed and had not been reduced when the fat was removed. Subsequently, because of the depression now existing between the lower palpebral and nasojugal sulci, the muscular bulge became more apparent.

In cases of hypertrophy of the tarsal portion of the orbicularis oculi muscle, when the hypertrophied muscle is erroneously saved and the volume of fat tissue is unduly reduced, the bulge of the muscle, besides persisting, is even more evident because of the depression existing between the lower palpebral sulcus and the nasojugal sulcus.

Transitory Hypertrophy of the Orbicularis Oculi Muscle

The bulge in these cases appears only during the contraction of the orbicularis oculi muscle (Fig. 3.47), and the face can acquire an expression of happiness. It is the so called "creasing" of the eyelids, which is observed in persons who "laugh with their eyes." This transitory hypertrophy can appear in persons whose orbicularis oculi muscle in the static position is perfectly normal (Fig. 3.48).

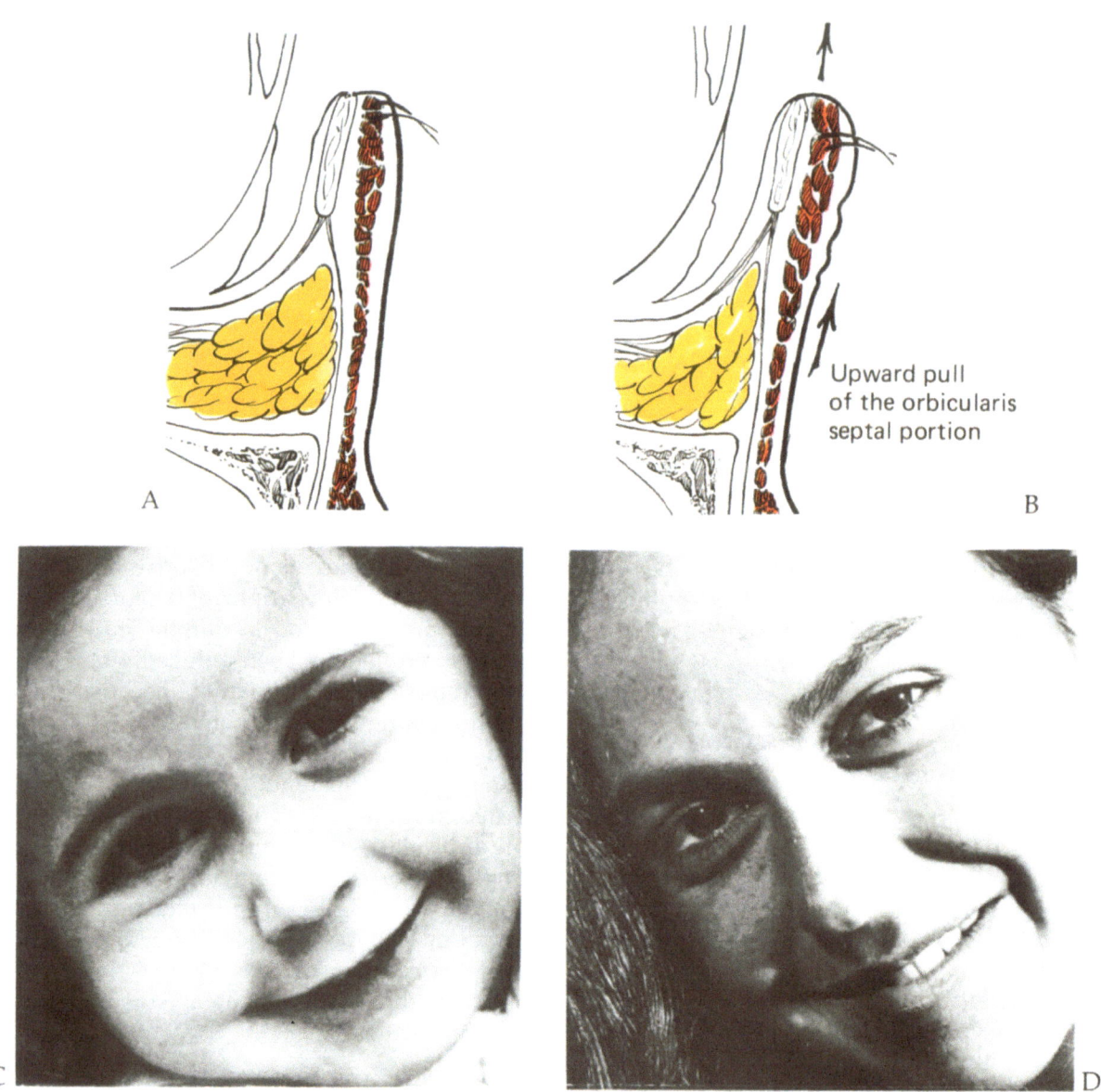

FIGURE 3.47. Transitory hypertrophy of the orbicularis oculi muscle. *A.* The hypertrophy does not exist when the muscle is at rest. *B.* It is only apparent when the muscle is contracted. In this condition the tarsal portion is increased by a sphincter type of contraction, and the upper septal portion of the muscle is added to the tarsal portion. *C.* Transitory hypertrophy of the orbicularis oculi muscle in a four-year-old girl. *D.* Transitory hypertrophy of the orbicularis oculi muscle is not unaesthetic and smiling accentuates the hypertrophy. Same girl, aged 16 (daughter of the author). (From Loeb, R: Necessity for partial resection of the orbicularis oculi muscle in blepharoplasties in some young patients. Plast and Reconstr Surg, 1977; 60(2):176–178.)

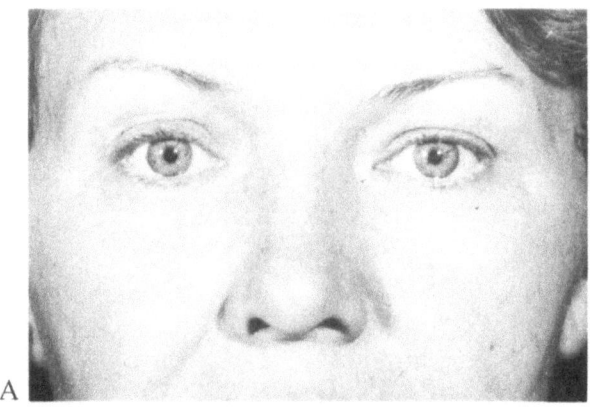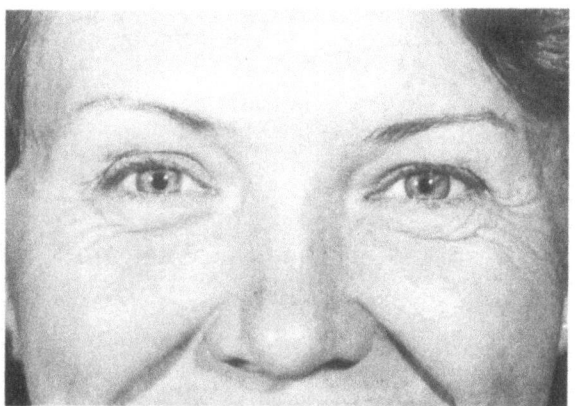

FIGURE 3.48. Transitory hypertrophy of the orbicularis oculi muscle. *A.* The hypertrophy does not exist when the muscle is at rest. *B.* The hypertrophy appears when the muscle is contracted, giving the appearance of happiness.

Treatment

Transitory Hypertrophy of the Orbicularis Oculi Muscle

In these cases there should be no surgical treatment because a reduction of this muscle could cause a depression in the tarsal region and by reducing the tonus of the muscle, favor a future scleral show or ectropion.

Hypertrophy of the Orbicularis Oculi Muscle

The surgery consists of diminishing the thickness of the superficial part of the pretarsal portion of the orbicularis oculi muscle. The surgical technique is described in Figures 3.49 and 3.50.

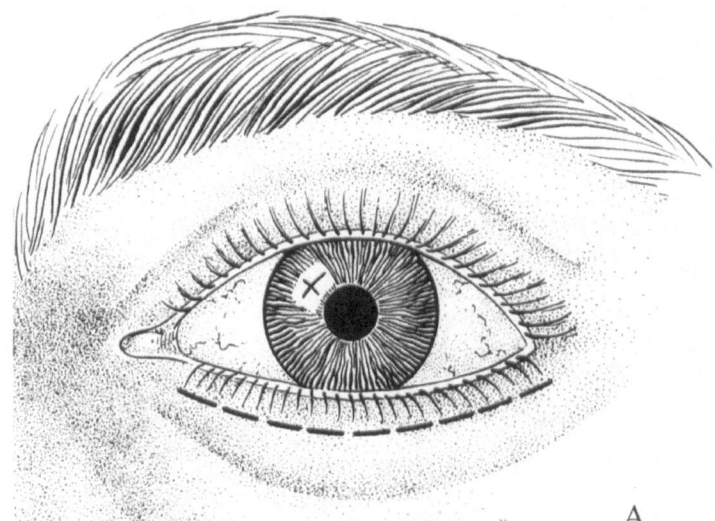

A

FIGURE 3.49. *A.* Correction of hypertrophy of the orbicularis oculi muscle. The dotted line is placed about 2 to 2.5 mm below the implantation of the eyelash from angle to angle of the eye. The resection is made along the pretarsal portion.

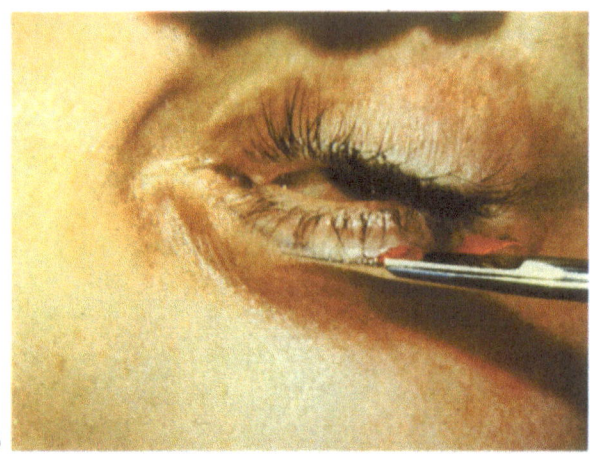

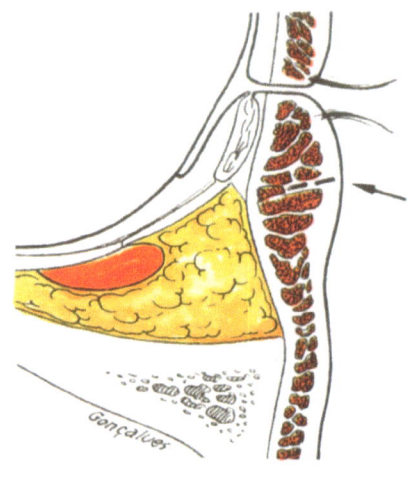

FIGURE 3.49. *B.* The incision is started with a scalpel and finished with scissors. It is made deeply, sectioning about half the thickness of the orbicularis oculi muscle in its tarsal portion. The diagram shows the relationship of the incision to the palpebral border.

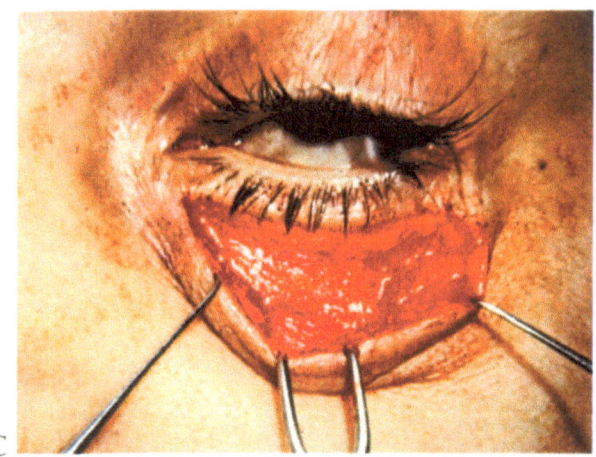

FIGURE 3.49. *C.* Skin-muscle flap showing the tarsal portion of the muscle in the upper part of the surgical field. Just below appears a flat area, which has reflected the light of the flash. This is septal and fat tissues.

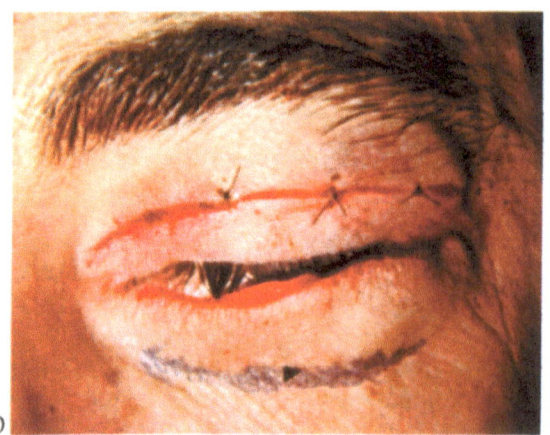

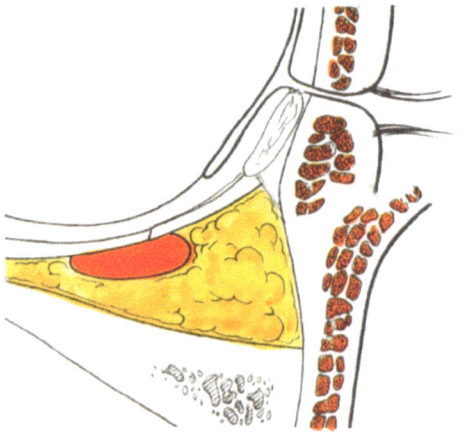

FIGURE 3.49. *D.* Sagittal diagram of the shortening of the skin muscle. After undermining, the flap is elevated in order to estimate accurately the amount of tissue to be resected.

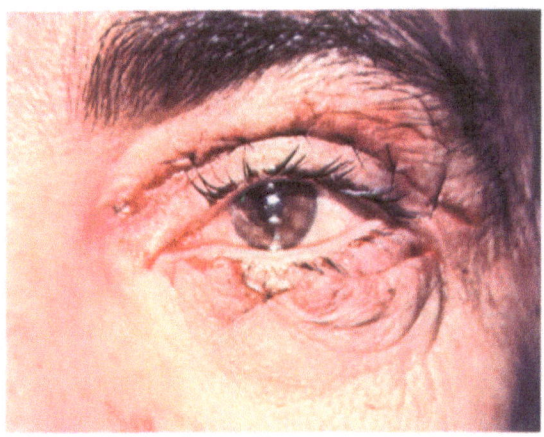

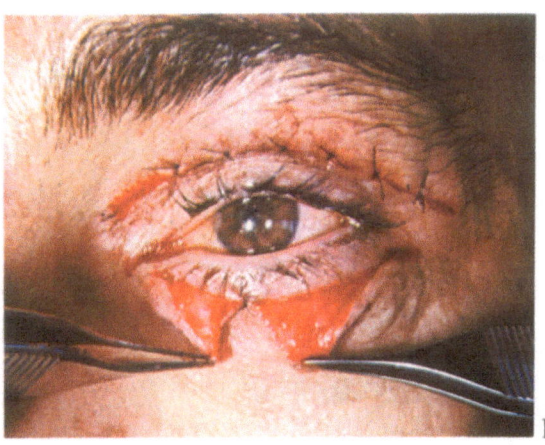

FIGURE 3.49. *E.* The amount of tissue to be resected is calculated carefully. The flap is sectioned and then fixed with a suture. The head of the patient is raised to verify the absence of scleral show or ectropion, and the amount of tissue to be resected is estimated.

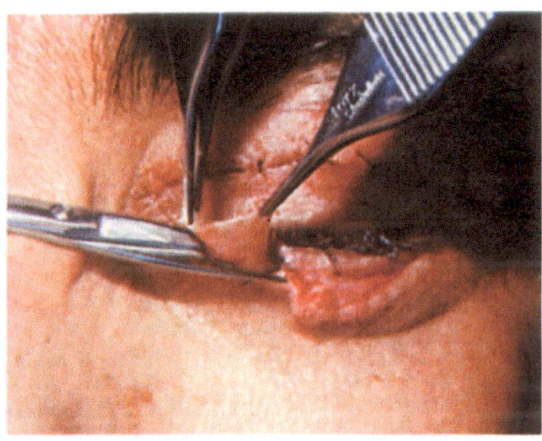

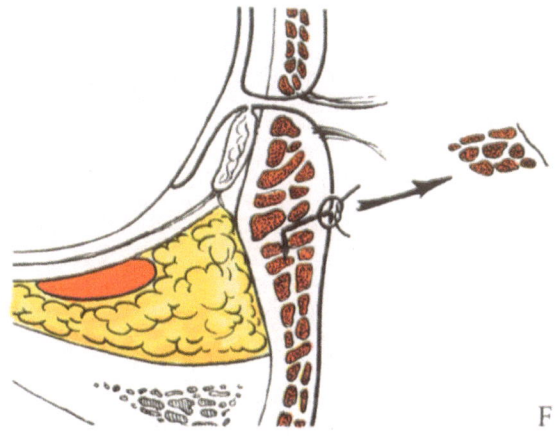

FIGURE 3.49. *F.* Shortening the skin-muscle flap. The excess tissue is resected and suturing is completed. In the majority of patients this resection serves to reduce the hypertrophied muscle sufficiently.

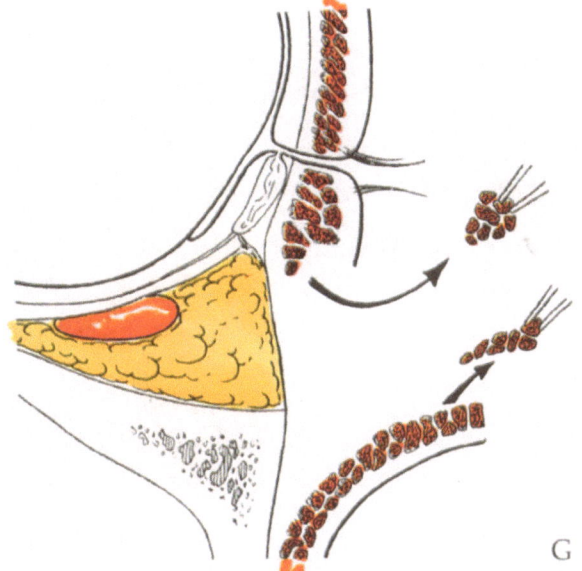

FIGURE 3.49. *G.* If an excess of muscular tissue should remain, more can be taken from both upper and lower flaps, always taking care not to create a muscular hypotonicity.

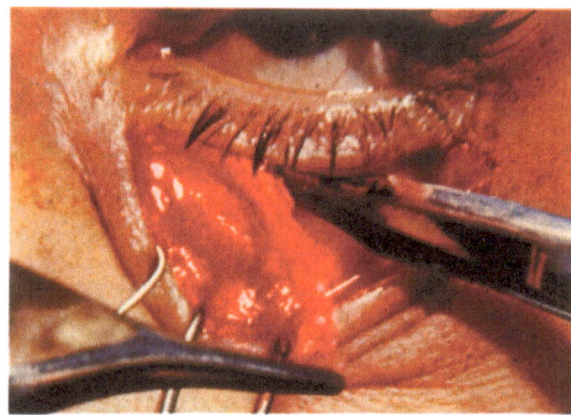

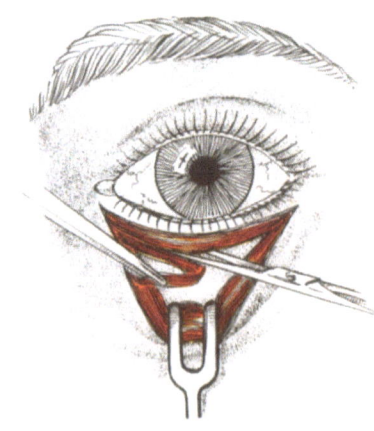

FIGURE 3.49. *H.* Removal of an extra strip from the tarsal portion of the muscle. Care must be taken in this step, particularly with aged patients, so as not to

reduce the tonus of the muscle. Such a weakening could favor scleral show or ectropion.

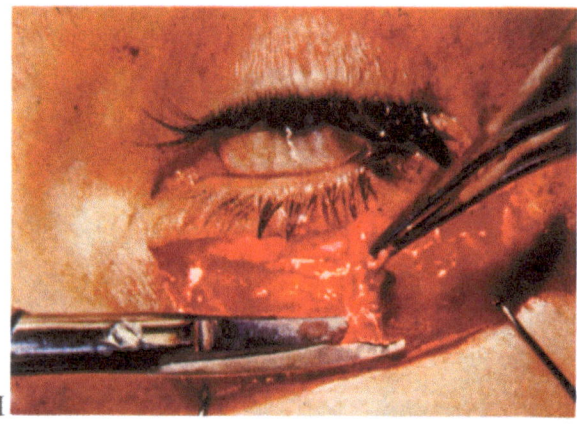

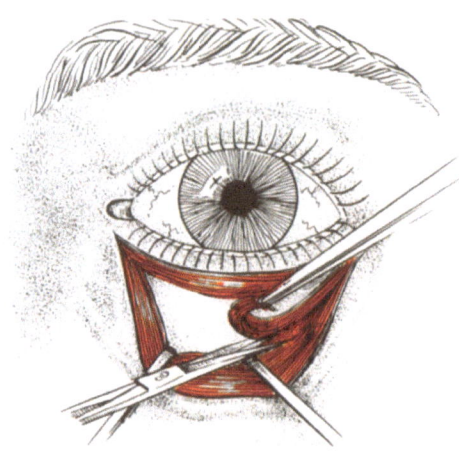

FIGURE 3.49. *I.* Same maneuver in the lower flap. (From Loeb R: Necessity for partial resection of the orbicularis oculi muscle in blepharoplasties in some

young patients. *Plast Reconstr Surg.* 1977; 60(2):176–178.)

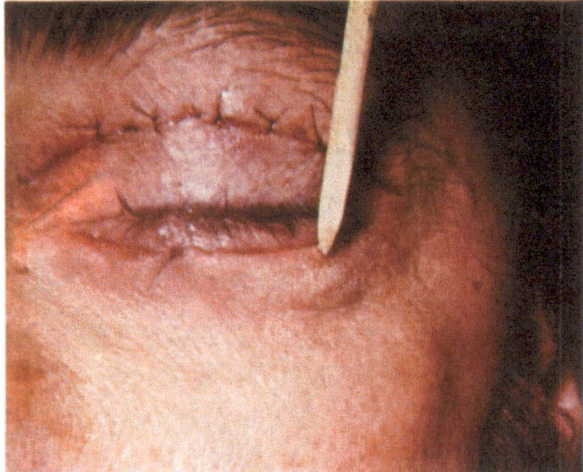

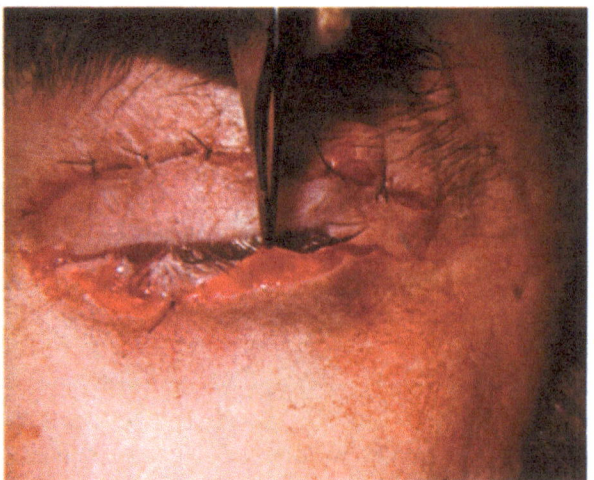

FIGURE 3.49. *J.* Sometimes an excess of muscle still remains. It must be corrected. *K.* The excess muscle is again evaluated and reduced.

FIGURE 3.49. *L*. Final results 48 hours postoperative.

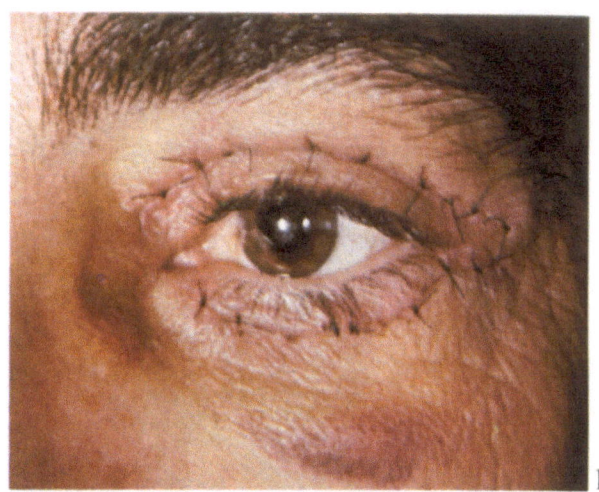

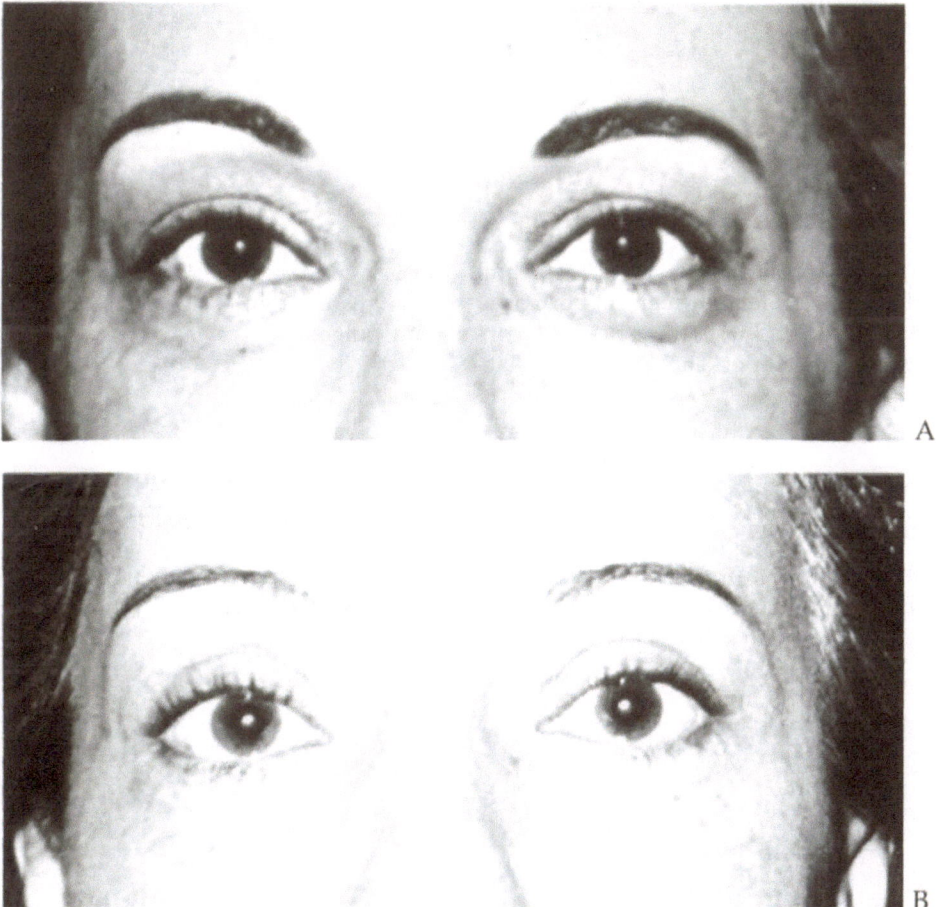

FIGURE 3.50. Hypertrophy of the orbicularis oculi muscle. The patient's appearance was such that she could have had either a muscular or a fat hypertrophy, and the differential diagnosis between the two was based on the excess volume being localized in the pretarsal portion, a condition that occurs only with muscular hypertrophy. This case was treated by resection of the superficial portion of the orbicularis oculi muscle. *A*. Preoperative view. *B*. Postoperative view. (From Loeb R: Necessity for partial resection of the orbicularis oculi muscle in blepharoplasties in some young patients. *Plast Reconstr Surg* 60 2, 1977; 60(2):176–178.)

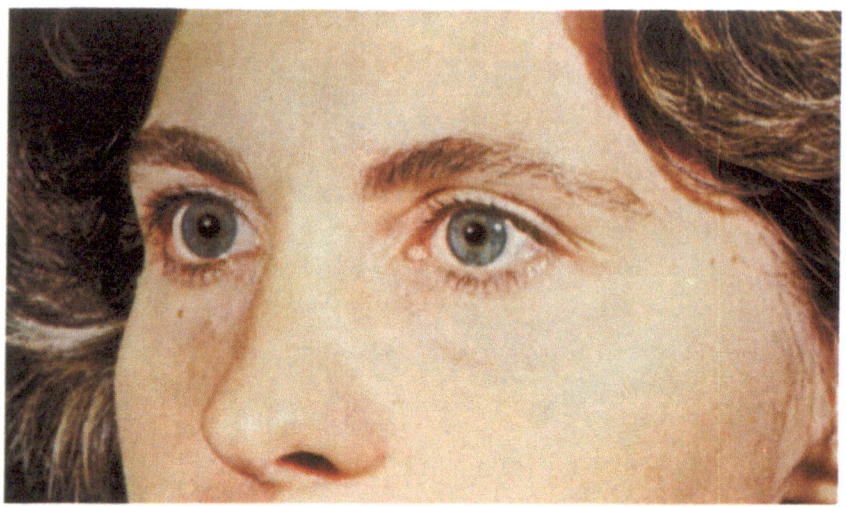

FIGURE 3.51. Patient presenting a bony palpebral bulge. Note the slight bulge at the central portion of the lower orbital border. These bulges can be confused with exaggerated fat pockets. An error in diag- nosis is serious, since resection of adipose tissue here may create a depression that would accentuate the bony bulge.

Bony Bulges

General Considerations

At times, patients present with a bulge in the central third of the lower orbital border that at first appears similar to an exaggerated fat pocket (Fig. 3.51) and is most apparent when the head is raised. Palpation immediately reveals it to be a solid bony hypertrophy. It can be removed surgically if necessary (Rees, 1980).

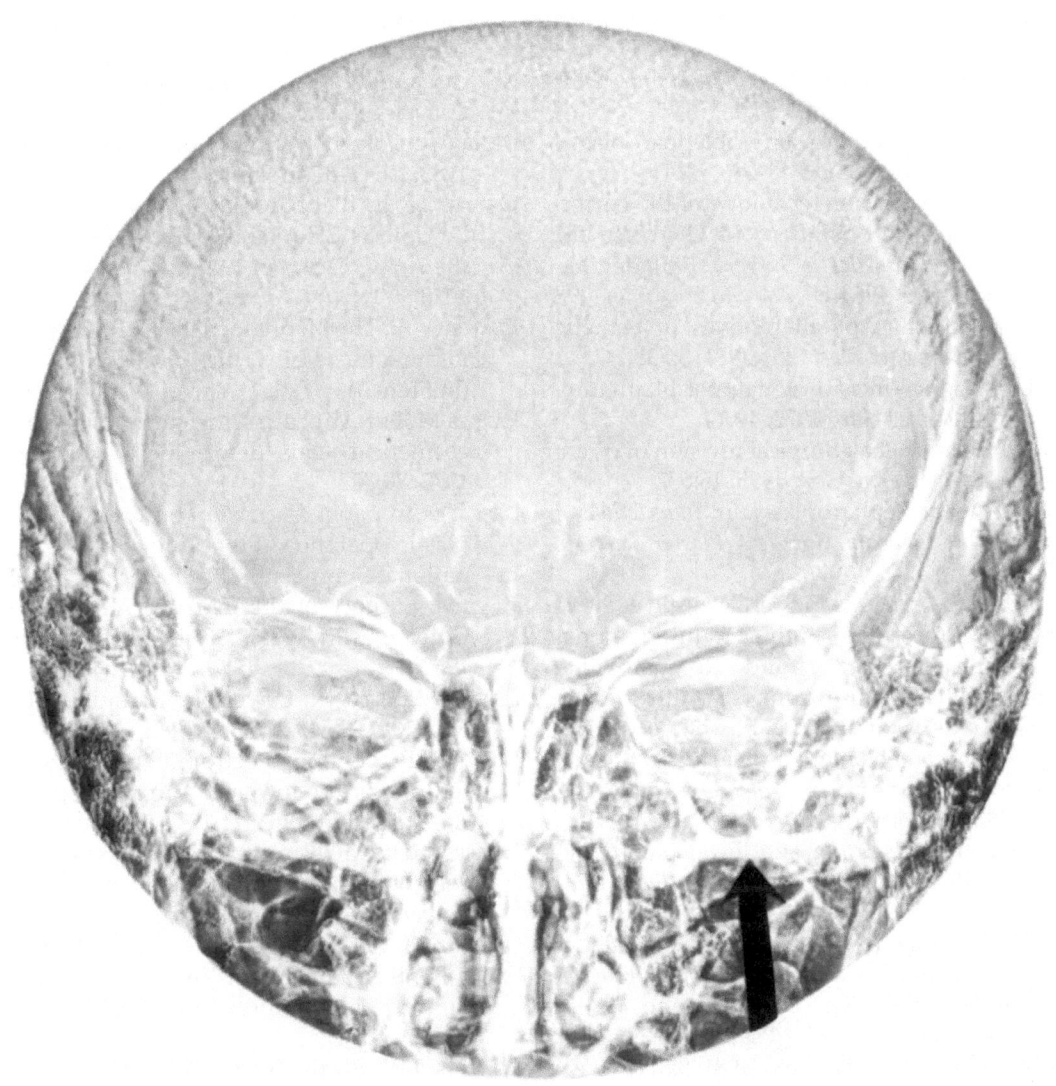

Xerography of patient shown in Fig. 3.51.

Additional Reading

Skin Bulges

ADAMSON JE, McCRAW JB et al: – Use of the muscle flap in lower blepharoplasty. *Plast Reconstr Surg* 1979; 63:359.

BACKER TJ: Upper blepharoplasty. *Clin Plast Surg* 1981; 8:635.

CHRIST JE: Cleansing eyelids after blepharoplasty. *Plast Reconstr Surg* 1985; 75:444.

CONVERSE JM: The Converse technique of the corrective eyelid plastic operation, in Converse JM (ed): *Reconstructive Plastic Surgery*. Philadelphia WB Saunders Co, 1964.

COURTISS EH: Selection of alternatives in esthetic blepharoplasty. *Clin Plast Surg* 1981; 8:739.

CRONIN TD: Marginal incision for upper blepharoplasty. *Plast Reconstr Surg* 1972; 49:14.

DOXANAS MT, SERRA F et al: Surgical revision of oriental eyelids. *Ophthalmic Surg* 1985; 16:657.

FLOWERS RS: Anchor blepharoplasty, in: *Transactions of the Sixth International Congress Plastic Surgery*. Paris, Masson et Cie, 1976.

GONZALEZ-ULLOA M, STEVENS EF: Senile eyelid esthetic correction. Proceedings of the 2nd International Symposium on Plastic and Reconstructive Surgery of the Eye and Adnexa, Smith B, Converse JM. (eds). St. Louis, CV Mosby Co, 1967.

GUERRA SILVA J: Aesthetic blepharoplasty, in: Sucena RC: Cirurgia Plastica, São Paulo, Livraria Rocca, vol 2, 1982. (in Portuguese)

GUY CL, LIVERETT DN: upper and lower blepharoplasty: Standard technique. *Clin Plast Surg* 1981; 8:663.

HINDERER U: The aging palbebral and periorbital region. *Transactions of the VII Congress of the International Plastic Reconstr Surg*, Rio de Janeiro, 1979.

HORNBLASS A: Ptosis and Pseudoptosis and Blepharoplasty. *Clin Plast Surg* 1981; 8:811.

KAYE BL: Two helpful technical aids in blepharoplasty. *Plast Reconstr Surg* 1983; 71:714.

KLASTSKY SA, MANSON PN: Separate skin and muscle flaps in lowerlid blepharoplasty. *Plast Reconstr Surg* 1981; 67:151.

LOEB R: Technical improvement for palpebral rhitidectomy. *Rev Latinoam Cir Plast* 1961; 5:93.

LOEB R: Surgical procedure to avoid paralysis of the occipital belly of the occipito-frontalis muscle in rhytidoplasty. *Transactions of the Fourth International Congress of Plastic and Rec. Surgery*, Rome, 1967, pp. 1116–1119.

LOEB R: Aesthetic blepharoplasties based on the degree of wrinkling. *Plast Reconstr Surg* 1971; 47:33.

LOEB R: La hipertrofia del músculo orbicular y su influencia en el relieve de las bolsas palpebrales. *Cirurgia Estética, Argentina* 1976; 1: pp. 7-8 (in Spanish).

LOEB R: Musculus orbicularis oculy hypertrophy – Different treatments depending on the clinical cases. *Abstracts of paper presented during the IX Congress of the* ISAPS, New York, 1987.

MOULY R: Cosmetic surgery of the eyelids. *Chirurgie* 1983; 109:248. (in French)

OWSLEY JQ Jr: Blepharoplasty variations, in Goulian D, Courtis EH (eds): Symposium on Surgery of the Aging Face, vol 19. St. Louis, CV Mosby Co, 1978.

PANNETON P: The blepharochalasis. Report of 51 cases in the same family. *Arch Ophthalmol* 1963; 53:725. (in French)

PARKES M, FEIN W et al: – Pinch technique for repair of cosmetic eyelids deformities. *Arch Ophthalmol* 1973; 89:324.

REES TD: In panel discussion on the cosmetic eyelid plastic operation. Proceedings of the 2nd International Symposium on Plastic and Reconstructive Surgery of the Eye and Adnexa, Smith B, Converse JM (eds). St. Louis, CV Mosby Co, 1967.

REES TD, TABBAL N: Lower blepharoplasty. *Clin Plast Surg* 1981; 8:643.

REES TD: Prevention of ectropion by horizontal shortenning of the lower lid during blepharoplasty. *Ann Plast Surg* 1983; 11:17.

ROGERS BO: An electrocauterization technique for cosmetic blepharoplasty, in: *Aesthetic Plastic Surgery*, vol II. Gonzales-Ulloa M and Meyer R Piccin, 1987.

SAYOC BT: Blepharochalasis in upper eyelids, including its classification. *Am J Ophthalmol* 1957; 43:970.

SHAGETS FW, SHORE JW et al: The management of eyelid laxity during lower eyelid blepharoplasty. *Arch Otolaryngol* 1986; 112:729.

SHEEN JH: Supratarsal fixation in upper blepharoplasty. *Plast Reconstr Surg* 1974; 54:424.

SHEEHAN JE: *Plastic Surgery of the Orbit*. New York, Macmillan, 1927.

SHIRAKABE Y, KINUGASA T et al: The double-eyelid operation in Japan: its elolution as related to cultural changes. *Ann Plast Surg* 1985; 15:224.

SKOOG T: *Plastic Surgery*. Philadelphia, WB Saunders Co, 1975.

SONG RY, SONG YG et al: Double eyelid operations. *Aesthetic Plast Surg* 1985; 9:173.

SPIRA M: Lower blepharoplasty – a clinical study. *Plast Reconstr Surg* 1977; 59:35.

STARK RB: Blepharoplasty, how I do it. *Ann Plast Surg* 1978; 1:58.

STEPHENSON KL: The history of blepharoplasty to correct blepharochalasis. *Aesth Plast Surg* 1977; 1:77.

TAYLOR DP, SALYER KE et al: Protecting the eye during surgery. *Plast Reconstr Surg* 1986; 77:684.

TOLEDO LS: Blepharoplasty with Fibrin seal. *Transactions VIII International Congress of Plastic and Reconstructive Surgery*, Canadá, 1983.

VOLFLEY D: Blepharoplasty: The ophthalmologist's view. *Otolaryngol Clin North Am* 1980; 13:237.

Fat Bulges

BAMES H: Baggy eyelids. *Plast Reconstr Surg* 1958; 22:264.

BARKER DE: Dye injection studies of intraorbital fat compartments. *Plast Reconstr Surg* 1977; 59:82.

CASTAÑARES S: Blepharoplasty for herniated intraorbital fat. Anatomic bases for a new approach. *Plast Reconstr Surg* 1951; 8:46.

CASTAÑARES S: Baggy eyelids. Physiological considerations and surgical technique. *Transactions of the 3rd International Congress of Plastic Surgery*. Excerpta Medica Foundation, 1964.

CASTAÑARES S: The lateral fat compartments of the lower eyelid. *Aesthetic Plast Surg* 1983; 7:27.

DUFOURMENTEL C, MOULY R: Surgical treatment of wrinkles and pouches of the eyelids. *Ann Chir Plast* 1958; 3:229. (in French)

GONZÁLEZ-ULLOA M, STEVENS EF: The treatment of palpebral bags. *Plast Reconstr Surg* 1961; 27:381.

JOHNSON JB, HADLEY RC: The aging face, in Converse JM (ed): *Reconstructive Plastic Surgery*. Philadelphia, WB Saunders Co, 1964.

OWSLEY JQ: Resection of prominent lateral fat pad during upper lid blepharoplasty. *Plastic Reconstr Surg* 1980; 65:4.

PITANGUY I, LESSA S et al: Subconjuntival fat herniation. *Rev Bras Cir* 1975; 65:151. (in Portuguese)

PSILLAKIS JM, ALBANO A: Surgical treatment of wrinkles and eyelid bulkiness. *Rev Asoc Med Bras* 1976; 22:97. (in Portuguese)

PUTTERMAN AM, URIST MJ: Baggy eyelids – a true hernia. *Ann Ophthalmol* 1973; 5:1029.

REES TD, DUPUIS C: Baggy eyelids in young adults. *Plast Reconstr Surg* 1969; 43:381.

REIDY JP: Swelling of eyelids. *Br J Plast Surg* 1960; 13:256.

SACHS ME, BOSNIAK SL et al: Correction of true periorbital fat herniation in cosmetic lower lid blepharoplasty. *Aesthetic Plast Surg* 1986; 10:111.

SCHWARZ F, RANDALL P: Conjunctival incision for herniated orbital fat. *Ophthalmic Surg* 1980; 11:276.

TESSIER P: The treatment of baggy eyelids through the conjunctival route in young patients, in: *Transactions First International Congress of the International Society for Aesthetic Plastic Surgery*, Rio de Janeiro, 1972.

TOBIN HA: Electrosurgical blepharoplasty: a technique that questions conventional concepts of fat compartmentalization. *Ann Plast Surg* 1985, 14:59.

SMITH JW: Blepharoplasty: Technical details. *Aesthetic Plast Surg* 1987; 2:95.

Muscular Bulges

ASTON SJ: Skin-muscle flap lower lid blepharoplasty: an easier dissection. *Aesthetic Plast Surg* 1982; 6:217.

BAKER TJ, GORDON HL et al: Upper lid blepharoplasty. *Plast Reconstr Surg* 1977; 60:692.

BEARE R: Surgical treatment of senile changes in the eyelids. The McIndoe-Beare technique, in: Smith B, Converse JM (eds): *Proceedings of the Second International Symposium on Plastic and Reconstructive Surgery of Eye and Adnexa*. Edited St. Louis, CV Mosby Co, 1967.

FURNAS DW: Festoons of orbicularis muscle as a cause of baggy eyelids. *Plast Reconstr Surg* 1978; 61:531.

FURNAS DW: The Orbicularis Oculi Muscle. *Clin Plast Surg* 1981; 8:687.

GORDON G: Observations upon the movements of the eyelid. *Br J Ophthalmol* 1951; 35:339.

KENNARD DW, GLASER GH: An analysis of eyelid movements. *J New Ment Dis* 1964; 139:31.

LOEB R: Orbicularis oculi muscle hipertrophie and its influence in the projection of palpebral pouches. *Cir Estét* 1976; 1:1. Buenos Aires. (in Spanish)

LOEB R: Necessity for partial resection of the orbicularis oculi muscle in blepharoplasties in some young patients. *Plast Reconstr Surg* 1977; 60:178.

SPINA V, KAMAKURA L et al: Surgical treatment of wrinkles of the lower eyelids associated with herniation of orbital fat: muscular-cutaneous flap technique. *J Int Surg* 1969; 52:400.

WALSH FB, HOYT WF: *Clinical Neuro-Ophthalmology*, vol 1, ed 3. Baltimore, Williams & Wilkins, Co, 1969.

Bony Bulges

LASSUS C: Osteotomy of superior orbital rim in cosmetic blepharoplasty. *Plast Reconstr Surg* 1979; 63:481.

LENTILHAC JP: Reduction of the supraorbital ridges. A new cosmetic operation?; Personal publication, Paris. (in French)

REES TD: Postoperative considerations and complications, in: *Aesthetic Plastic Surgery*. Philadelphia, WB Saunders Co, 1980, p.536.

4

Depressions of the Eyelids

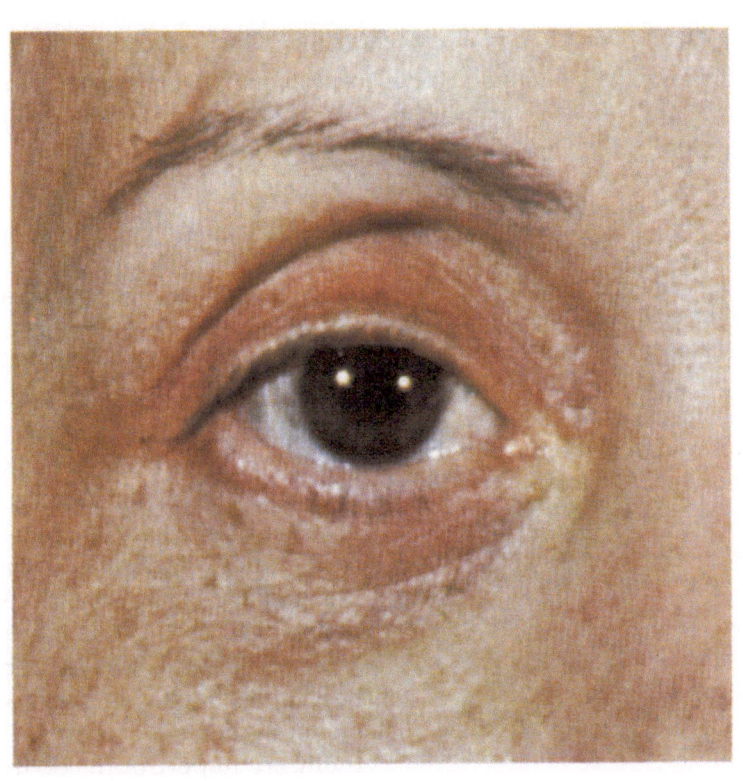

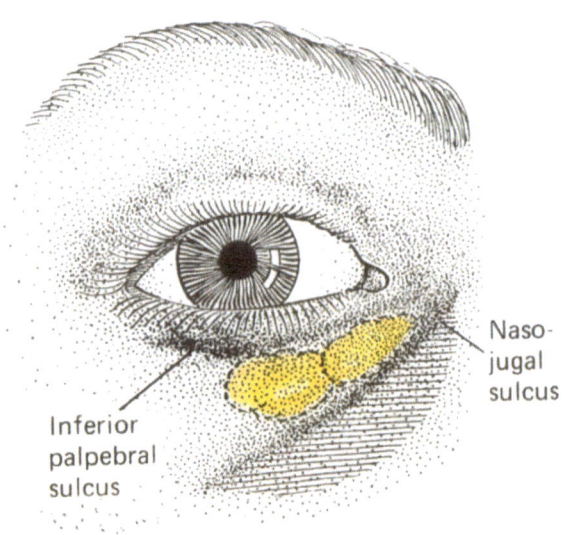

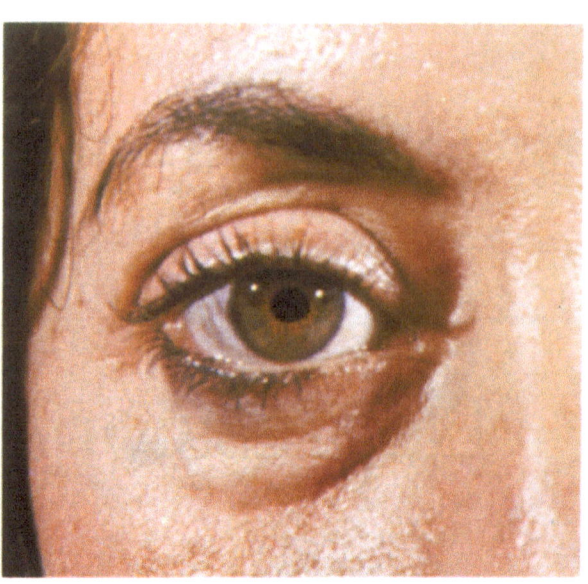

FIGURE 4.1. Nasojugal and lower palpebral sulci made evident by the hypertrophy of the medial and intermedial fat pockets. (From Loeb R: Fat pad sliding and fat grafting for leveling lid depressions. *Clin Plast Surg*, October 1981; vol 8, No 4.)

Introduction

Based on the principle that the eyelids should exhibit a flat surface (Fig. 1.1), depressions of the eyelids can be considered defects in the appearance and just as undesirable as bulges. They are morphological alterations caused by a reduction in the volume of tissue, and thus are the opposite of bulges, where excess tissue exists. As we will show in this chapter, palpebral depressions can be a causative factor in scleral show and ectropion.

Etiology

Palpebral depressions are caused by insufficient volume of muscular or fat tissue subjacent to the skin. The sunken surface of the skin then contrasts with the neighboring palpebral regions. The deepest part of the depression usually has a coloration that contrasts with that of the rest of the eyelid and that varies with the quantity, quality, and bloodsupply of the tissue over which it lies. Added to these factors is the naturally lesser incidence of light in the depths of the depression, resulting in shading.

The best example of a palpebral depression is the sunken septal portion of the lower lid, resulting from a reduced volume of fat beneath it. Another good example is the depression of the tarsal portion of the lower lid as a consequence of an exaggerated reduction of the orbicularis oculi muscle. These two types of depressions, adipose and muscular, can cause or contribute to scleral show and/or ectropion (see Chapter 6).

Other types of depressions are caused by the deepening of the principle natural sulci: the lower palpebral, the palpebro-malar, and the nasojugal. Such depressions as these are most evident when they contrast with fat pockets near them. A hypertrophy of the orbicularis oculi muscle or an enlarged volume in the cheek region can also cause these sulci to appear excessively deep. The best examples of depressed sulci are those of the nasojugal and lower palpebral, limiting the central and medial fat pockets (Fig. 4.1).

Palpebral depressions can be distressing to some patients and of major importance to others, mostly when they are very exaggerated. In these cases, correction is necessary (Fig. 4.2).

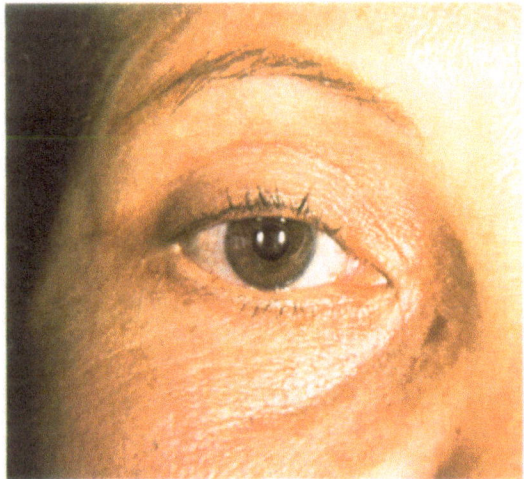 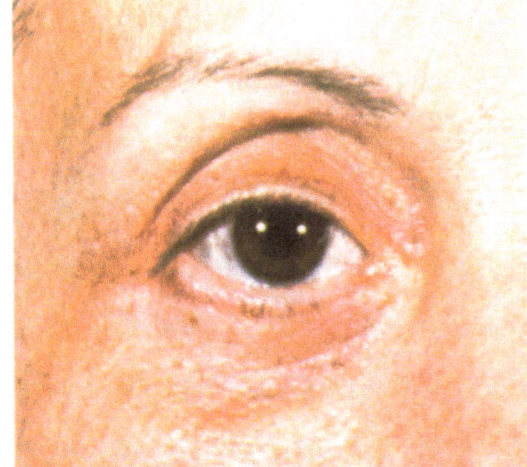

FIGURE 4.2. Patient showing iatrogenic depression caused by overreduction of fatty tissue in the mesial third of the septal portion of the upper and lower lids. Excessive removal of fat tissue from the lower lid also contributed to the occurrence of scleral show.

FIGURE 4.3. Palpebral depression giving a morbid appearance.

In extreme examples, they can give the eye an unaesthetic or morbid appearance (Fig. 4.3), and their correction is imperative since they are at times accompanied by scleral show or ectropion.

It is evident that palpebral depressions should receive special care and attention, equivalent or superior to that given to bulges.

Because of the frequency of depressions and because of the aesthetic and functional problems that they cause, they will be analyzed in detail. Particular attention will be given to their correction by means of fat grafts.

Fat Grafts – a Historical Perspective

It is axiomatic that tissue should be substituted with like tissue. For many years the correction of depressions in the tissues of the most diverse areas of the body were made with autogenous fat or derma-fat grafts. There have always been problems with soft-tissue transplantation, however, and as Peer (1959) stated: "The literature on free fat transplantation during the 30 years between 1925 and 1958 gives evidence of waning enthusiasm for clinical use of the tissue."

Absorption, uncertainties of overcorrection, replacement by fibrous tissue, and infection were constant problems. But not all fat grafts failed. A careful analysis of both literature and personal experience revealed that the earliest investigator, Neuber, was correct when he stated in 1893 that "pieces of fat that exceed the size of a bean or an almond do not heal in, and the smaller the piece, the more certain will be the result."

Considering that the tissue necessary for the correction of a palpebral depression is, at the maximum, the size of an almond or a bean, we adopted Neuber's principles. As long as the grafts do not exceed such sizes and as long as the site is favorable, these fat grafts do not show problems of rejection or absorption.

Between 1955 and 1970, a period before our systematic correction of depressions of the eyelids, we had some experience with small fat grafts. When we reduced fat pockets during routine blepharoplasties, we always kept the resected fat available until almost the end of the surgery. Should the final observation indicate that an excess amount had been removed, some of the retained fat was replaced in the cavity in the form of a free transplant. The portion of fat

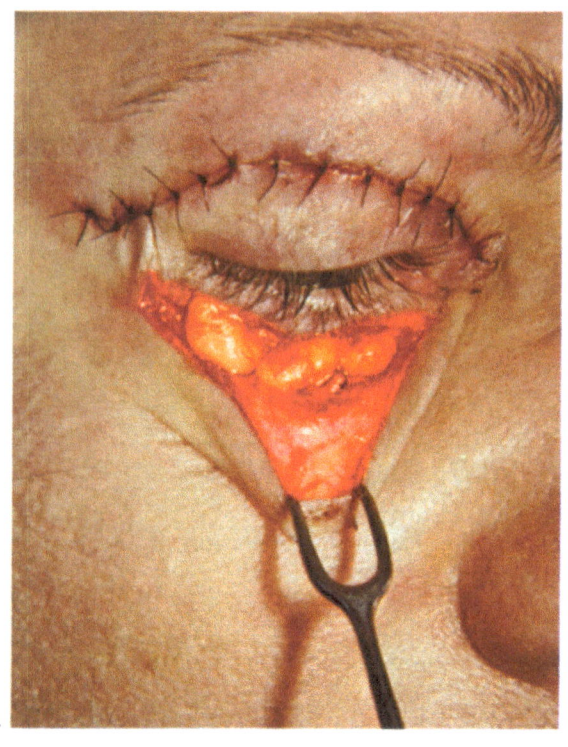

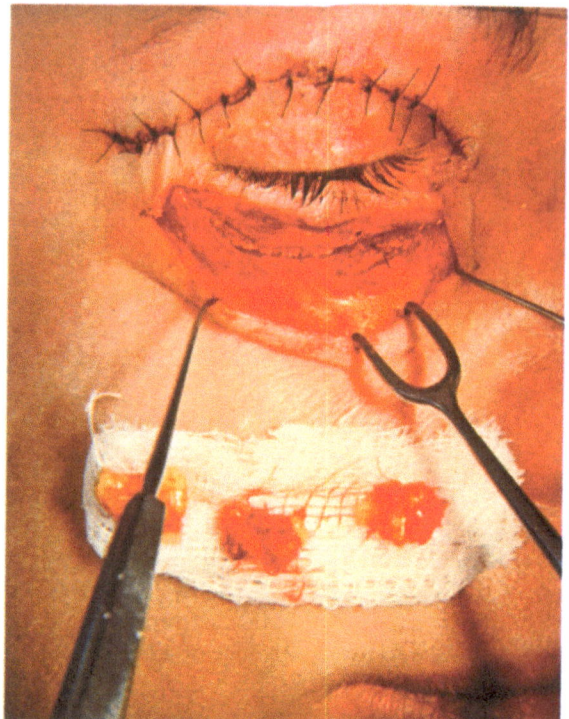

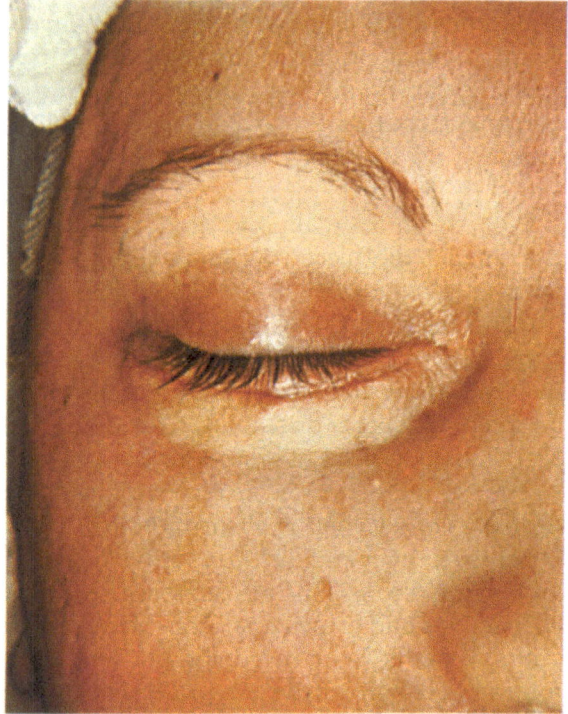

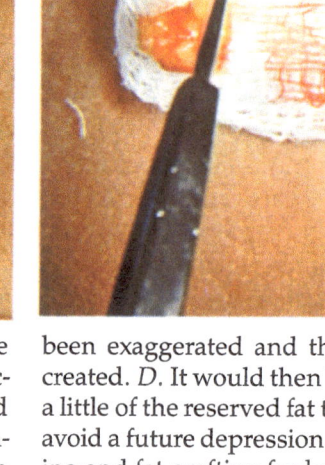

FIGURE 4.4. How we began the use of fat grafts in the eyelids. *A.* Exposure of the three palpebral fat pockets. *B.* The excess fat was removed and retained until almost the end of the surgery. *C.* Always concerned about the amount of fat tissue removed, we would sometimes conclude that the resection had been exaggerated and that a depression would be created. *D.* It would then become necessary to return a little of the reserved fat to its original site in order to avoid a future depression. (From Loeb R: Fat pad sliding and fat grafting for leveling lid depressions. *Clin Plast Surg,* October 1981; vol 8, No 4.)

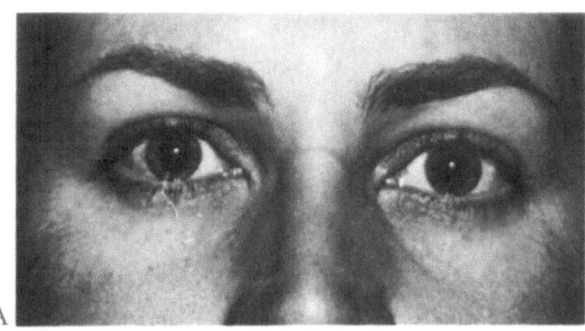

A

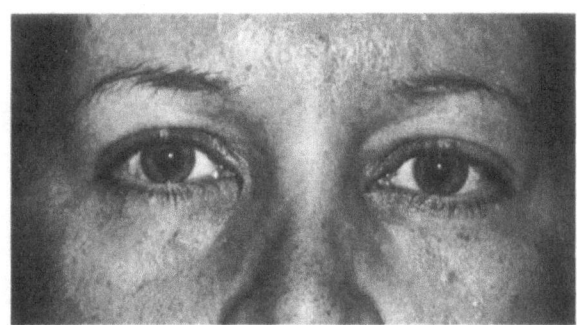

B

FIGURE 4.5. Patient seeking help because of depression of the lower eyelids. This was the first patient in which we placed free fat grafts. She told us: "Doctor, could you fill the sunken place a little? It makes me look tired, and I am not tired. Could you put a little fat there?" Because of the success that we had observed with fat replacement, we accepted the idea and used a small free fat graft taken from under her chin. A. Preoperative view showing dark circles under the eyes. B. View 10 years after fat graft surgery. The patient has a more mature aspect, but observe how the left lower eyelid depression was eliminated.

returned was generally subdivided into small fragments to be distributed throughout the length of the eyelid and below the orbicularis oculi muscle (Fig. 4.4).

Because these immediate fat grafts were only the correction of a future, potential depression, they did not appear at the time to merit much importance. We must report, however, that in these small fat grafts, we never observed any rejection or absorption worthy of note. Since 1970 we have confidently used these fat grafts, returning part of the fat resected from the palpebral pockets to its original site. Errors of calculation can always happen and we have to become accustomed to living with them, and to learn, in time, how to contend with them.

As a result of our observations of the success of these grafts, it occurred to us that we might use this same concept to augment a depressed eyelid in cases where no excess orbital fat was available. Using the same principles, we took small autogenous free fat grafts, first from the submental and later from the abdominal area, and used them to build up depressed lower eyelids (Fig. 4.5). The only difference is that the fat grafts are taken from the submental or abdominal regions and not from the eyelids themselves. These fat grafts evolve very favorably, as long as the necessary requisites are respected. Biopsies, some as long as 10 years later, have shown good integration of the graft (Fig. 4.6).

General Considerations

The correction of depressions (Fig. 4.7A) is exactly the opposite of the fat resections done during the reduction of hypertrophied fat pockets: instead of removing the fat, it is grafted in place (Fig. 4.7B). In determining the volume of fat to be used for the graft, it is important that it be small: too much will produce a surprisingly exaggerated bulge in the lid in the future (see Chapter 6). The experienced specialist, accustomed to the reduction of fat pockets, knows how to evaluate critically the quantity of fat to be used in these cases since, we repeat, grafting is the opposite of reduction (Fig. 4.7C).

When reducing fat pockets in the lower lid, some surgeons accept and even create a certain degree of septal concavity between the lower palpebral sulcus and the nasojugal sulcus, although they recognize the risk of causing scleral show or ectropion. We believe that these depressions should not exist, but should be filled sufficiently to obtain the flat plane, which is the aesthetic ideal.

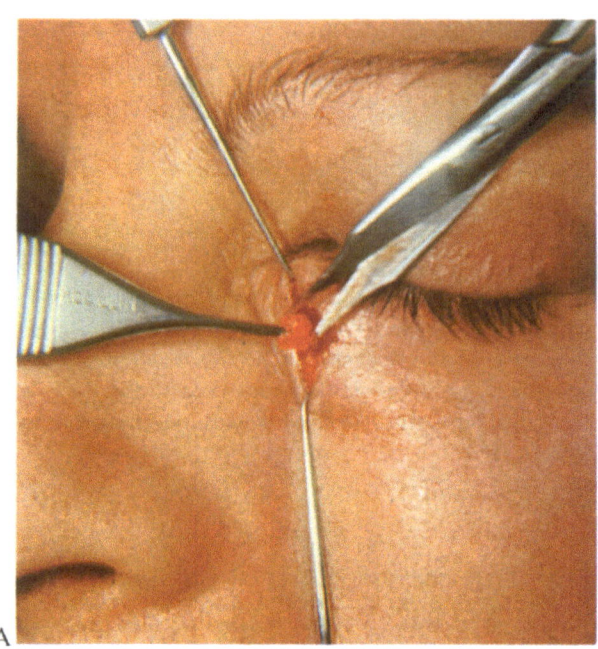
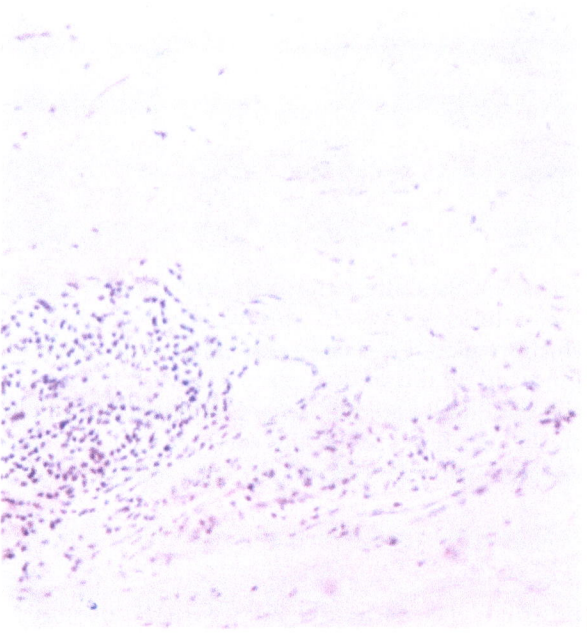

FIGURE 4.6. *A.* Same patient as in Fig. 4.5. Biopsy being taken from the preseptal region through a small incision 10 years after the operation. *B.* Photomicrograph of the fat tisue taken in the biopsy, showing fat tissue surrounded by mature fibrous tissue. There is no inflammatory cellular infiltrate. Hemoto- xylin and eosin, 200 ×. (From Loeb R: Correction of subpalpebral depressions with small free fat grafts, in: Transactions of the Seventh *International Congress of Plastic and Reconstructive Surgery.* São Paulo, Sociedade Brasileira de Cirurgia Plástica, 1979, pp 361–364.)

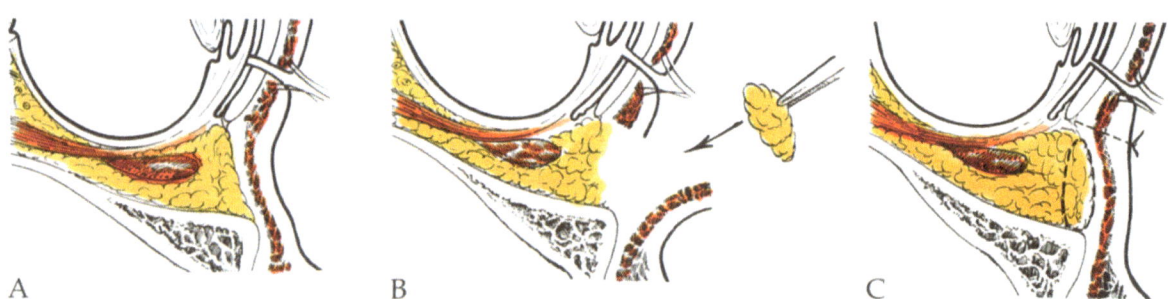

A   B   C

FIGURE 4.7. *A.* Sagittal section showing the lower lid with its septal portion depressed because of a reduced volume of fat tissue. *B.* Placing a small fat graft. Its size should be about that of a bean, *in no case larger than an almond.* The graft is placed in contact with the orbital fat for better integration. *C.* Fat graft (*dotted oval*) inserted and in contact with the adipose tissue of the orbital region. The orbital fascia and the orbicular muscle must cover it without any tension. A single routine cutaneous suture is placed, generally 6-0 nylon. The surface of the lower eyelid should be flat at this point. (From Loeb R: Fat pad sliding and fat grafting for leveling lid depressions. *Clin Plast Surg,* October 1981; vol 8, No 4.)

In Occidentals, depressions of the upper lids are not very noticeable, since the upper palpebral sulcus is normally evident. However, depressions of the lower lids, commonly called "dark circles under the eyes," are conspicuous and confer an expression of tiredness and/or aging. Fat grafts are indicated in these cases. To correct these depressions, appropriately sized fat grafts should be inserted under the depressions. The graft bed should be ideal, or the graft will not integrate correctly.

The implant site should have the following attributes:

1. It should be well vascularized. This is normally not a problem in the eyelids. However, fibrous tissue in the orbital region (generated by previous surgery, perhaps) can interfere with otherwise good circulatory conditions.
2. It should have orbital fat present. A fat graft placed in direct contact with fat already present in the orbital region is more easily integrated. This continuity is usually possible because the fat is placed below the orbicularis oculi muscle, exactly where what fat may be present is situated.
3. It should be dynamic The constant movement of the eyelids, brought about by the orbicular and other nearby muscles of the eye, is of great help in the neovascularization and consequent integration of the fat graft.

Classification and Treatment of Palpebral Depressions

There are three principal types of eyelid depressions: (1) congenital – depressed septal region, (2) developmental – depressed nasojugal and palpebro-malar sulci, and (3) iatrogenic – various locations.

Congenital Depressions (Depressed Septal Region)

Some young individuals have depressions in the septal region of the eyelid. Such depressions are congenital aberrations and are most evident in the lower eyelids. Because they are caused by the small volume of fat tissue present in the orbit, they appear above the area where the palpebral fatty tissues normally exist. This defect is accentuated because of the difference in level between the sunken septal area and the normal projection of the tarsal portion of the orbicularis oculi muscle.

These septal depressions are permanent, even with aging, since these patients have never been observed to experience, over time, the usual tendency toward an increase in the volume of the orbital fat. Therefore, these atrophied pockets are not going to suffer pressure from inside, and the defect is not going to correct itself. Correction with free fat transplants is indicated in these cases of congenital depressions. In our experience there is no need to undercorrect or overcorrect. *The graft should be the exact size needed to compensate for the defect.*

Treatment

It is customary to do this type of fat graft under local anesthesia and with sedation. An incision similar to that used for a routine blepharoplasty is made approximately 2 mm below the inferior palpebral border (Fig. 4.8).

The orbicularis oculi muscle is sectioned longitudinally with curved scissors, crossing the orbital septum at the level of the septal region. On examining the interior of the cavity existing below the orbicularis oculi muscle, it is always surprising to observe the empty space (Fig. 4.8C), caused by the small volume of fat tissue. In the deep area, however, some orbital fat can be seen (Fig. 4.8C).

Careful hemostasis should be maintained since hematomas can prejudice good integration of the graft. After the amount of fat needed is determined, it is taken from the submental or abdominal regions, with the submental preferred. Using a technique similar to that utilized for the treatment of double chin, the fat is removed through a small incision near and parallel to the submental sulcus and is then carefully inserted below the orbicular muscle of the eye and in direct contact with the orbital fat (Fig. 4.8D).

After the graft is in place, the palpebral appearance should be normal, that is, equiva-

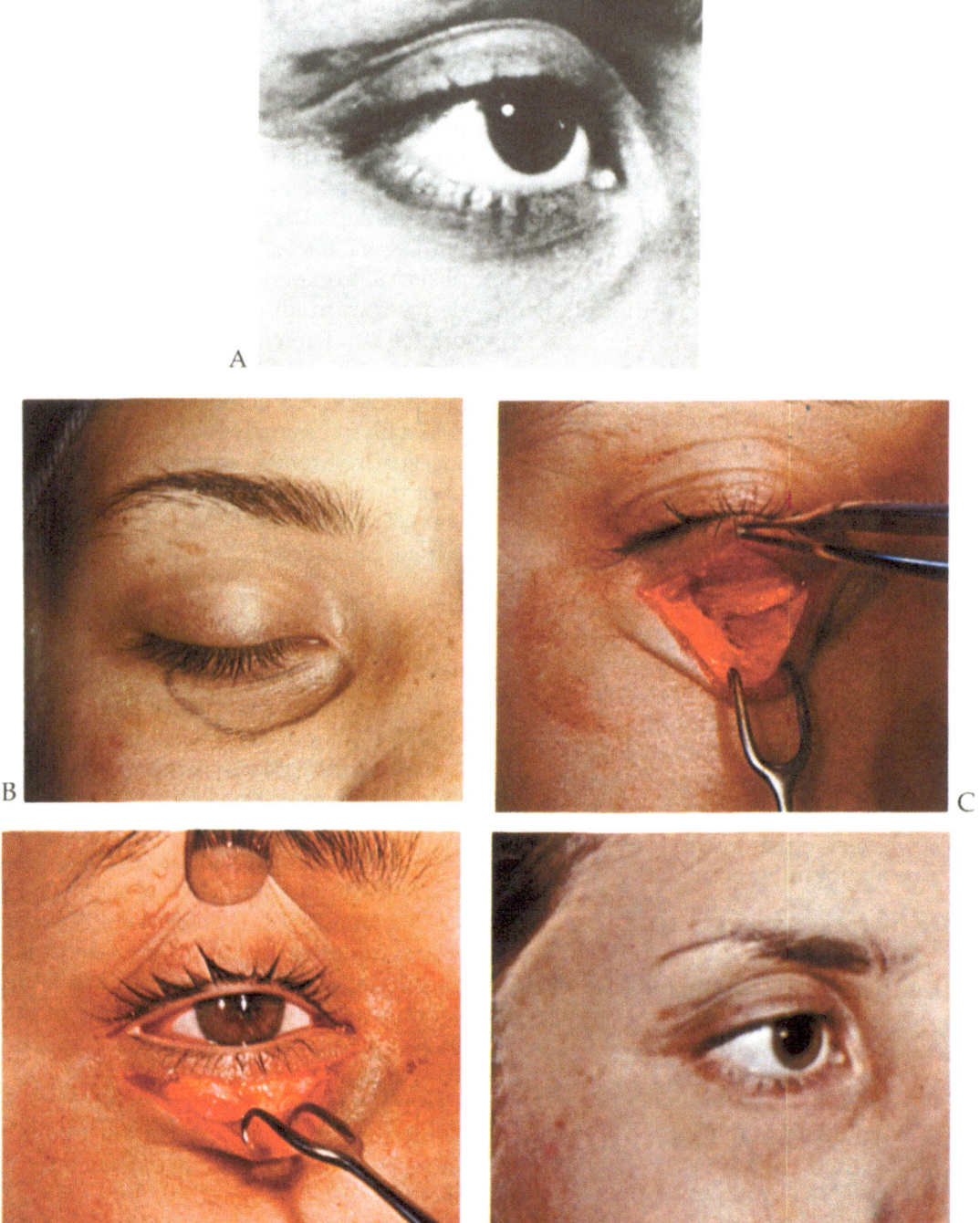

FIGURE 4.8. *A.* Young patient with depression of the septal portion of the lower lid and scleral show. *B.* Demonstration of the depressed area to be grafted. *C.* It is always surprising to observe the cavity caused by the absence of the normal adipose tissue. *D.* Fat graft inserted. *E.* Postoperative view showing the correction of the palpebral depression by means of a fat graft. Note the improvement in the scleral show. This was brought about by the leveling of the preseptal portion. (From Loeb R: Correction of subpalpebral depressions with small free fat grafts, in: *Transactions of the Seventh International Congress of Plastic and Reconstructive Surgery.* São Paulo, Sociedade Brasileira de Cirurgia Plástica, 1979, pp 361–364.)

lent in all ways to a palpebral fat pocket that has been correctly reduced. The fat graft should not give the impression of "wanting to jump out" of where it was inserted. The orbicular muscle and the fascia should be able to cover the graft easily without suturing, nor are they themselves sutured.

The head of the patient is then elevated to a vertical position in order to observe the effect of the graft. This guarantees that the degree of augmentation is adequate. If the objective has not been reached, more fat tissue can be inserted or removed at this time.

The cutaneous suturing is done with 6-0 nylon separated sutures. Hematomas are avoided by good hemostasis and compression of the area.

Developmental Depressions (Depressed Nasojugal and Palpebro-Malar Sulci)

Some patients have a nasojugal sulcus more marked than normal, forming a groove that separates the lower eyelid from the cheek and nasal regions and giving a tired look to the eye (Fig. 4.9). This defect should not be confused with a depression of the lower palpebral septal region itself (described on page 81) because their placements are different (Figs. 4.10 and 4.11).

Treatment

There are two ways to correct a depressed nasojugal sulcus: transplant free fat from the

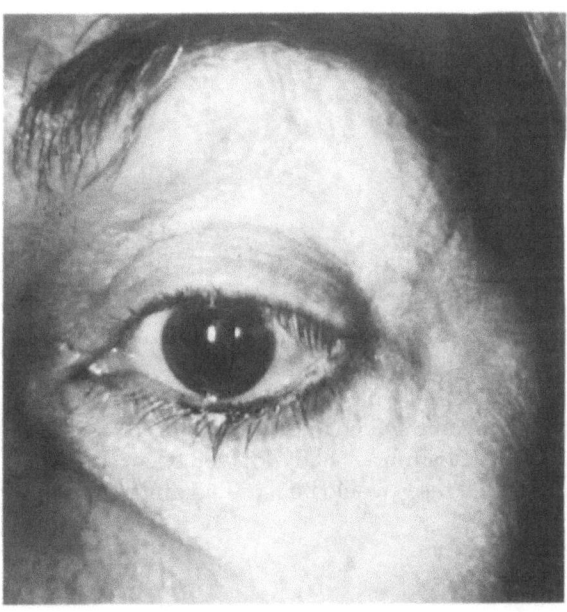

FIGURE 4.9. A 30-year-old patient with depressed nasojugal sulcus. Note that the depression is below the septal portion of the eyelid.

submental or abdominal area, or slide fat from the mesial and central fat pockets.

Transplant Free Fat from the Submental or Abdominal Area

If there is no excess fat in the medial or central fat pockets, the depressed nasojugal sulcus can be leveled by implanting a free fat graft. The graft is introduced through a small incision in the septal region, parallel to and a few milimeters above

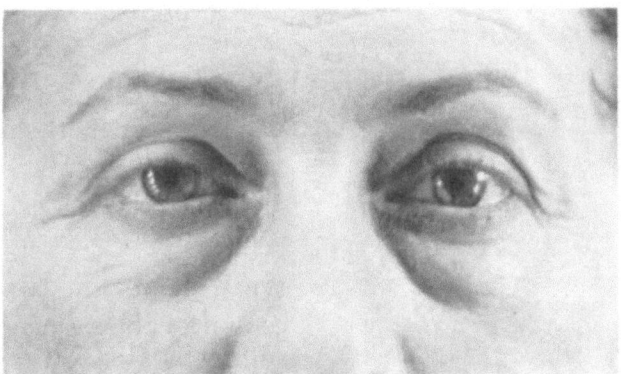

FIGURE 4.10. Depressed nasojugal sulci. These grooves confer a "tired" look to the face and are popularly called "dark circles under the eyes." Such areas are more subject to shadows (*the dark areas*), which then constrast with the bulges (*the light areas*) of the mesial and central fat pockets.

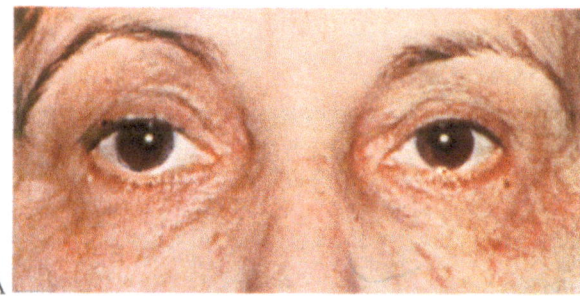
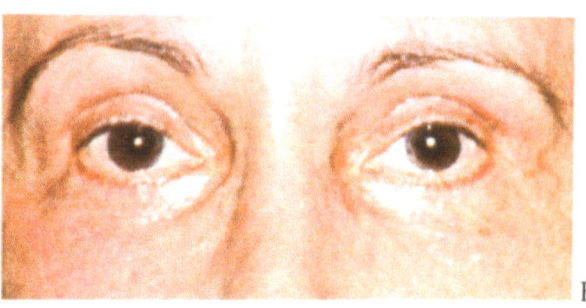

FIGURE 4.11. Persistence or evidence of depressed nasojugal sulci in patients operated on in the past. The results of the blepharoplasties shown here were considered at the time to be satisfactory: the concept of the "flat surface" had not yet been conceived. Today such cases would be handled differently. More attention would be paid to the nasojugal sulci, avoiding excessive resections in the medial and central pockets so as not to accentuate the sulci. To repair these cases it would be necessary to reoperate, implanting fat tissue to fill out the depressed areas.

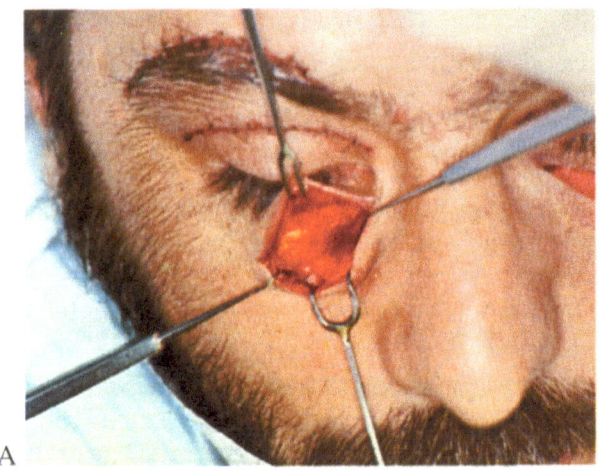
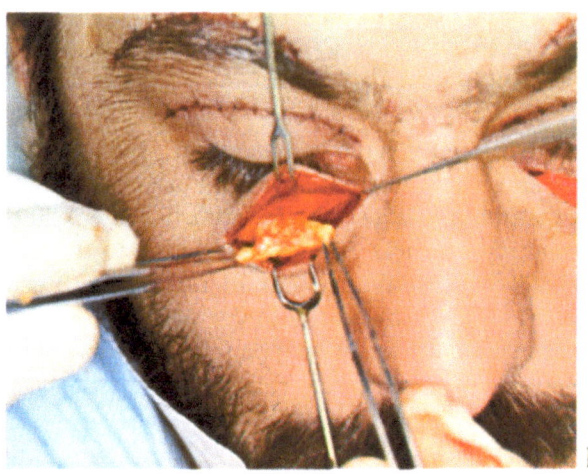

FIGURE 4.12. Typical case of depression of the nasojugal sulcus, with absence of hypertrophic fat pockets. In these cases a free transplant of fat tissue is used to level the depression. A. Preoperative view. B. The graft being inserted.

the nasojugal sulcus. The quantity of fat tissue needed is generally small (Fig. 4.12).

Slide Fat from the Medial and Central Fat Pockets

When there is hypertrophy of the mesial and central fat pockets next to a depressed nasojugal sulcus, the best way to level the sulcus is to slide the fat from the pockets in the form of a pedicle graft. Precise technical details are given in Figures 4.13A – K.

FIGURE 4.13. *A.* Anatomical concepts for the correction of a depressed nasojugal sulcus by sliding fat from the medial and central fat pockets. Here are shown the principal sulci of the lower eyelid: lower palpebral and nasojugal. Between these are the fat pockets. The excess fat from the medial and central pockets is slid over the angular muscle and sutured to its anterior-superior face.

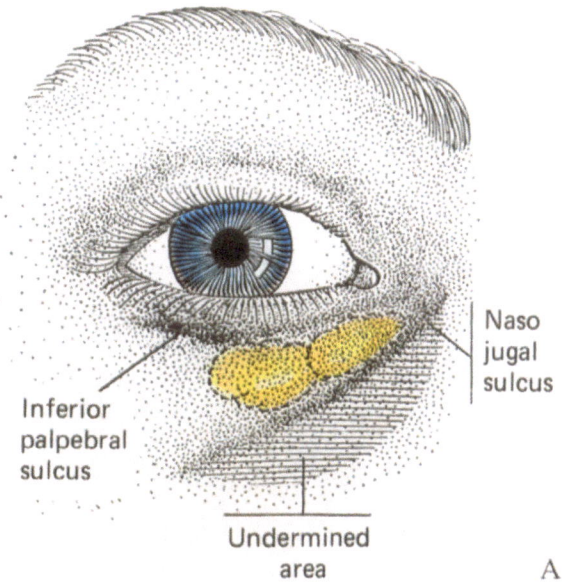

A

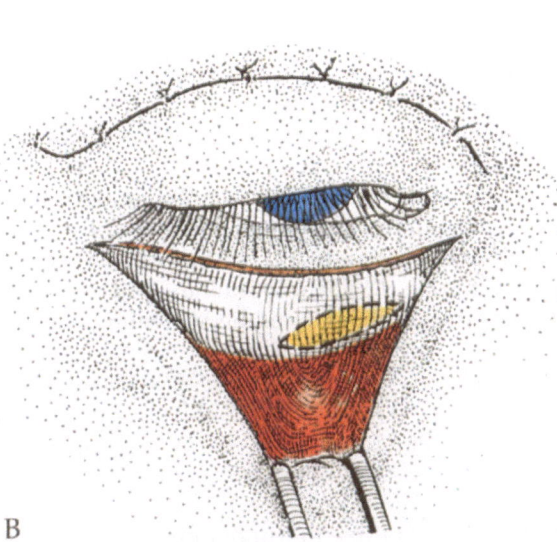

B

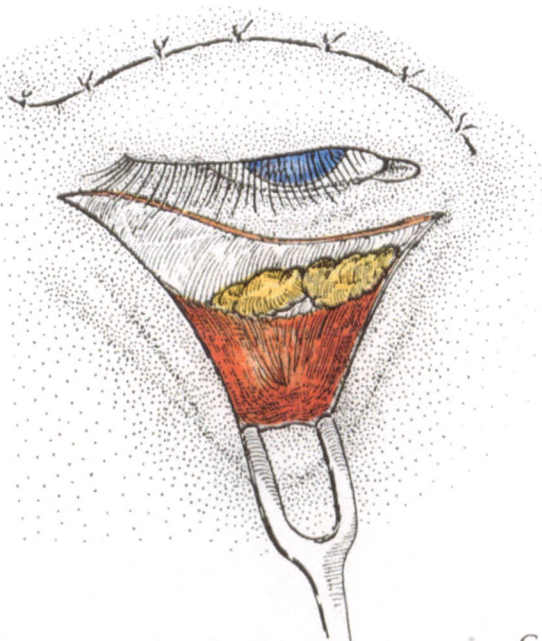

C

FIGURE 4.13. *B.* A low incision is made a few milimeters below the ciliary border. The skin-muscle flap is undermined, exposing the orbital septum, which covers the medial and central fat pockets. Instead of sectioning the anterior part of the septum, as is usual, we section its anterior-inferior portion in such a manner that the fat herniates downward toward the nasojugal sulcus and the angular muscle. At times we include a partial resection of the fascia to facilitate the herniation. *C.* The medial and central fat pockets have herniated downward in the direction of the angular muscle, and we can now accurately determine the volume of excess tissue. If necessary, some fat can be resected. (From Loeb R: Fat pad sliding and fat grafting for leveling lid depressions. *Clin Plast Surg,* October 1981; vol 8, No 4.)

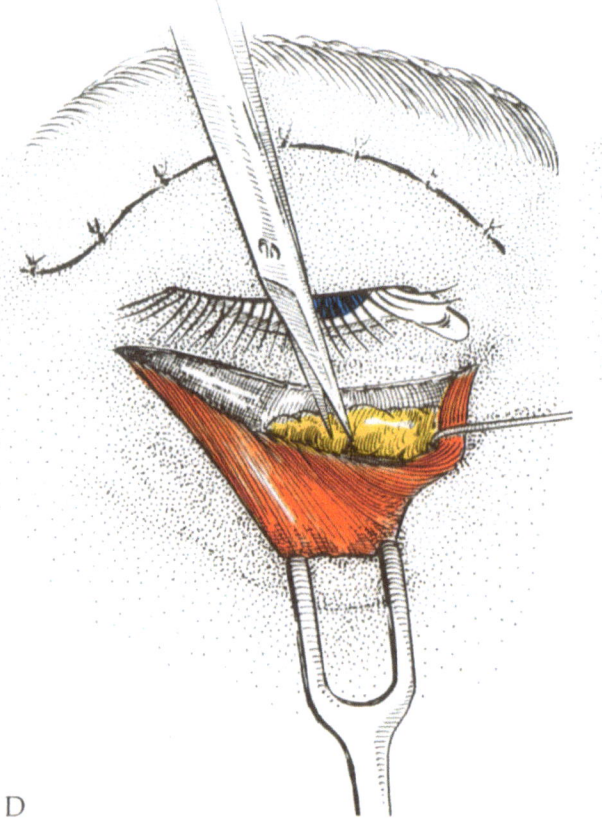

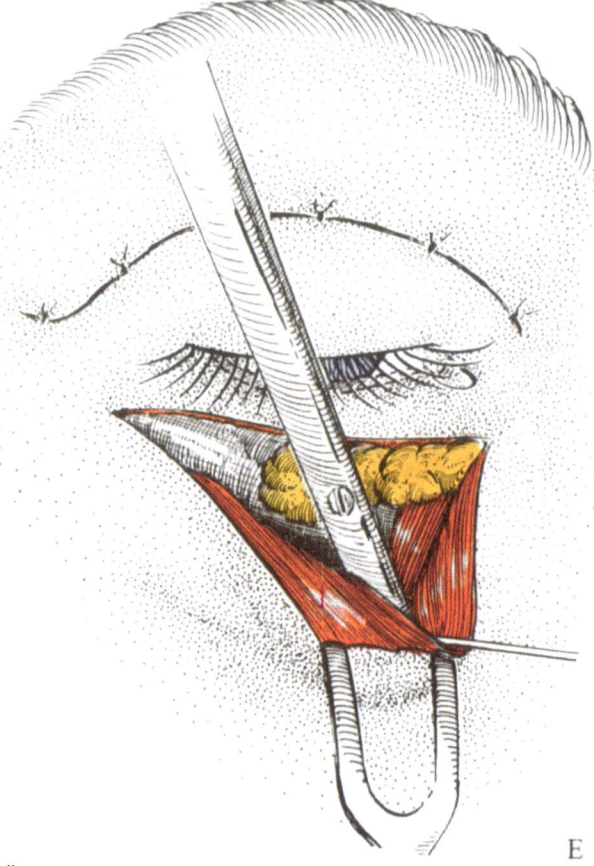

D

E

△
FIGURE 4.13. D. The undermining in the direction of
the angular muscle is begun with scissors, sectioning
the orbital septum, which is at this level inserted in
the orbital border separating the orbit from the nasal
and cheek regions. This will make it possible to slide
the adipose tissue so that it can be brought over the
angular muscle. E. The undermining proceeds, pas-
sing over the anterior face of the angular muscle.

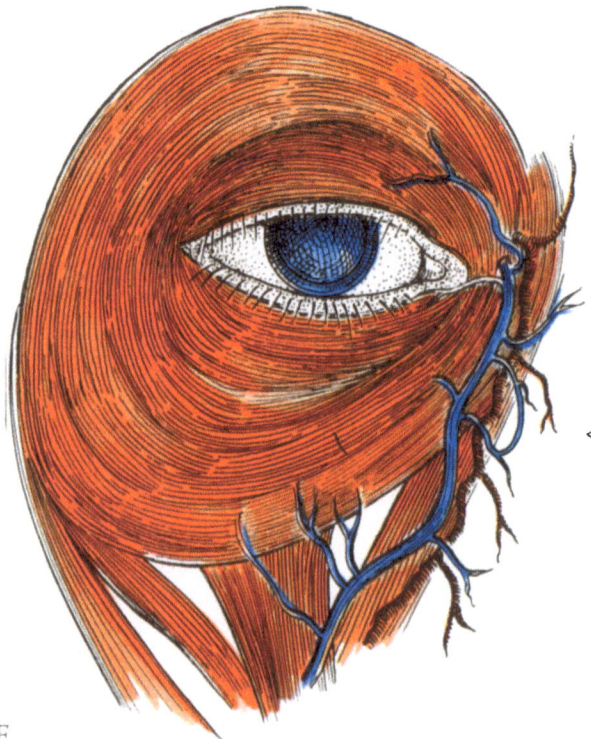

F

◁ FIGURE 4.13. F. During the undermining, great care
should be taken to preserve the blood vessels in the
region, among which are the angular and nasal veins
and arteries. Cutting these provokes much bleeding,
and in this region the vessels are deep, making it difficult to determine where the bleeding is. Careful
hemostasis should be maintained. When we en-
counter such bleeding, we initially press the soft tissues against the deep bony plane to attain hemostasis
by simple manual compression. After some minutes
we relax the compression, and only then do we
coagulate or ligate the compromised vessels.

FIGURE 4.13. *G.* To reduce the possibility of damaging the blood vessels, we continue the undermining with hemostatic forceps.

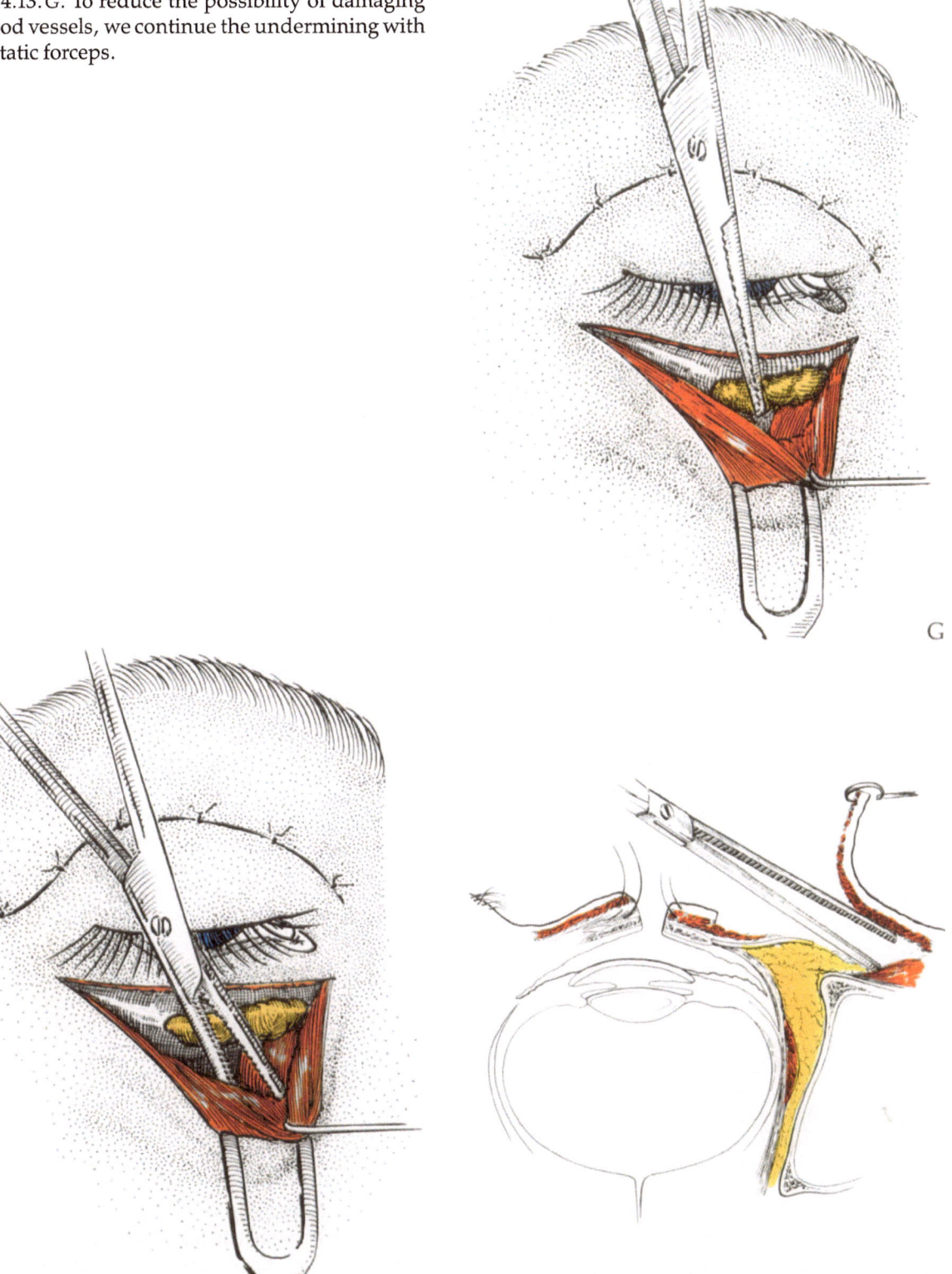

G

H

FIGURE 4.13. *H.* (*LEFT*) Undermining is done up to the anterior-superior border of the angular muscle, including its anterior face. (*RIGHT*) Sectioning of the orbital septum has been done. Fat tissue of the medial and central pockets herniates in the direction of the angular muscle, covering part of it.

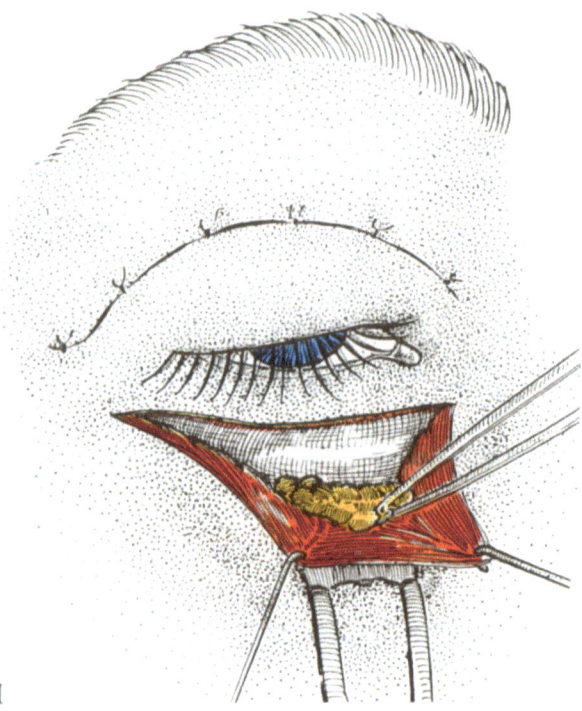

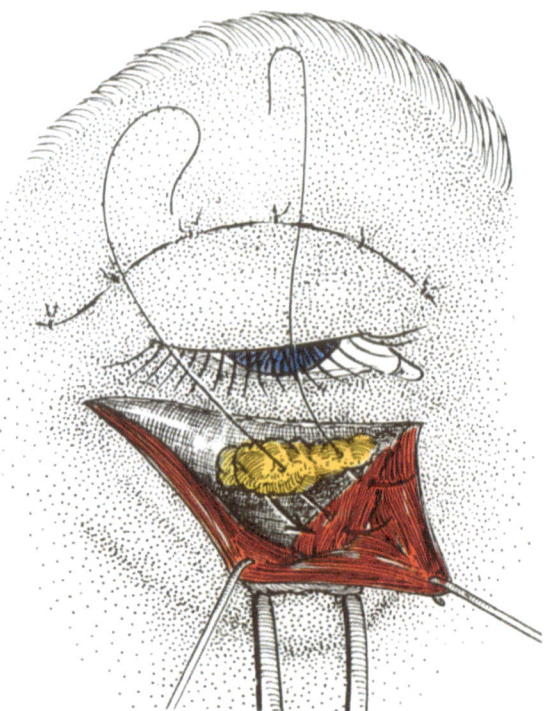

I   J

FIGURE 4.13. *I.* We now evaluate the quantity of fat tissue coming from the mesial and central pockets and slide the excess over the anterior face of the angular muscle, thus bringing the fat flap across the area where the depression of the nasojugal sulcus had been. The volume of fat should be such that it can be mobilized easily without causing any depression of the septal region. If the quantity of fat tissue is excessive, it can be reduced at this time. *J.* We then suture the fat tissue over the surface of the angular muscle with 6-0 Nylon, thus filling the depression that had formed the exaggerated sulcus.

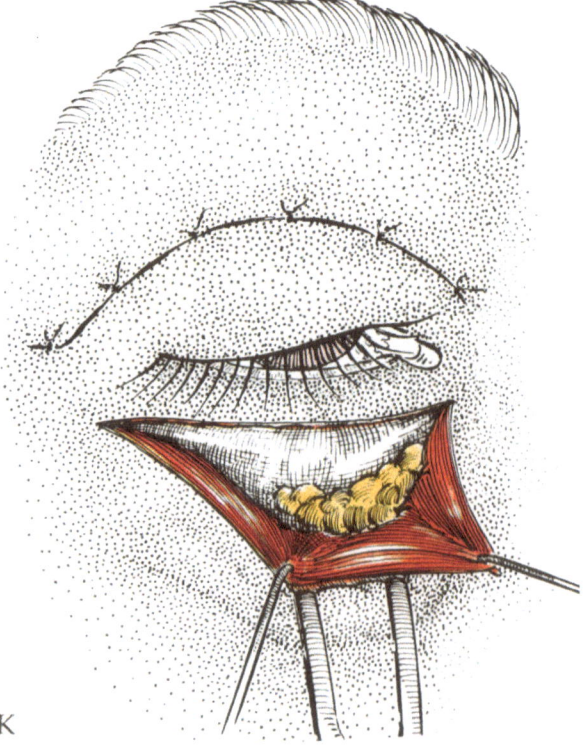

K

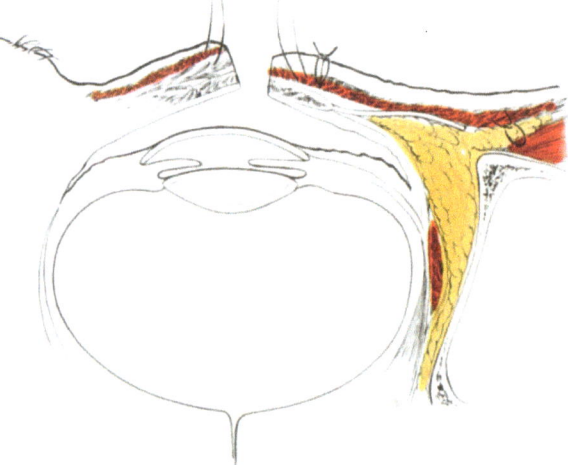

FIGURE 4.13. *K.* The flap should adapt itself perfectly to the region to which it has been transferred. (*LEFT*) Anterior view. (*RIGHT*) Profile section showing the orbital septum that was sectioned at the level of the inferior orbital arch. Fat tissue from the medial and central pockets has been sutured to the angular muscle.

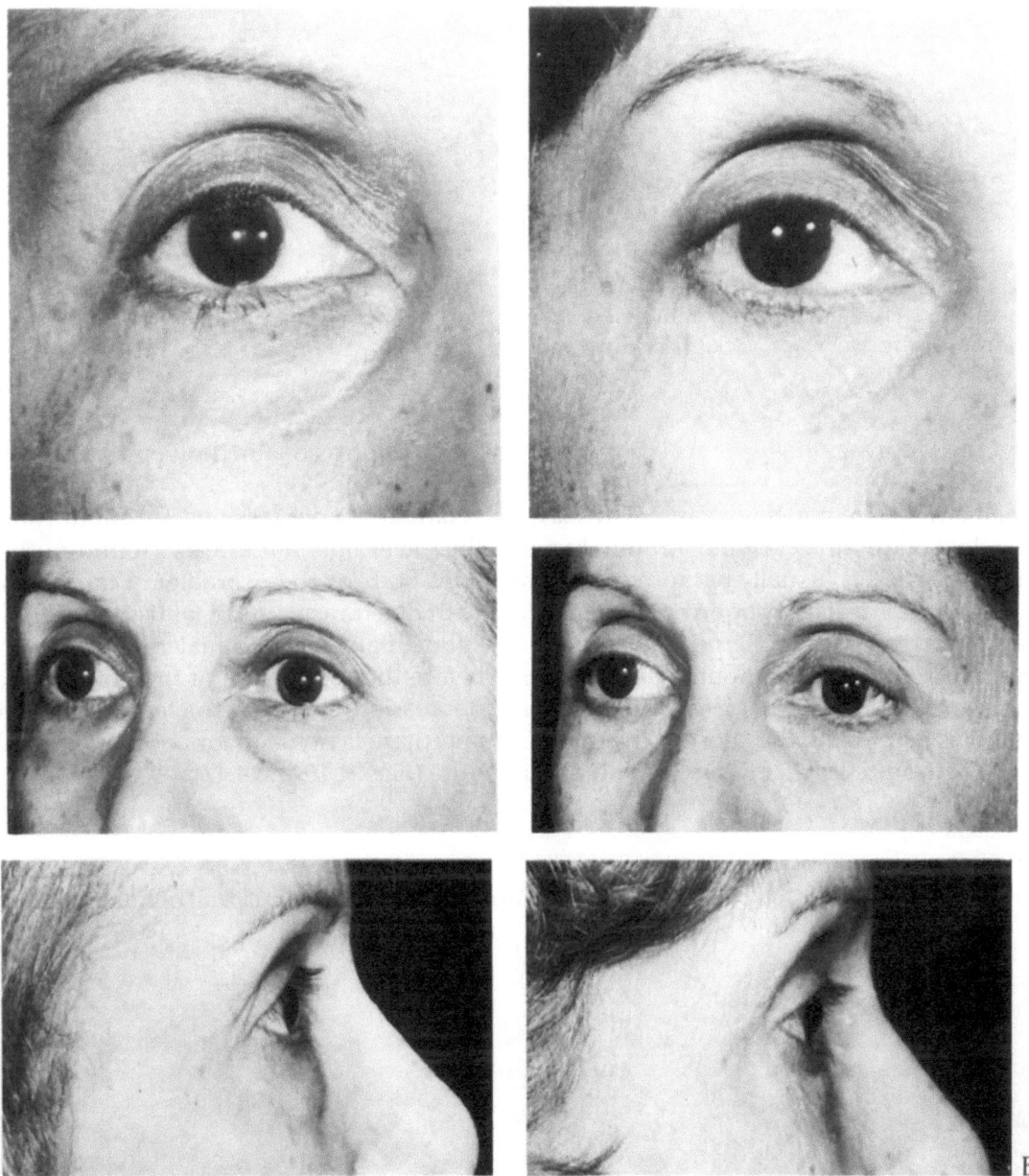

FIGURE 4.14. Exacerbated nasojugal sulcus. A. The depression of the nasojugal sulcus appears deep because of the bulging of the mesial and central fat pockets. B. Patient after the reduction of the bulges and the sliding of the remaining fat as described above.

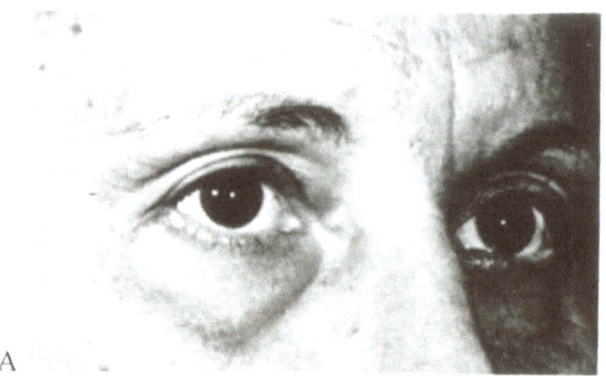
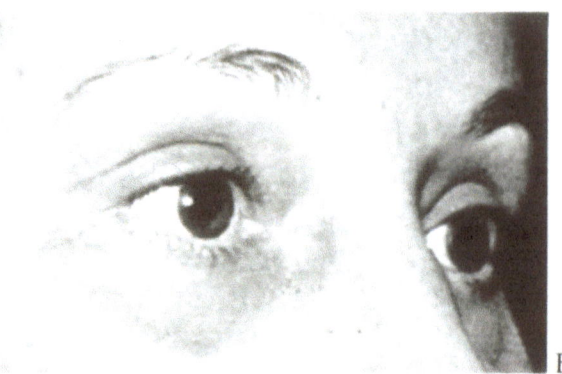

A   B

FIGURE 4.15. Correction of the nasojugal sulcus using the fat-sliding technique. *A*. Preoperative view showing a drop of the eyebrows, facial flaccidity, and a deep nasojugal sulcus. *B*. Correction by fat sliding and a temporal face lift.

Iatrogenic Depressions

Iatrogenic cases are generally caused by excessive reduction of the volume of the hypertrophied fat pockets, usually because of qualitative or quantitative diagnostic error. It can occur, for example, in cases of hypertrophy of the orbicularis oculi muscle without hypertrophy of the fat pockets. In these cases, the surgeon should only reduce the thickness of the muscle, but if he instead resects fat tissue, he will gener-

ate a depression in the septal portion of the eyelid.

Iatrogenic depressions are more common in the lower lids, but are also found in the upper lids. Both of these problems can be corrected with free transplants of fat tissue taken from the submental or abdominal regions. If observed before the completion of the initial surgery, the depression can be corrected with its own fat, and there is no need for another surgical procedure (Figs. 4.16 and 4.17).

Iatrogenic Depression of the Lower Eyelid Corrected with a Free Transplant of Adipose Tissue

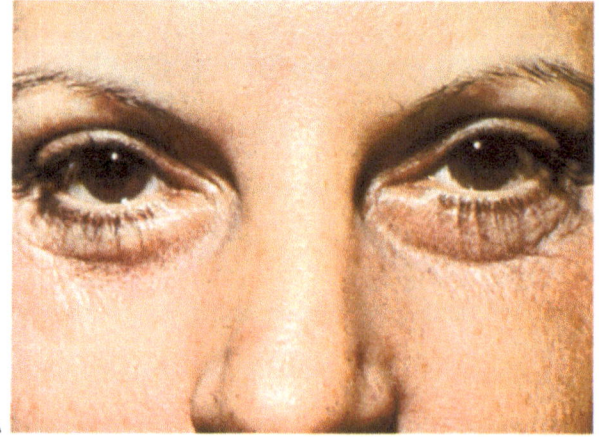
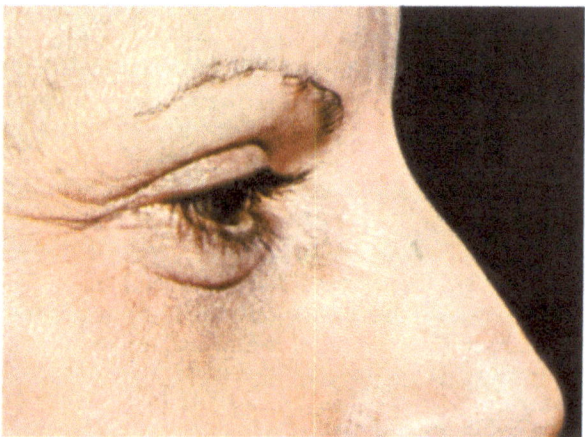

A

FIGURE 4.16. *A*. A 35-year-old patient with iatrogenic depression of the lower lids at the level of the septal region and nasojugal sulci caused by excessive resection from the fat pockets. (From Loeb R: Correction of rings under the eyes or lid depressions with fat grafts. Cir Estét Argentina, 1978; 2:68–71.) (in Spanish)

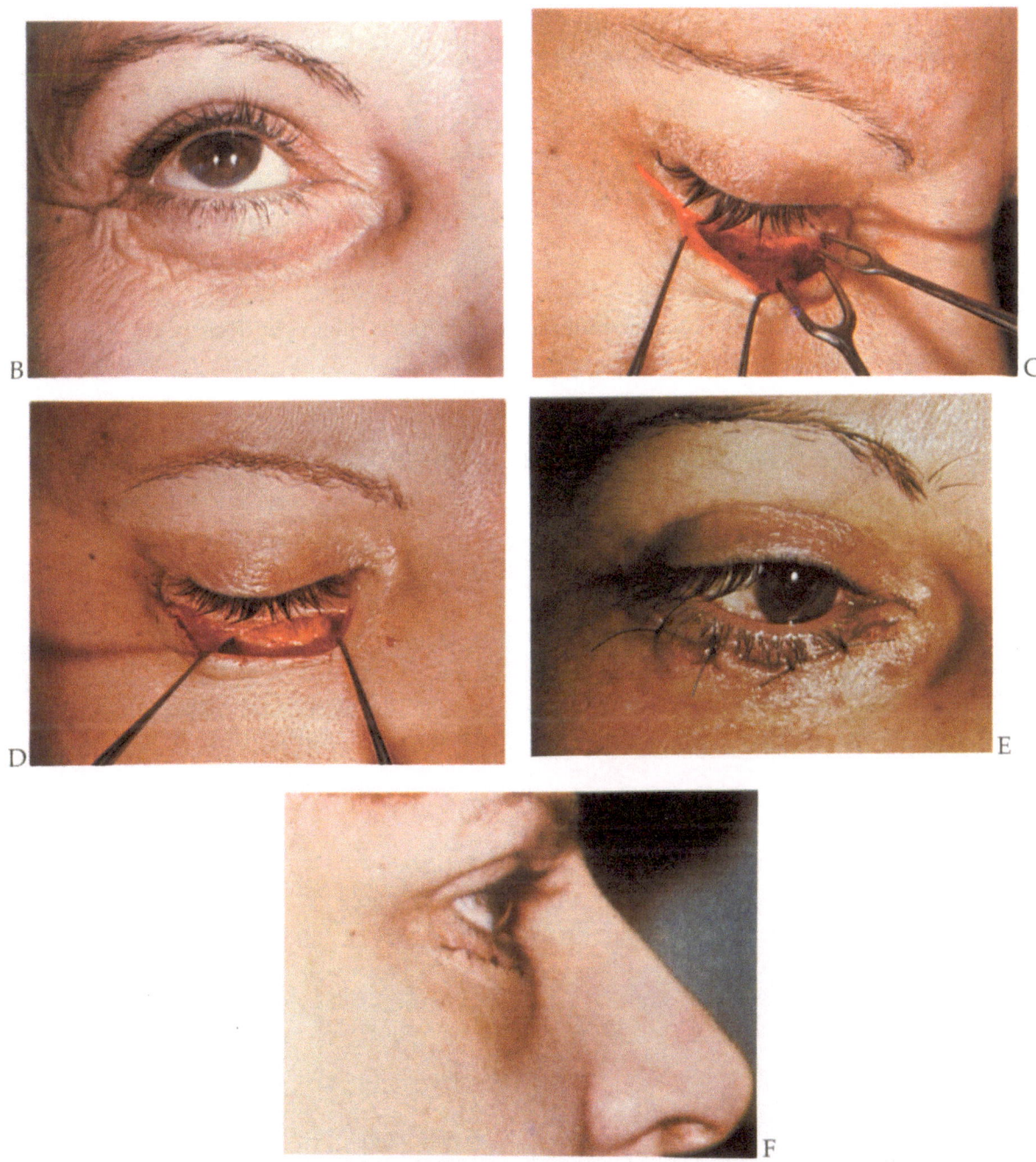

Figure 4.16. *B*. Preoperative close-up view. Septal portion depressed, particularly near the nasojugal sulcus. *C*. After the skin incision, skin-muscle undermining was done. Note cavity caused by lack of fat in preseptal region. *D*. View of septal region showing the graft inserted in the cavity. It should be in contact with the remaining orbital fat tissue. *E*. Skin sutured with 6-0 nylon. *F*. Three-day postoperative profile view. Residual edema can be seen.

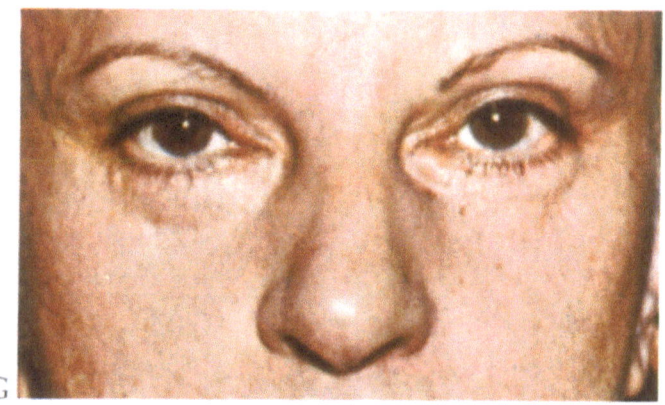
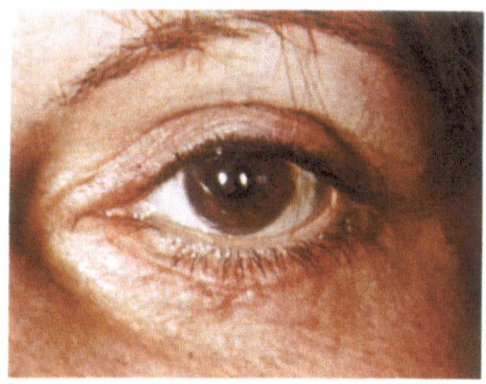

FIGURE 4.16. *G.* Six months after fat grafting. (*LEFT*) Front view. (*RIGHT*) Close-up.

Iatrogenic Depression of the Upper and Lower Eyelids Corrected by Free Fat Grafts

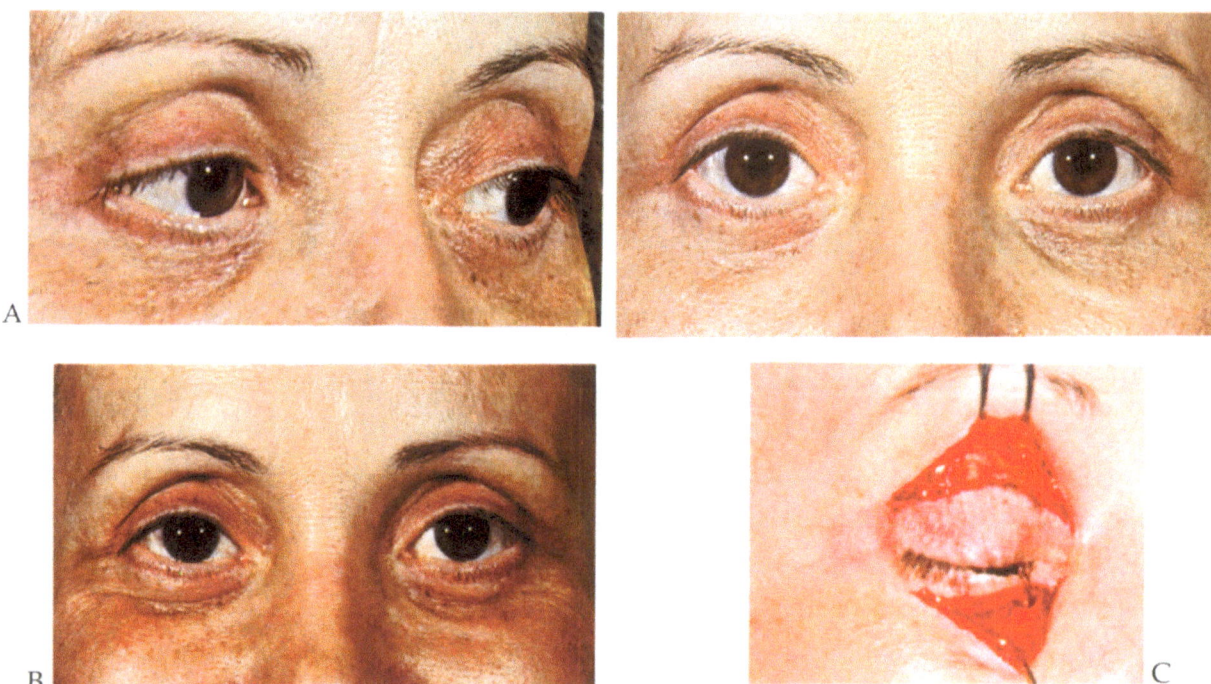

FIGURE 4.17. *A.* Bilateral iatrogenic depressions in the preseptal portions of the upper and lower lids resulting from excessive removal of fat tissue during aesthetic blepharoplasty. (From Loeb R: Free fat grafted under lower lid depressions and subsequent slid to level deep nasojugal folds. *Transactions of the VIII International Congress of Plastic Surgery.* Montreal, June-July 1983, pp 480–481.) *B.* When the patient laughs, the preseptal portions are deepened even more because the orbicularis oculi muscle bulges in the pretarsal region, thereby increasing the difference in level between the pretarsal and preseptal areas. *C.* Over-reduction of the fat tissue in both upper and lower lids.

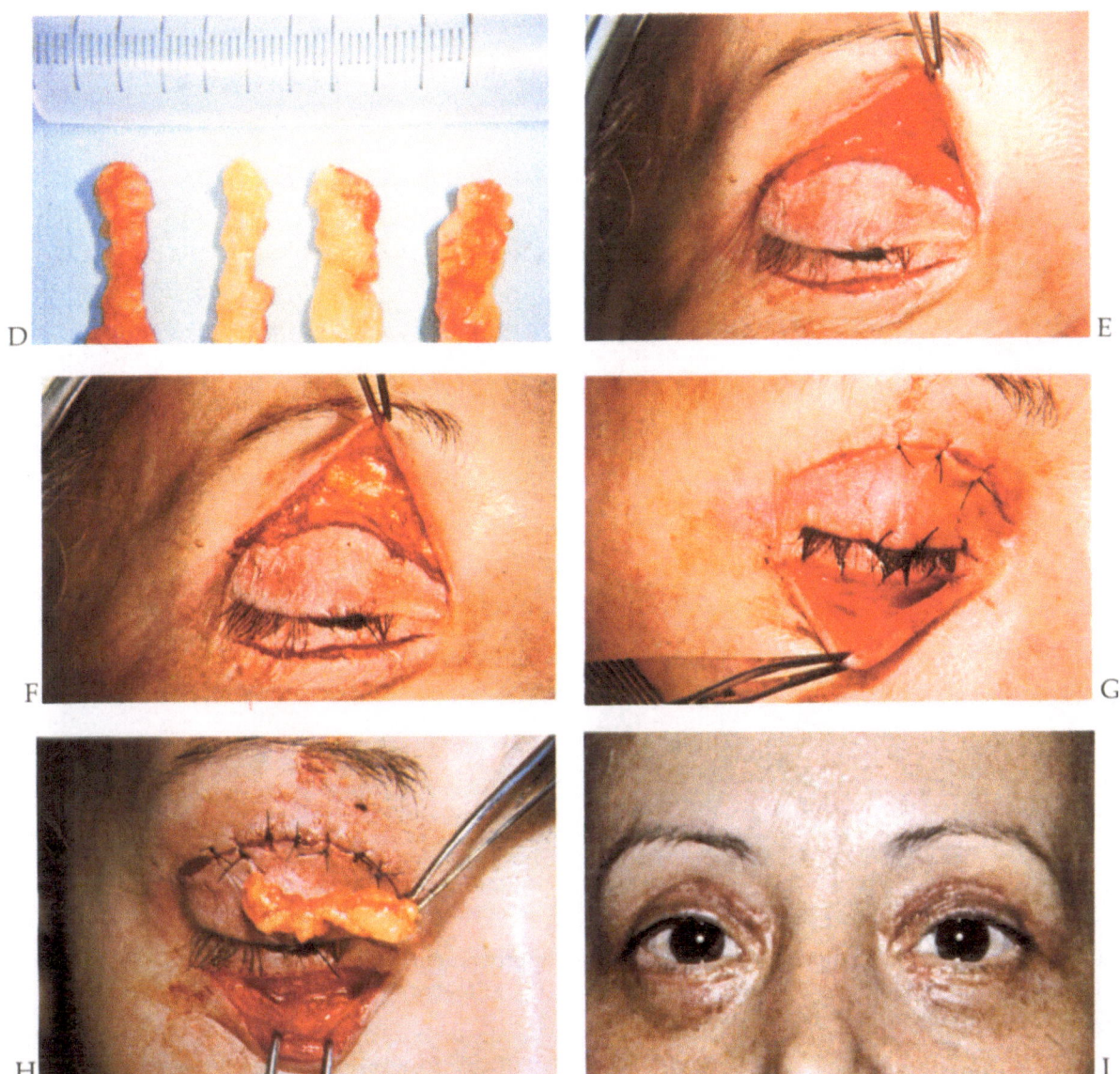

FIGURE 4.17. *D.* Portions of fat tissue to be used as grafts. The patient did not have sufficient submental fat, so it was necessary to obtain it from the abdominal region. It was subdivided into four portions, as shown. *E.* Close-up view of upper eyelid showing absence of fat tissue. *F.* Fat graft introduced. Excess volume should be avoided. *G.* Upper eyelid tem-porarily sutured. Once the tarsorrhaphy has been made, which is important in these cases, we can evaluate the projection of the eyelid. The absence of fat tissue in the lower lid is obvious and shows the need for the graft. *H.* Graft being introduced. *I.* About 1 month after surgery.

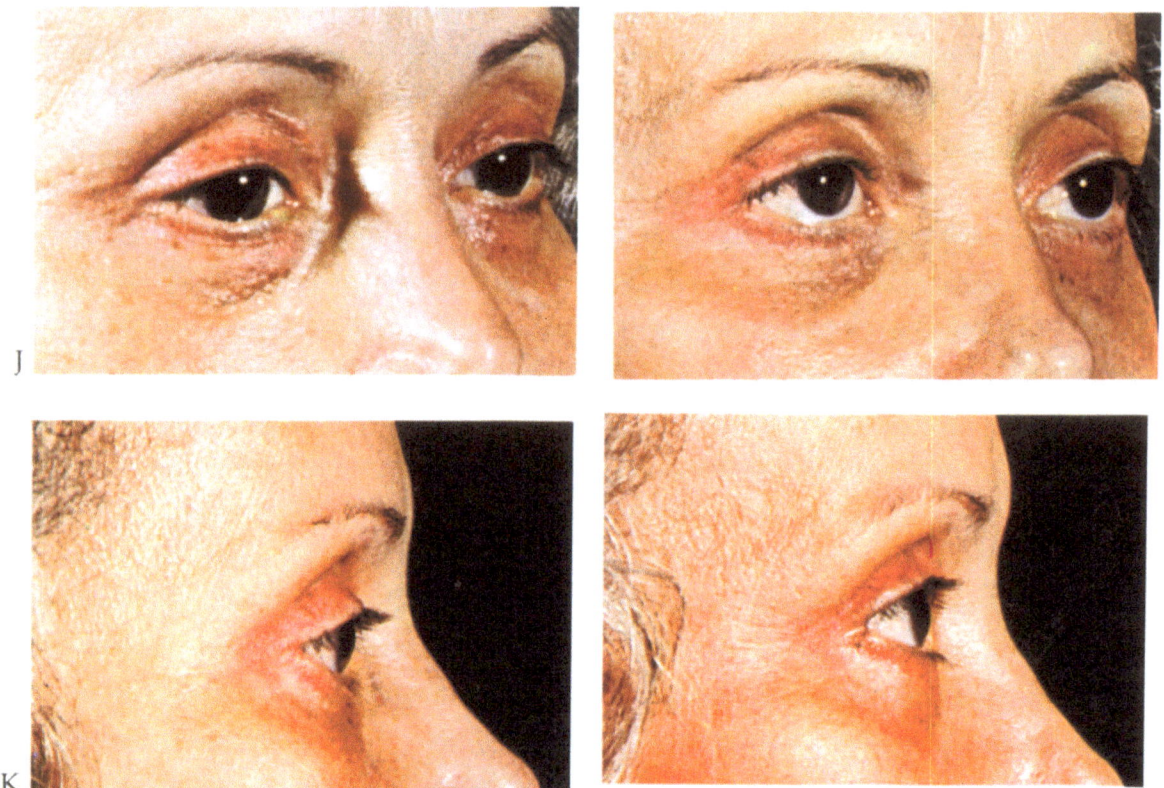

FIGURE 4.17. *J.* Correction of palpebral depression with fat graft in the septal region. (*LEFT*) Preoperative view. (*RIGHT*) Postoperative view after 1 year. Note the improvement of the depression. *K.* Profile view: (*LEFT*) Preoperative; (*RIGHT*) Postoperative.

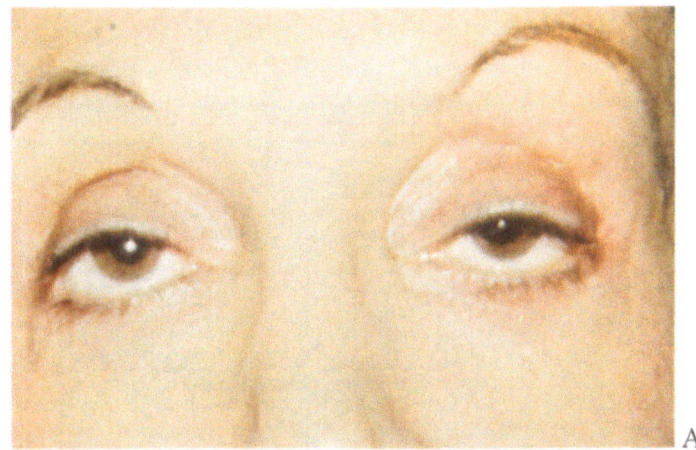

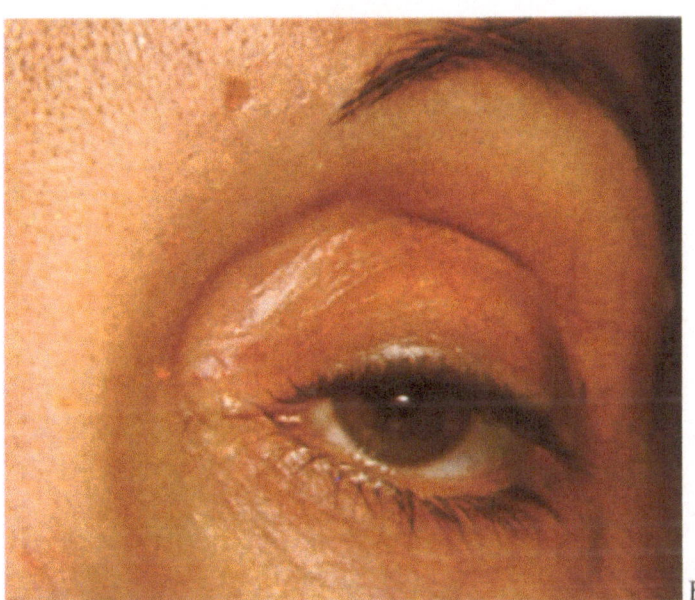

FIGURE 4.18. *A.* Iatrogenic depressions in the upper eyelids due to excessive removal of fat tissue. The defect is localized mainly in the mesial and central thirds. Observe also that there is a marked scleral show of both lower lids. *B.* Close-up of the same defect. (From Loeb R: Fat pad sliding and fat grafting for leveling lid depressions. *Clin Plast Surg,* October 1981; vol 8, No 4.)

Iatrogenic Depressions of the Upper Eyelids.

Just as in the lower eyelids, exaggerated resections of fat tissue during aesthetic blepharoplasty in the upper lids can generate depressions in the septal portions. We have corrected these defects with fat grafts taken from the submental region (Fig. 4.18).

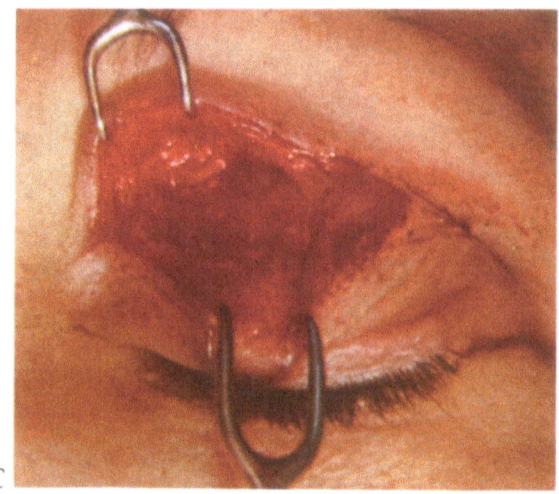

FIGURE 4.18.C. After incision and undermining, the remaining orbital fat is seen.

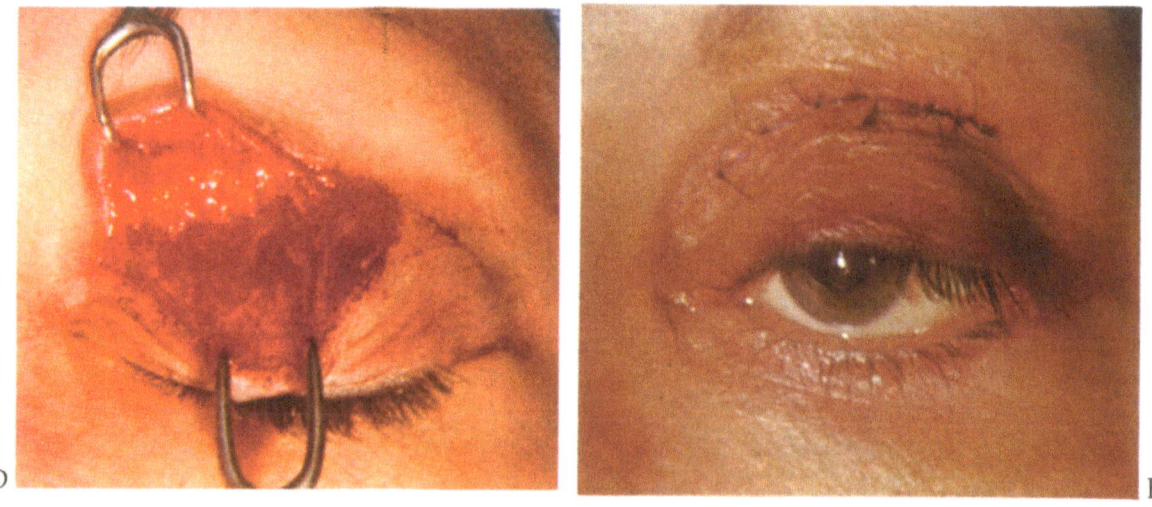

FIGURE 4.18.D. Same region showing the graft in contact with the remaining orbital fat. The graft is about the size of an almond. E. Result five days after surgery; close-up view.

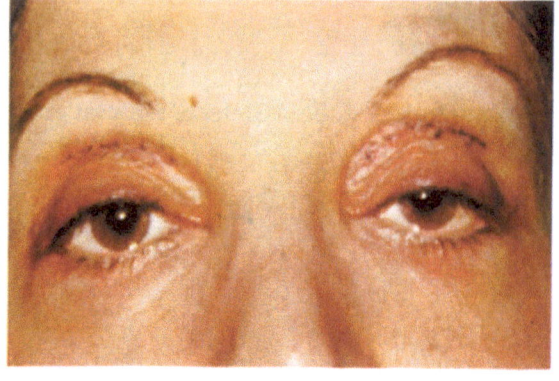

FIGURE 4.18.F. Result five days after surgery.

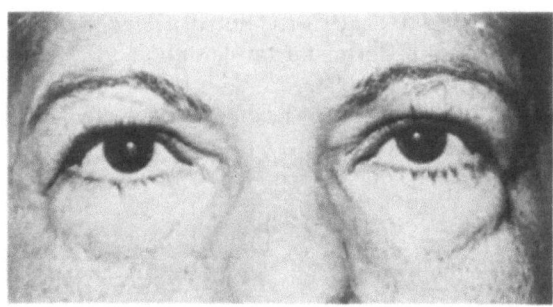 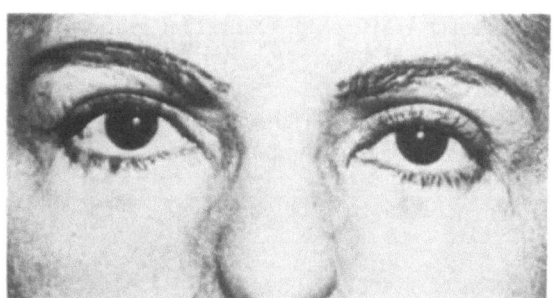

FIGURE 4.19. Typical case of depressed palpebro-malar sulcus.

Depressed Palpebro-Malar Sulcus

Treatment of a depressed palpebro-malar sulcus can be performed either by reducing the volume of the lateral fat pocket or by elevating the tissues of the face by means of a temporal face lift. It should be remembered, however, that raising the tissues of the malar region could lead to a surplus of skin in the lateral third of the lower eyelid. This excess skin should be reduced. In these cases the incision is extended beyond the lateral angle of the eye. This permits the removal of more skin and still reduces the possibility of a future ectropion (Fig. 4.19).

Additional Reading

BERINI G: Fatty tissue graft in total mastoid removal – findings, results and statistics. *Acta Otorinolaryngol Iber Am* 1957; 8:620. (in Spanish)

CARDOSO ÁLVARO D: Blepharoplasty by Folding of the Orbicularis Muscle, in: *Transactions of the VII International Congress of Plastic and Reconstructive Surgery.* Rio de Janeiro, Cartgraph, 1979. (in Portuguese)

CARDOSO ÁLVARO D: Blepharoplasty avoiding fat pad resection for correcting the depressed lower palpebral sulcus. *Rev Asoc Méd Bras* 1980; 26:377. (in Portuguese).

ELLENBOGEN R: Free autogenous pearl fat grafts in the face. – A preliminary report of a rediscovered technique. *Ann Plast Surg* 1986; 16:179.

IVERSON RE, et al: Correction of enophthalmos in the anophthalmic orbit. *Plast Reconstr Surg* 1973; 51:545.

LOEB R: Correction of eyelid depressions with free fat grafts. *Cir Esté* 1978; 3:68. (in Spanish)

LOEB R: Correction of subpalpebral depressions with small free fat grafts, in: *Transactions of the VII International Congress of Plastic and Reconstructive Surgery.* Rio de Janeiro, Cartgraft, 1979.

LOEB R: – Improvements in blepharoplasty: Creating a flat surface for the lower lid, in: *Transactions of the VII International Congress of Plastic and Reconstructive Surgery.* Rio de Janeiro, Cartgraft, 1979.

LOEB R: Fat pad sliding and fat grafting for leveling lid depressions. *Clin Plast Surg* 1981; 8:4.

LOEB R: Free fat grafted under lower lid depressions and subsequent slid to level deep nasojugal folds. *Transactions of the VII International Congress of Plastic Surgery, Montreal,* 1983: pp. 480–481.

MÉLEGA JM: The adquired and contracted anophthalmic orbit. *Rev Asoc Méd Bras* 1974; 20:437. (in Portuguese).

MUTOU Y: Use of a silicone bag-gel prosthesis to fill in a supra-tarsal depression of the upper eyelid. *Plast Reconstr Surg* 1978; 62:862.

NEDER A: Use of buccal fat for grafts. *Oral Surg* 1983; 53:348.

NEUBER H: Fat transplantation. *Verh Dtsch Ges Chir* 1893; 1:66. (in German)

NEUBER H: Fat grafting. *Chir Kongr Verh Dtsch Ges Chir* 1910; 39:188. (in German)

PEER LA: Loss of weight and volume in human fat grafts., *Plast Reconstr Surg* 1950; 5:217.

PEER LA: The neglected free fat graft. *Plast Reconstr Surg* 1956; 18:233.

PEER LA: Transplantation of fat, in: *Transplantation of Tissues,* vol 2. Baltimore, Williams & Wilkins Co, 1959.

REGNAULT P: Correction of the infrapalpebral depression. *Aesthet Plast Surg* 1978; 2:311.

SAUNDERS MC: Survival of autologous fat grafts in humans and mice. *Connect Tissue Res* 1981; 8:85.

Spina V, Ferreira MC et al: Dermo fat grafts in the repair of facial defects. *Rev Paul Med* 1972; 80:19. (in Portuguese).

Urzua R: Fat grafts for facial scarring. *Rev Asoc Méd Argent* 1939; 53:647. (in Spanish)

Van Gemert JV et al: Correction of a deep superior sulcus with dermisfat implantation. *Arch Ophthalmol* 1986; 104:604.

Wells HG: Adipose tissue: a neglected subject. *JAMA* 1940; 1114:2177.

5
Complementary Surgeries

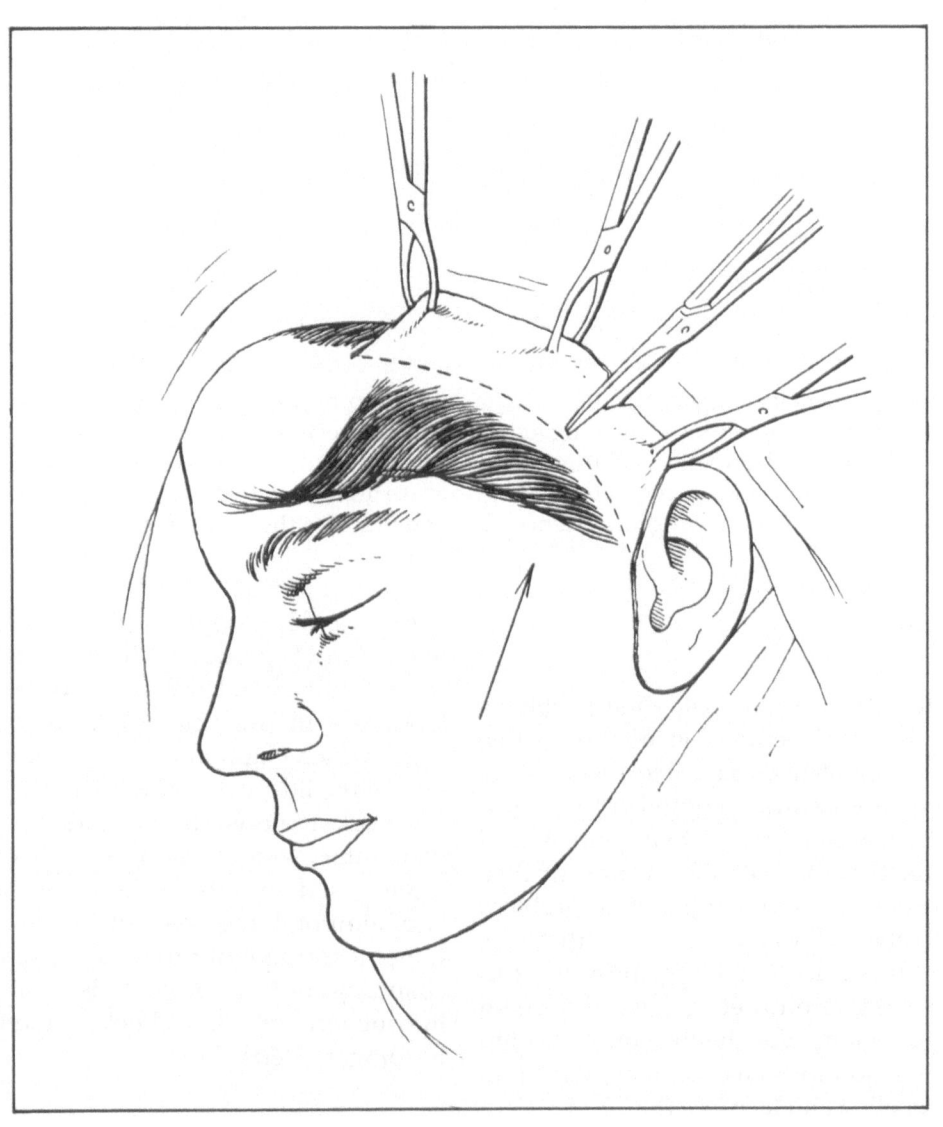

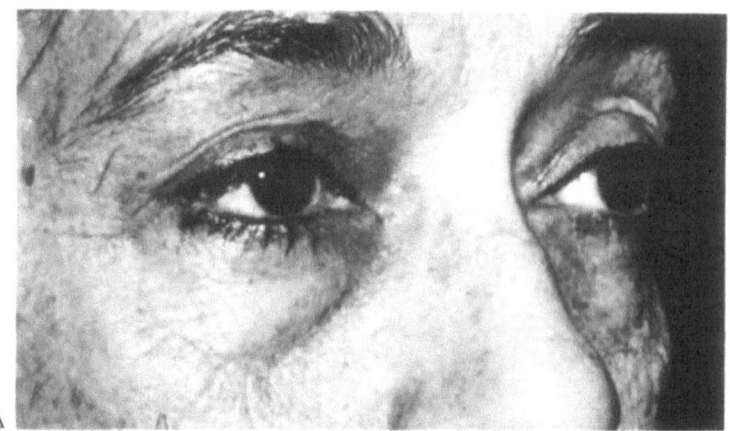

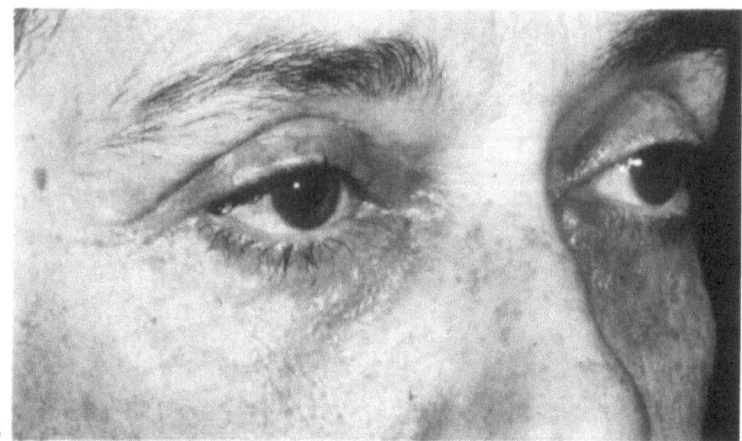

FIGURE 5.1. Complementary surgery needed after a blepharoplasty. *A.* Preoperative view showing looseness of the eyelids, with a drop in the lateral and central thirds of the eyebrows, plus accentuated crow's-feet. *B.* Postoperative view showing persistence of the drop of the eyelids and looseness of the upper lids. Correction solely by a blepharoplasty was not possible, and it was necessary to complement it with a face lift to elevate the lateral thirds of the upper lids and to soften the crow's-feet.

Introduction

The patient with aesthetic palpebral problems generally comes to the initial consultation with a desire for a blepharoplasty. However, such surgery does not always accomplish the anticipated aesthetic results, and the surgeon should make certain that the patient is aware of this. There is always, of course, the eternal problem of unattainable expectations, but there is another problem also: a blepharoplasty can unveil other, hitherto unrecognized, defects in neighboring regions. For this reason it is often necessary to resort to such complementary procedures as peeling and face lifts (Fig. 5.1).

After a blepharoplasty the principal residual defects are (1) ptotic eyebrows, principally in the central and lateral thirds, with persistent skin looseness in the upper lids; and (2) "crow's-feet," which begin in the central and lateral regions of the lids, extending to the zygomatic and/or cheek regions. In both these cases, complementary surgery is needed. The most commonly used are lifts of the forehead, eyebrows and temporal regions, and chemical peeling. Other less frequent procedures are division and suspension of the orbicularis oculi muscle and liposuction of the cheek region near the nasojugal sulcus.

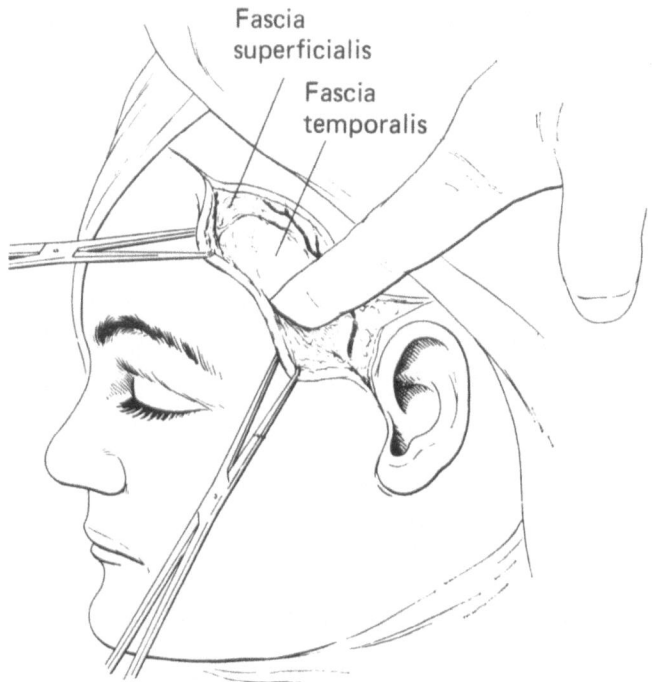

Fascia
superficialis

Fascia
temporalis

FIGURE 5.2. Undermining begins at the level of the temporofrontal region, using first a scalpel and then scissors. The rising portion of the superficial temporal artery is seen at the level of the lateral portion of the zygomatic arch. Using only blunt dissection with the fingers, the undermining continues medially over the temporal fascia, and stops anteriorly at the line where the temporal fascia meets the superficial fascia, reaching almost to the level of the supero-lateral portion of the orbital arch. It is important not to force those soft parts that show resistance to the fingers, since one wants to avoid damage to the frontal branch of the facial nerve, which emerges here to the surface. The blunt dissection is limited inferiorly, near the zygomatic arch, by the line where the temporal fascia joins the superficial one.

The Temporal Face Lift

Sometimes called a cheek-temporal lift, this is the technique by which the skin of the cheek, lateral third of the forehead, eyebrow, eyelid, and other neighboring regions are lifted. It is widely used, since it gives the following results:

1. lifting of the lateral third of the forehead, as well as of the eyebrows, principally in their lateral and central thirds;
2. reduction of the skin looseness in the central and lateral thirds of the upper eyelids;
3. reduction of the "crow's-feet" in the palpebral, zygomatic, and/or cheek regions;
4. lifting of the skin of the lateral and central thirds of the lower lids, thus reducing the possibility of an eventual scleral show.

Technique

An incision is made in the scalp extending from the temporal region to the lobe of the ear, followed by undermining of the temporal, cheek, and masseteric regions.

Limited undermining does not permit good mobilization of the flaps. On the other hand, excessive undermining close to the orbit may section the frontal branch of the facial nerve, with subsequent paralysis of the frontal muscle. For this reason, we have standardized a technique that preserves branches of this particular cranial nerve. The details are given in Figures 5.2 to 5.17.

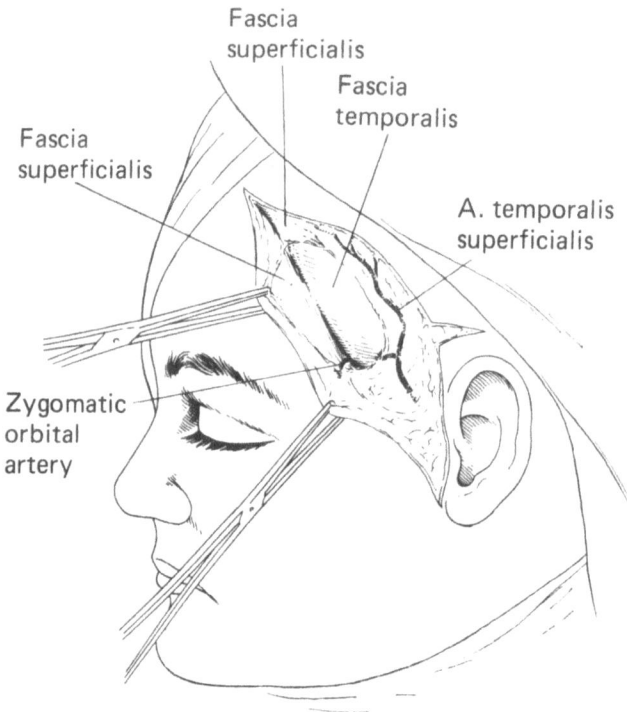

FIGURE 5.3. The suprafascial undermining continues from the posterior extremity of the zygomatic arch to the zygomatic orbital artery, which is tied and sec-tioned. (From Loeb R: Ritidoplasties – General Considerations. Monography. São Paulo, Brasil, Gráfica Saraiva, June 1966. (in Portuguese).)

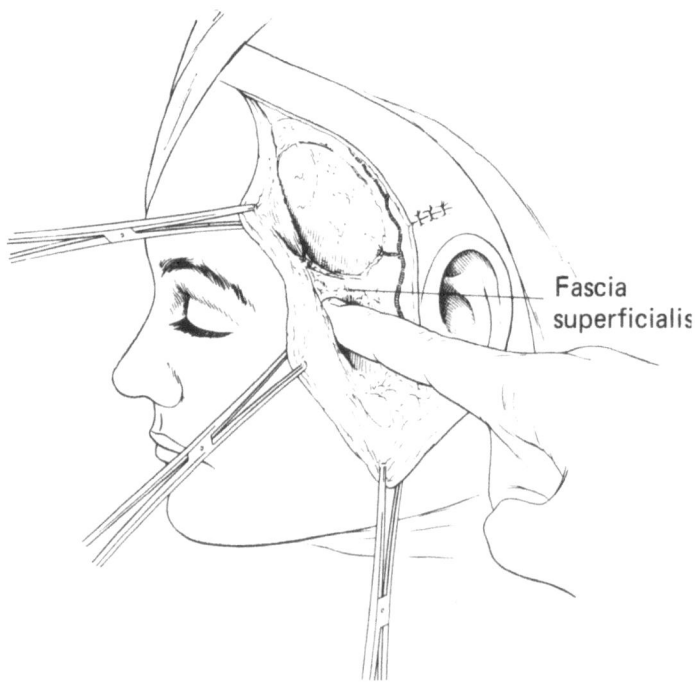

FIGURE 5.4. Using blunt dissection, the undermining continues medially in the zygomatic region, over the subjacent superficial fascia, in order to separate the latter from the skin.

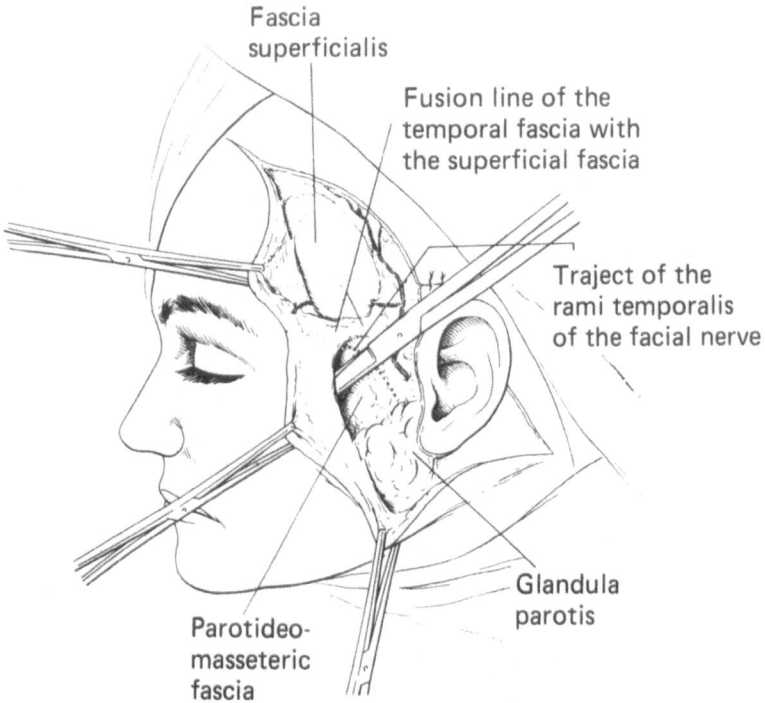

FIGURE 5.5 The undermining is continued, using scissors, below the zygoma in the buccal region, over the superficial fascia, to approximately the anterior border of the parotideo-masseteric fascia. At the level of the zygomatic arch, normally there is a septum with a vascular-nervous bundle, located at the level of the implantation of the superficial fascia in the zygoma. This bundle is composed of a motor branch of the facial nerve and branches of the superficial temporal artery. *It should never be sectioned; it deserves the utmost respect and care.*

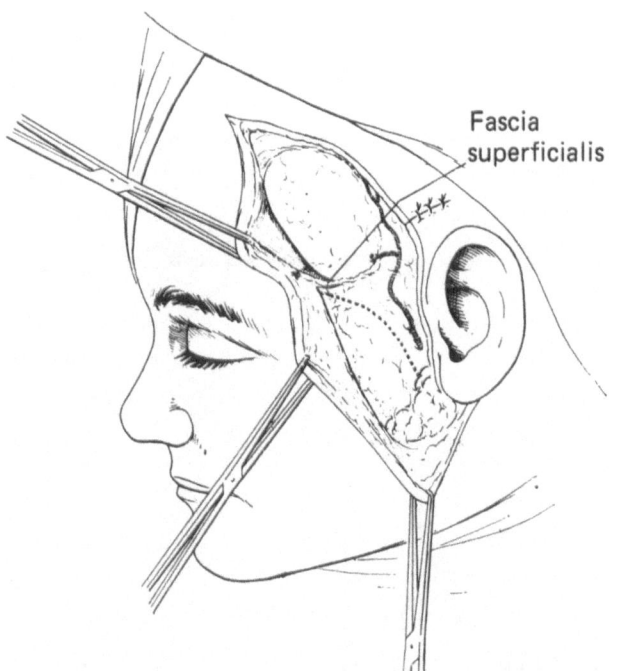

FIGURE 5.6. With these precautions observed, an adequate undermining is performed, and the superficial fascia is isolated near its implantation in the zygoma. The temporal branches of the facial nerve at this level are in the subcutaneous tissue.

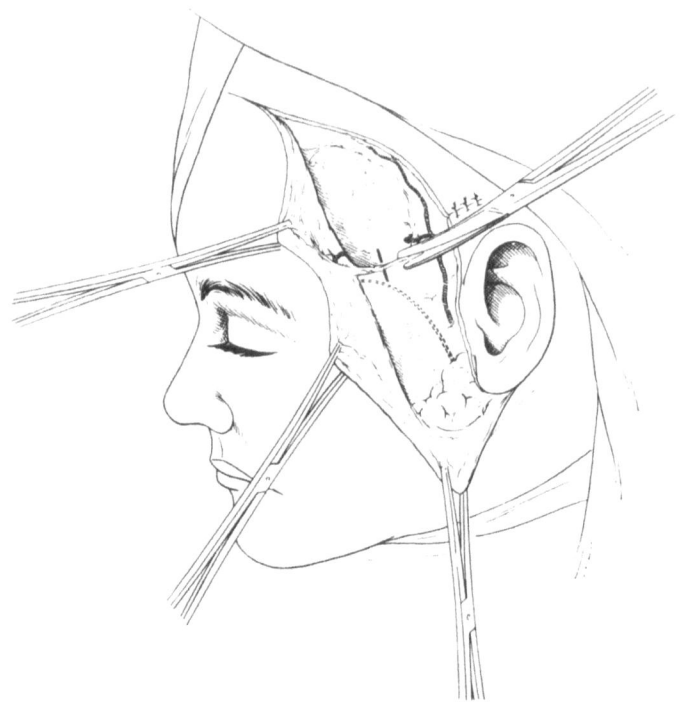

FIGURE 5.7. To facilitate the mobilization of the temporal flap, the line of fusion between the superficial and temporal fascia is freed just above the zygomatic arch. This section of the fascia should have a maximum extension of 3 cm, starting from the posterior border of the zygoma. The dotted line shows the limit of the undermining. (From Loeb R: Technique for preservation of the temporal branches of the facial nerve during face-lift operations. *Br J Plast Surg* 1970; 23(4):390–394.)

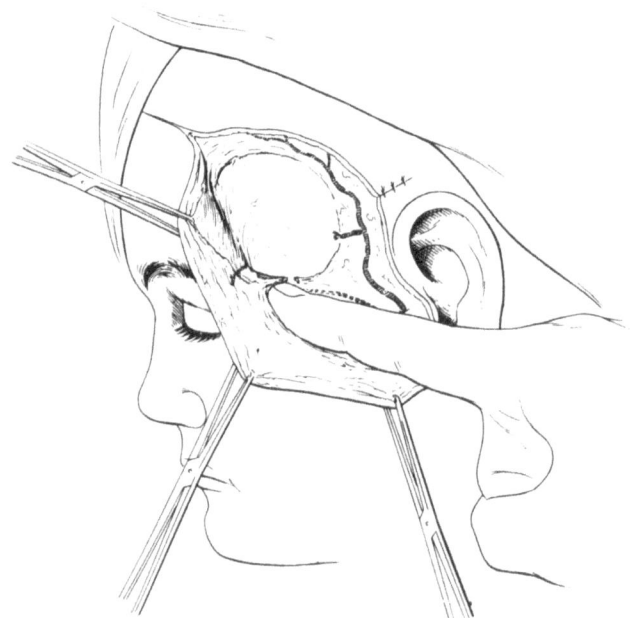

FIGURE 5.8. After having sectioned the superficial fascia at its site of implantation in the zygomatic arch, it is sometimes necessary to liberate more soft tissue, using careful digital pressure to avoid compromising superficial nerve branches.

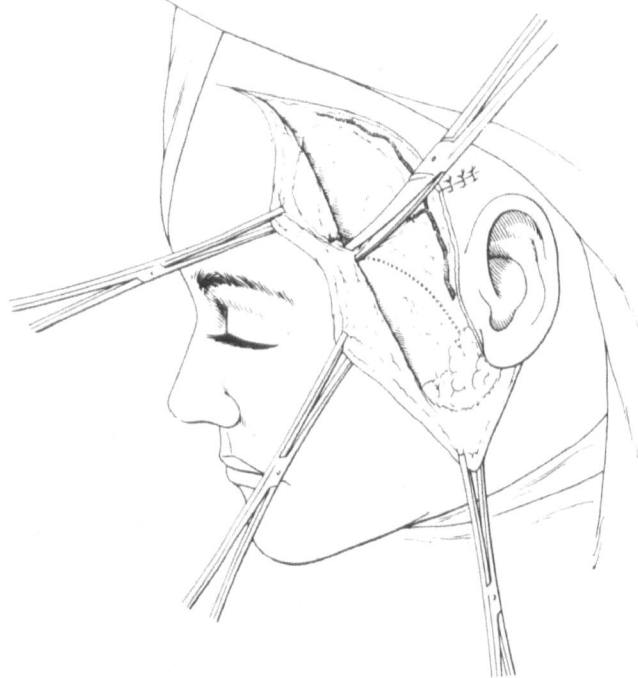

FIGURE 5.9. Reckless sectioning of the soft parts close to the orbit may severe nerves. *The undermining shown here should never be done* because there is danger of severing the frontal branch of the facial nerve.

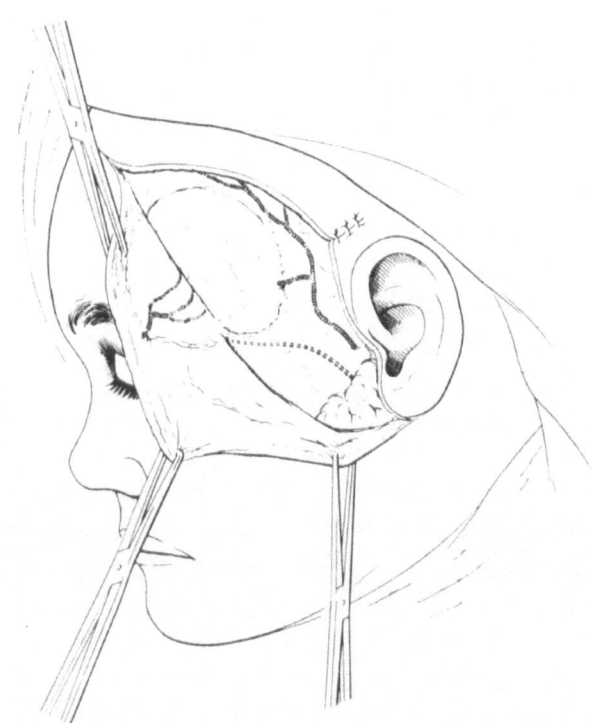

FIGURE 5.10. Near the orbital arch, the frontal branch of the facial nerve is in close proximity to the zygomatic orbital artery, a branch of the superficial temporal artery. Sectioning this artery should never happen because in so doing the temporal nerve branch is also affected. If it is necessary to section and/or distend the orbicularis oculi muscle, it should be done at this moment.

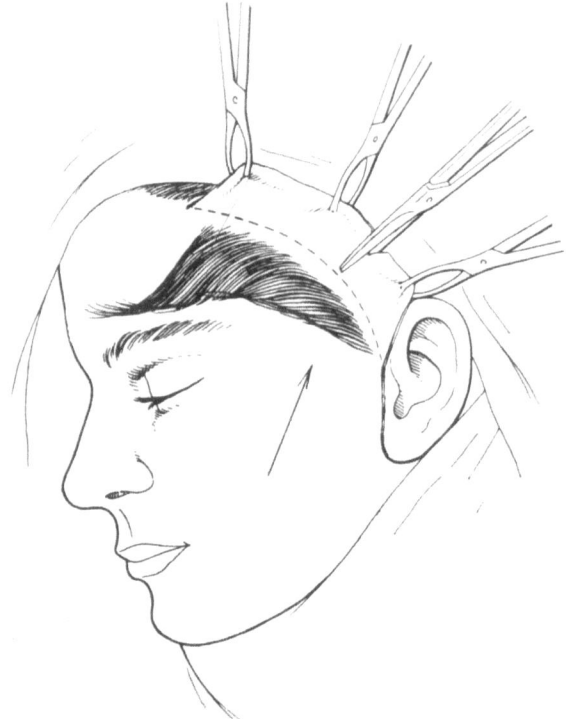

FIGURE 5.11. When the undermining is completed, the flap is pulled back, and the skin of the face and scalp is resected, using the quadrangular flap resection technique. In doing so, excess tension on the suture line is avoided. (From Loeb R: Ritidoplasties – General Considerations: Monography. São Paulo, Brasil, Gráfica Saraiva, June 1966. (in Portuguese).)

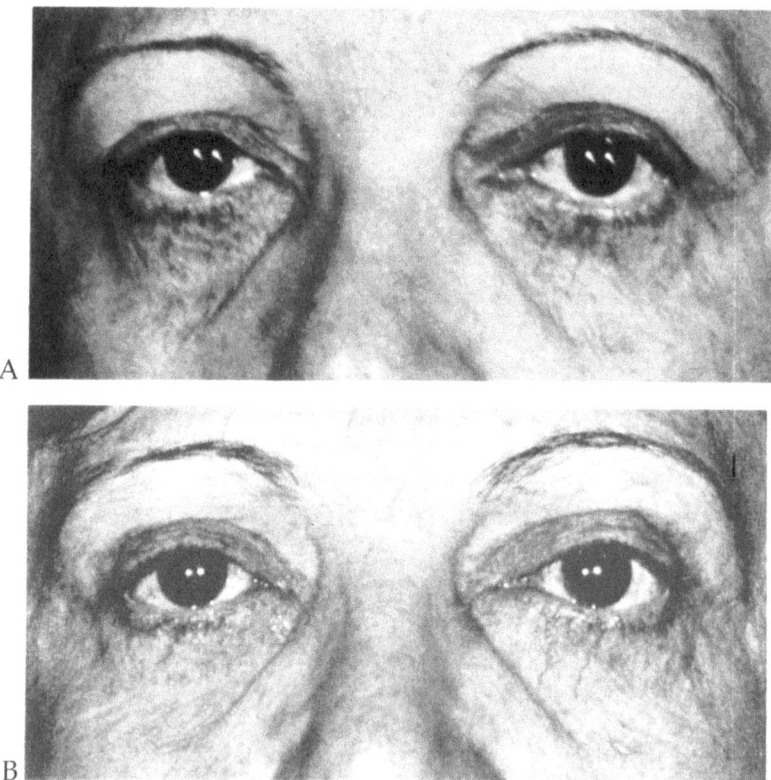

FIGURE 5.12. A temporal face lift used in the correction of scleral show. *A.* Scleral show caused by cicatricial retraction after an unsuccessful facial peel. *B.* Correction by means of a cheek-temporal face lift. The results were not rewarding.

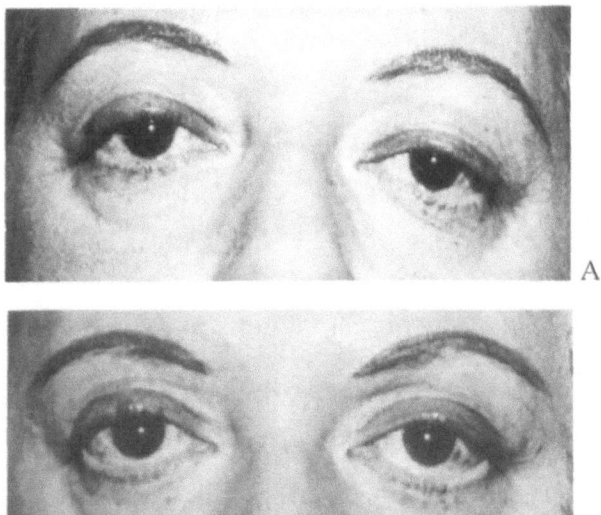

FIGURE 5.13. A. Preoperative view. This case shows the unsuccessful result following blepharoplasty and temporal face lifts. Palpebral rim directed out and down. This anatomical defect confers a sad look to the eyes and causes a slight scleral show. Correction was by means of a blepharoplasty and a cheek-temporal face lift. B. Postoperative view showing improvement in the direction of the palpebral rim. There was, however, exacerbation of the scleral show at the level of the lateral and central protions of the globe, probably due to excessive skin resection from the lower lid.

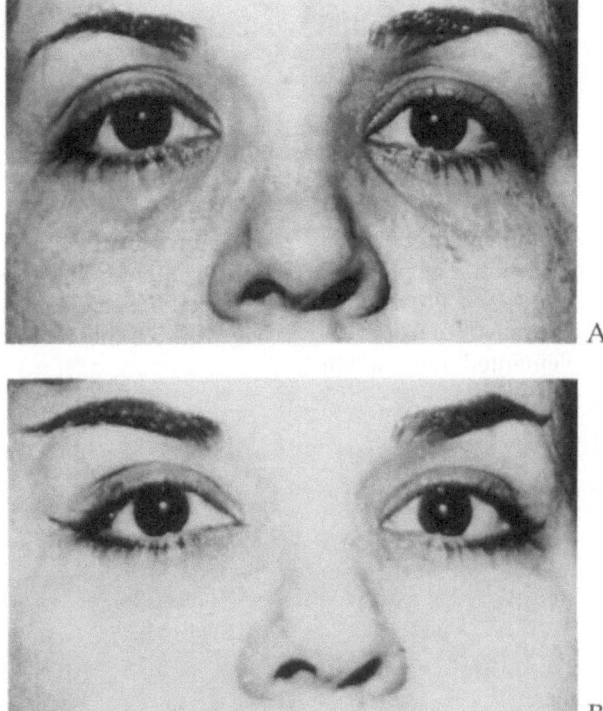

FIGURE 5.14. Temporal lift. A. Preoperative view showing tissue looseness in the lateral third of the lids, especially in the upper left lid, giving a sad look to the face. B. Postoperative view. The excess tissue of the lids has been corrected, improving the facial expression.

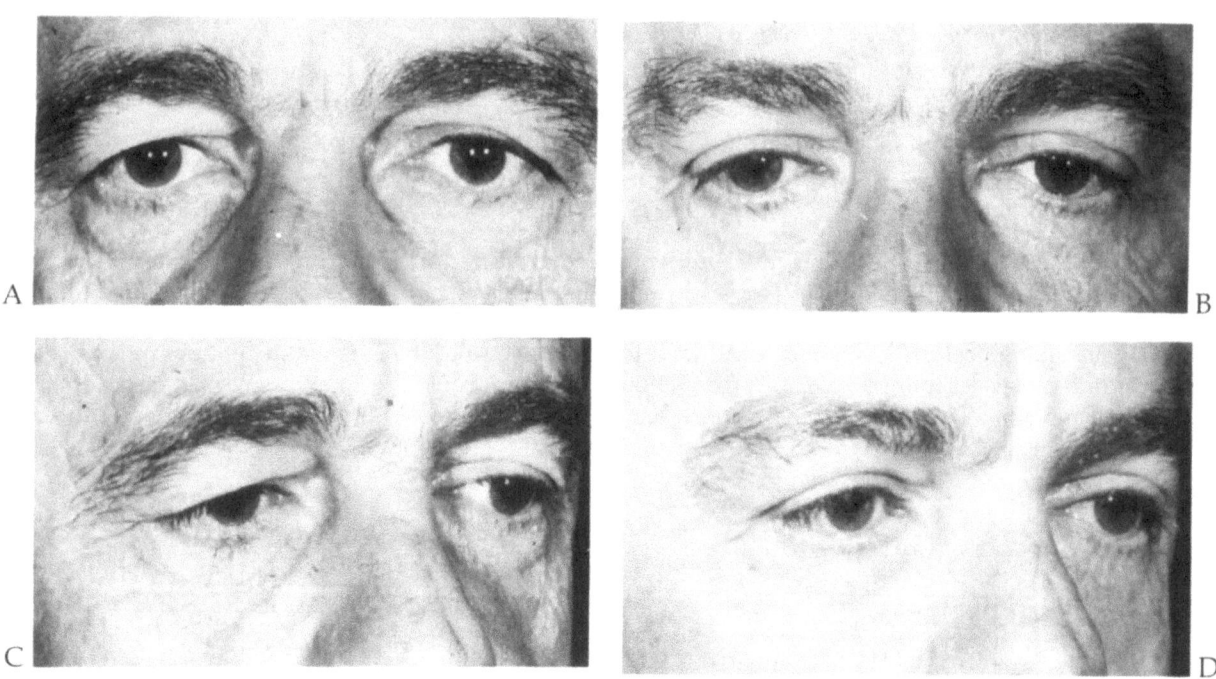

FIGURE 5.15. Blepharoplasty complemented with a temporal lift. Patient with loose skin and palpebral bulges, mostly in the upper right, and ptosis of the eyelids. Correction was done by means of upper and lower blepharoplasty, complemented with a tem-poral lift. Observe the elevation of eyebrows and the improvement in the appearance of the palpebral rim. (For skin resection, see page 47; fat resection, see pages 57–59; cheek-temporal lift, see pages 101–102.)

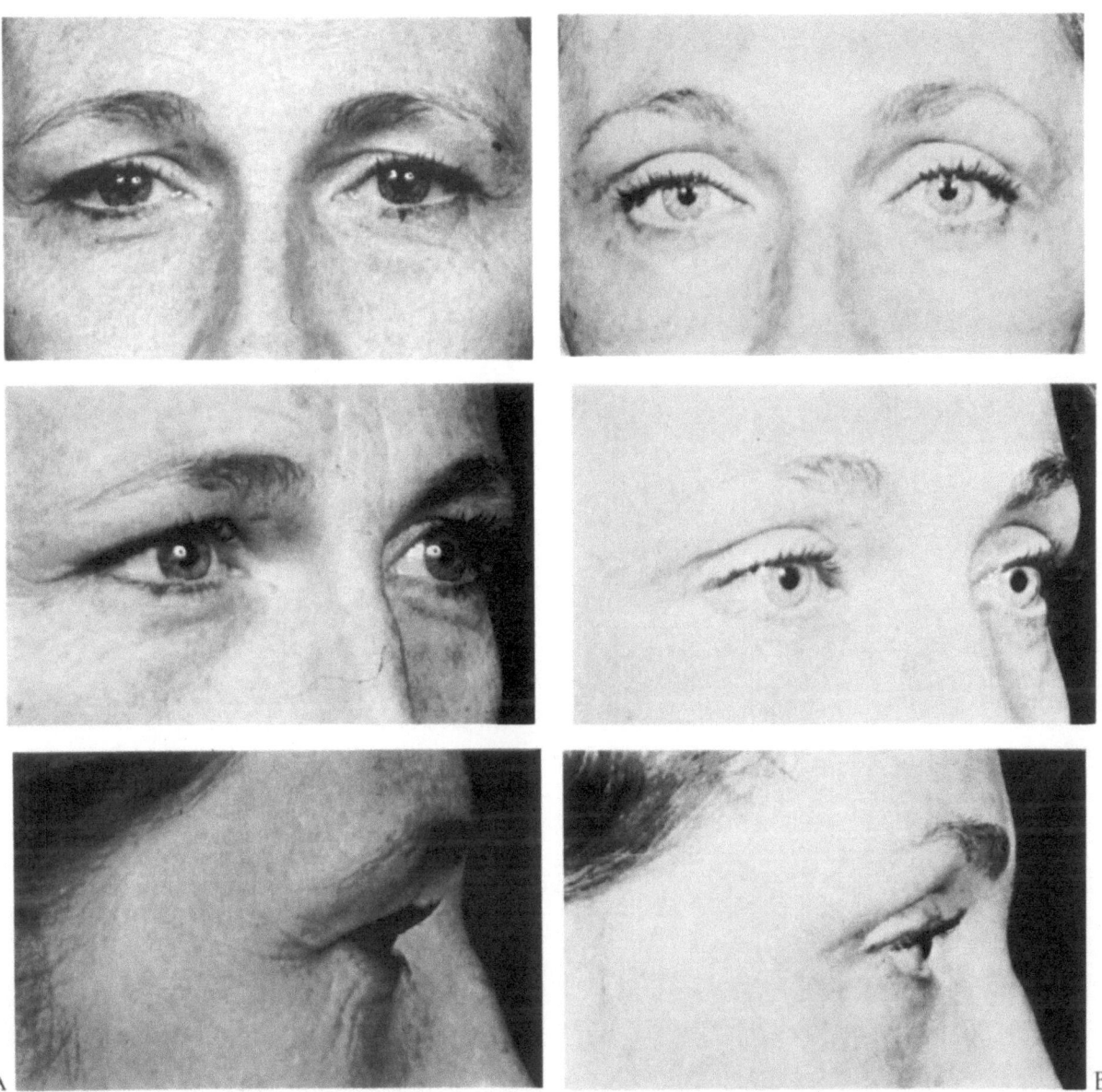

FIGURE 5.16. Blepharoplasty with face lift and peel. *A*. Preoperative view showing patient with loose palpebral skin, fat pockets, and ptosis of the eyebrows. *B*. Postoperative view after correction of looseness and fat pockets by a blepharoplasty, elevation of the eyebrows by a temporal face lift, and correction of the crow's-feet by a skin peel in the malar and zygomatic regions.

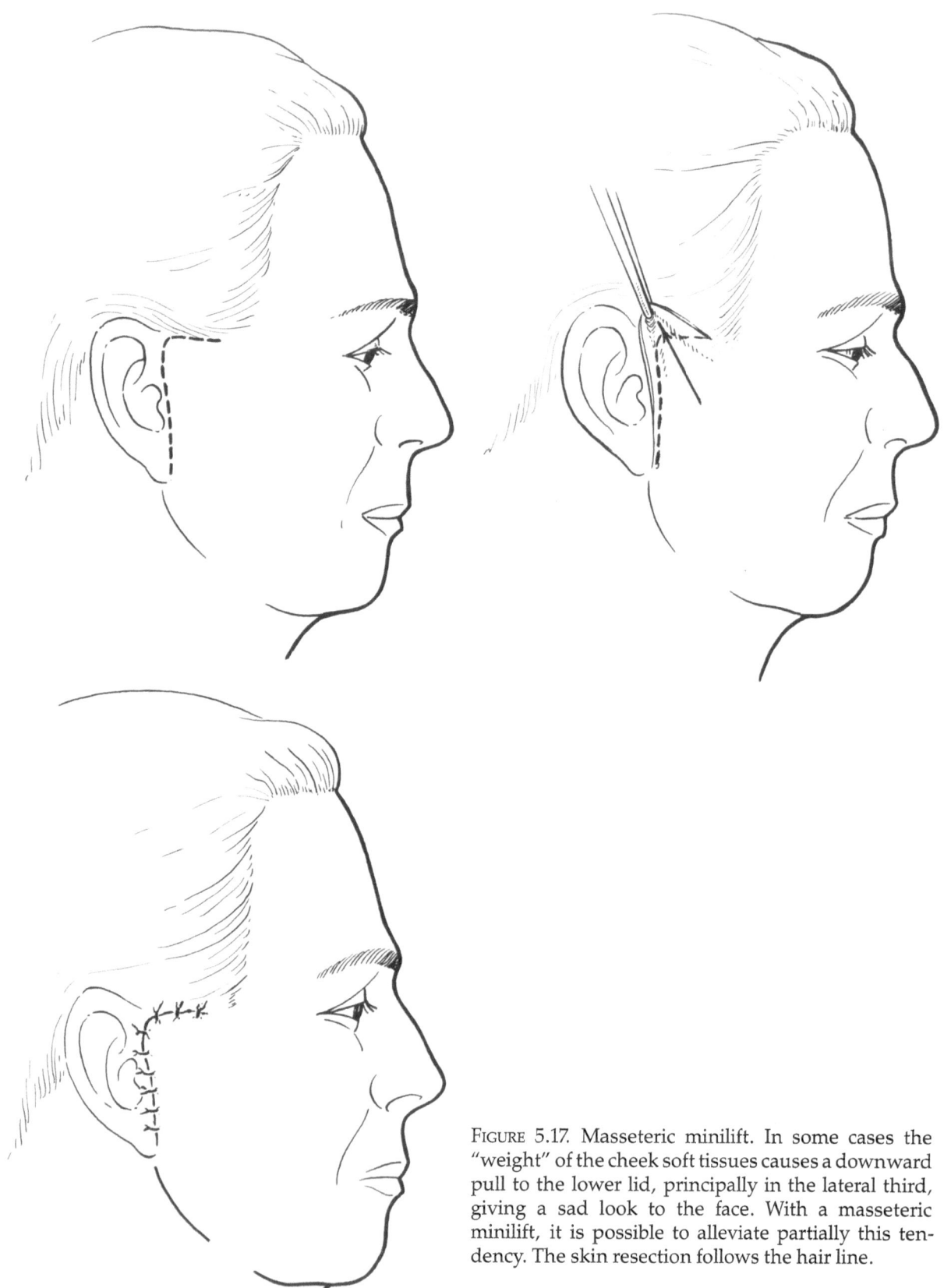

FIGURE 5.17. Masseteric minilift. In some cases the "weight" of the cheek soft tissues causes a downward pull to the lower lid, principally in the lateral third, giving a sad look to the face. With a masseteric minilift, it is possible to alleviate partially this tendency. The skin resection follows the hair line.

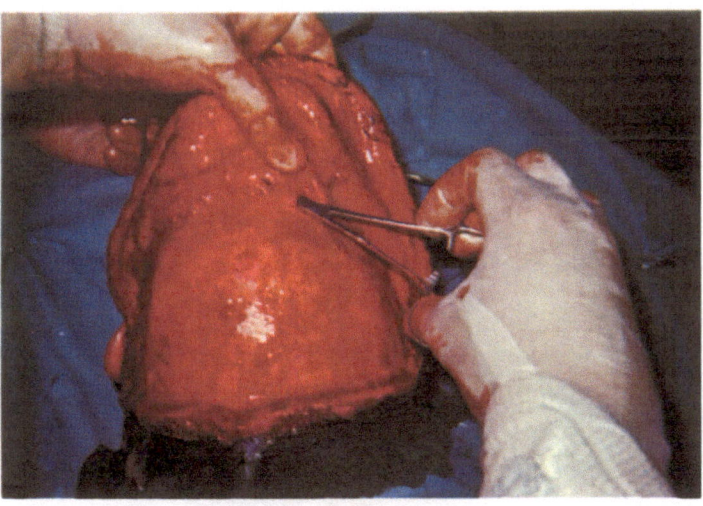

FIGURE 5.18. Frontal lift. After incision and subaponeurotic undermining, the thickness fo the corrugator muscle is reduced.

The Forehead Lift

This is the procedure by which the tissues of the upper third of the face are elevated (Dingman and Peled, 1979); it acts directly upon the frontal, eyebrow, and eyelid regions, and indirectly on the cheek and zygomatic areas. We have observed the following esthetic benefits from a frontal face lift:

- elevation of the tissues of the forehead;
- elevation of the mesial, central, and lateral portions of the eyebrows;
- elevation and distension of the skin of the upper lids;
- improvement of the crow's-feet;
- elevation of the lateral angles of the eyes;
- elevation and improvement of the palpebromalar sulcus.

When performing this type of lift, part of the corrugator muscle and of the frontal belly of the occipitofrontal muscle can be resected if necessary. There are two basic techniques for placing the incision line: The first, which we rarely use, is to place it coincident with the hairline; the second is to make a coronal incision about 3 to 4 cm behind the hairline.

Technique

A coronal incision is made in the scalp about 3 to 4 cm behind the hairline. Supraperiosteal undermining is done to the superior orbital border and the glabellar region. Laterally, the undermining extends as far as the zygoma, even at times to the buccal, cheek, and masseteric regions. The thickness of the corrugator muscle is reduced surgically.

The frontal muscle is sectioned with a scalpel into squares approximately 2 cm on a side. The thickness of these squares is reduced almost by half with scissors.

After careful hemostasis, the scalp is pulled back and the excess is resected. Generally we use the technique of quadrilateral resection to guarantee homogeneous stresses at the traction points. It is sutured with 4-0 nylon (Fig. 5.18 to 5.24).

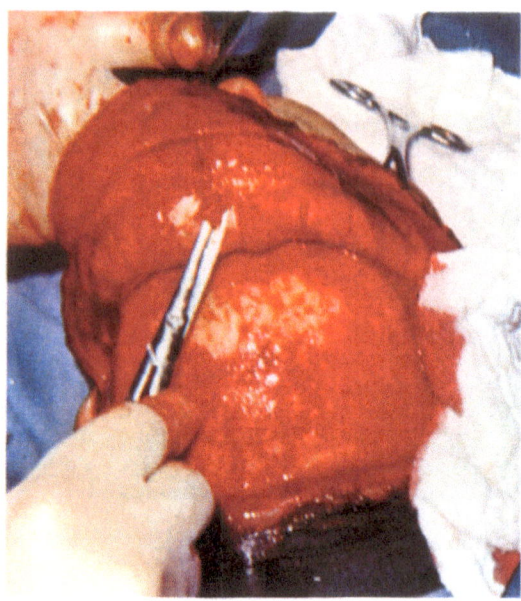

FIGURE 5.19. The frontal muscle is sectioned in practically its entire thickness. Part of the thickness of the resulting squares is reduced with scissors.

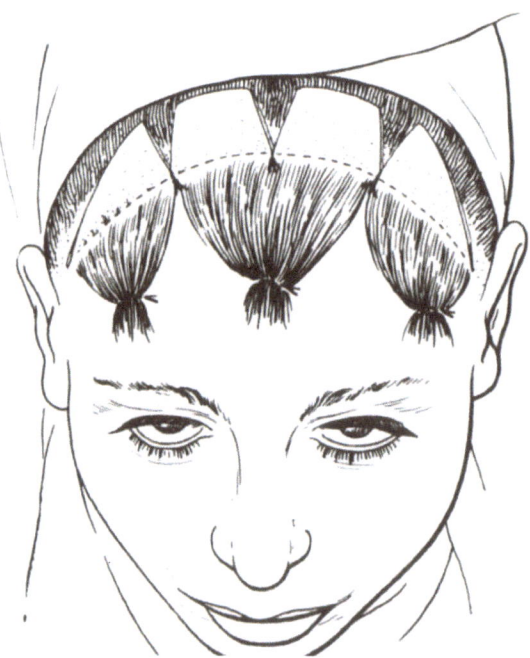

FIGURE 5.20. The frontal lift is made through a coronal incision in the scalp. For the purpose of avoiding undue stress at the suture line, the area to be resected is subdivided into square segments, over which the traction can be applied homogeneously. (From Loeb R: Ritidoplasties–General Considerations. Monography. Gráfica Saraiva, São Paulo, Brasil, June 1966.) (in Portuguese)

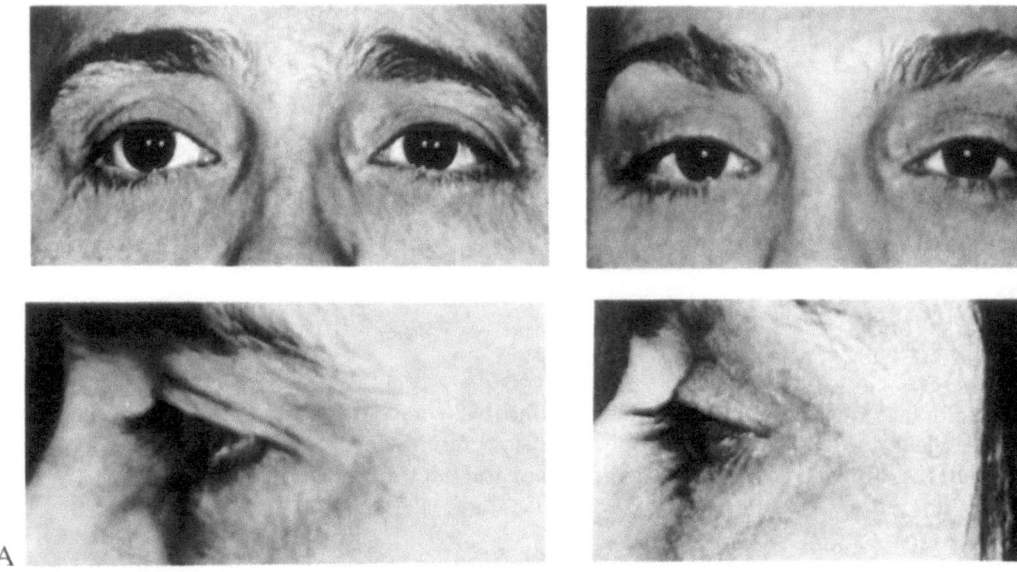

A

B

FIGURE 5.21. Blepharoplasty with temporal and brow lifts. *A.* Preoperative view: patient with palpebral looseness and an accentuated droop in the right eye-brow region, causing upper eyelid assymetry. *B.* Post-operative view: correction was by means of a blepharoplasty with temporal and brow lifts.

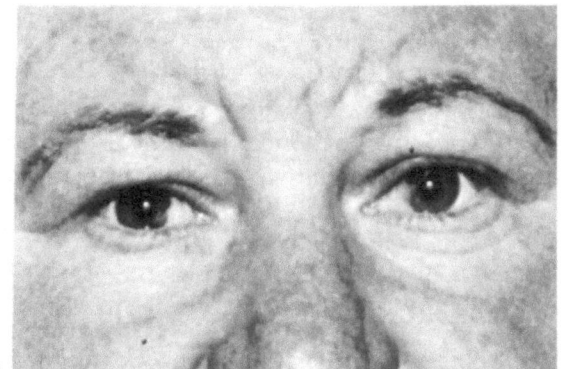

A

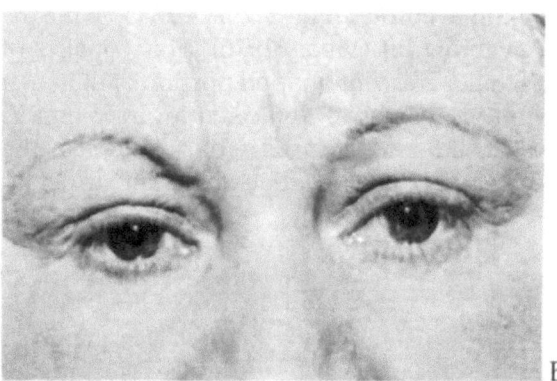

B

FIGURE 5.22. Temporofrontal lift. *A.* Preoperative view: patient with blepharochalasis, low forehead, and crow's-feet. *B.* Postoperative view: patient after a blepharoplasty and a forehead lift. The frontal region has benefited by the distension.

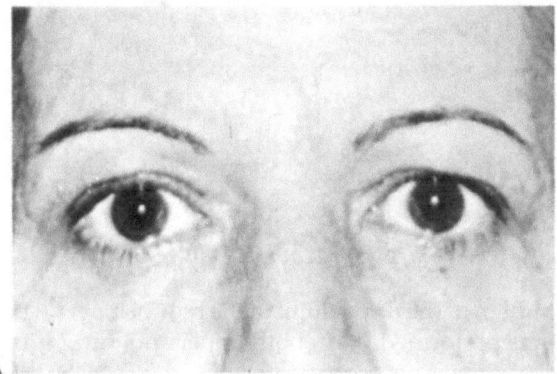

A

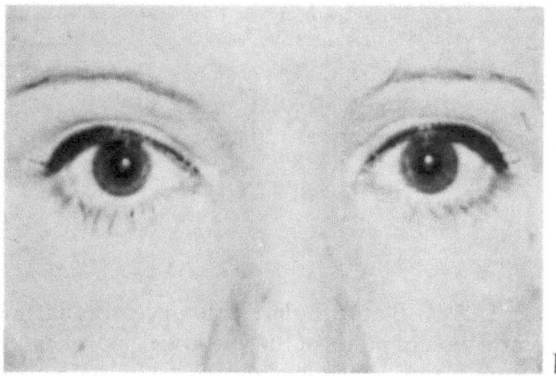

B

FIGURE 5.23. Blepharoplasty with a frontal lift. *A.* Preoperative view: loose skin of the upper lid and ptosis of the eyebrows. *B.* Postoperative view: after skin resection in the lids and a forehead lift.

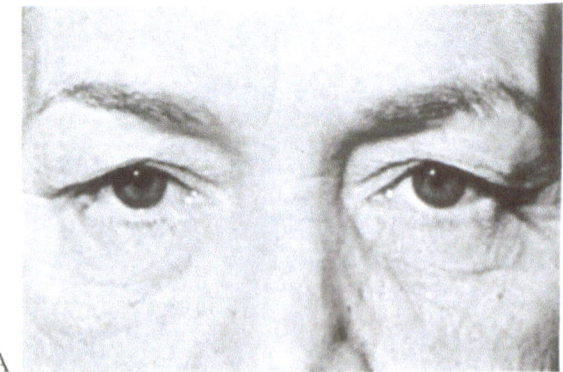
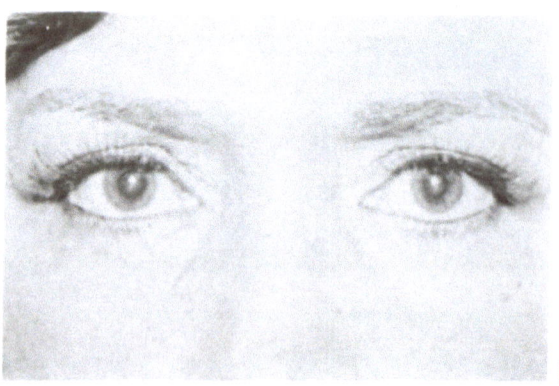

FIGURE 5.24. Blepharoplasty with a temporofrontal lift. *A.* Preoperative view: loose tissue in the upper and lower eyelids. In the upper lids the excess skin almost covers part of the iris, impairing vision. *B.* Postoperative view: patient after reduction of excess skin and a temporofrontal lift.

The Eyebrow Lift

The most direct and efficient way to correct drooping eyebrows (Fig. 5.25A – E) is by means of a eyebrow lift (Vinas, 1976). This consists of removing a crescent-shaped portion of skin just above the eyebrows. The resulting raw area is then closed and sutured, thus reducing the looseness of both the forehead and the upper lid and improving the crow's-feet. The scar should be hidden in the upper border of the eyebrows.

Technique

The procedure is generally done under local anesthesia. The width of skin to be resected

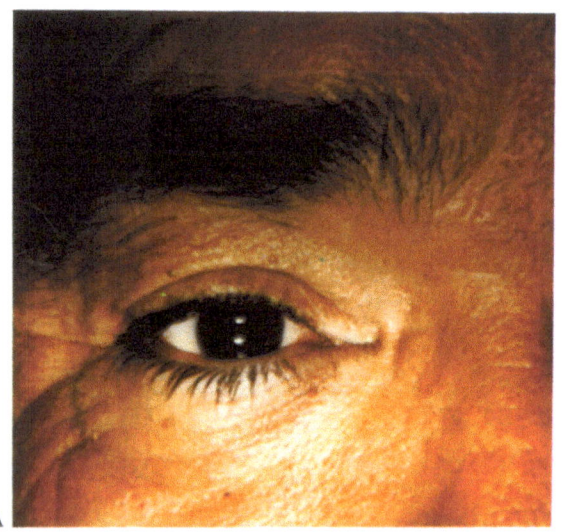
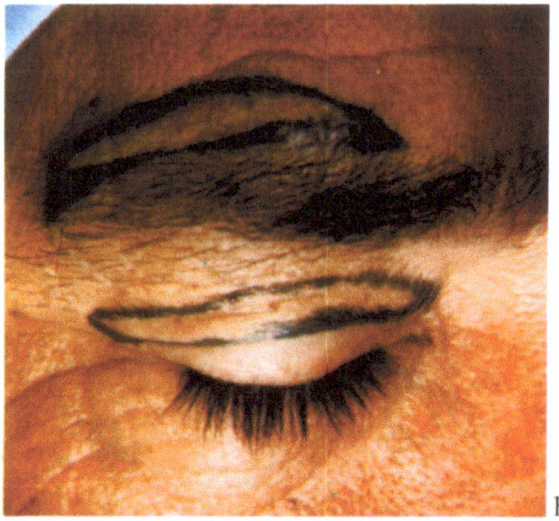

FIGURE 5.25. *A.* Blepharoplasty plus eyebrow lift for the correction of ptosis of the eyebrows, looseness of the upper and lower eyelids, and crow's-feet. *B.* Markings placed. *C.* Resulting raw area consequent to the supraciliary skin ressection. *D.* The suture is hidden in the upper limit of the brow. Upper lid markings performed. *E.* In both upper and lower lids it is sometimes necessary to extend the resection laterally, in order to contribute to the elevation or the soft tissues lateral to the lids.

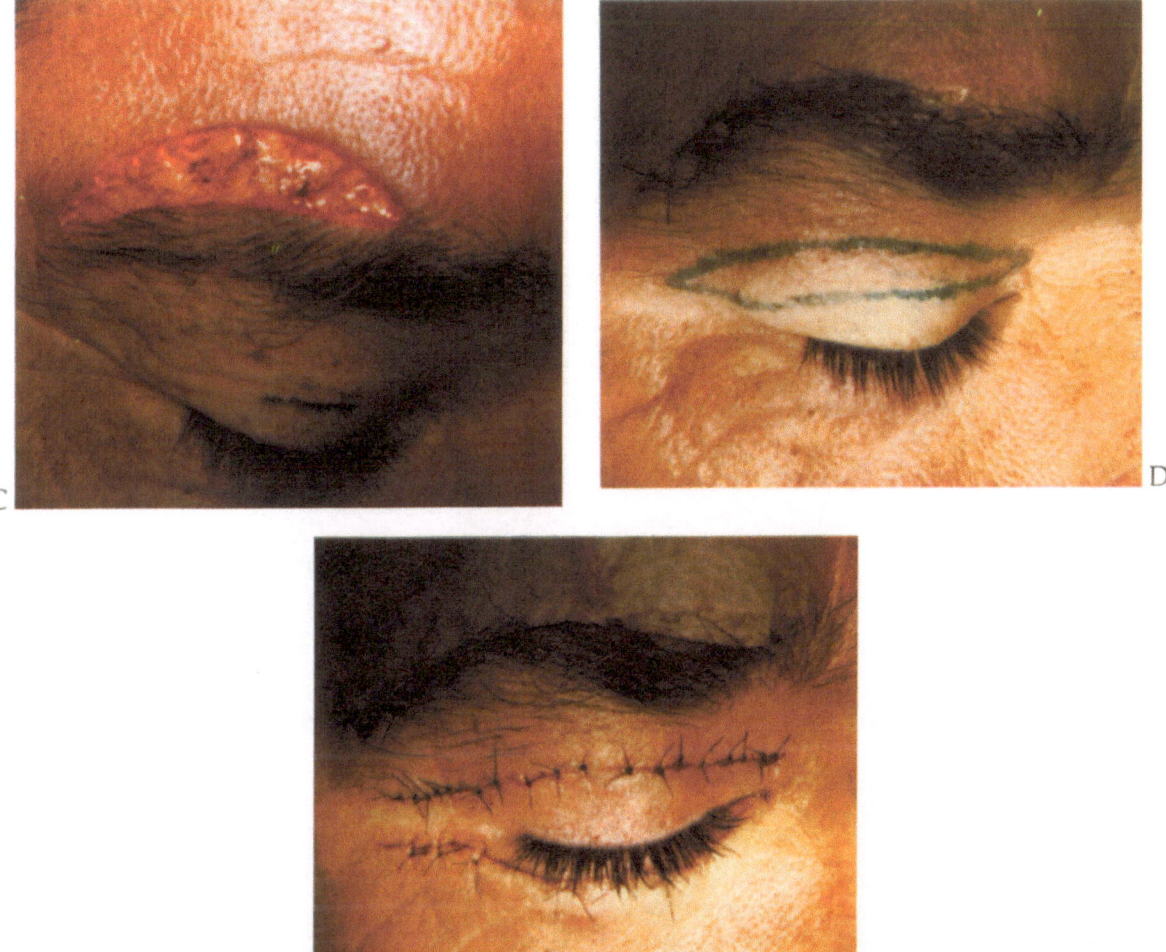

FIGURE 5.25

should be evaluated carefully because any over-resection will elevate the eyebrows excessively and give an expression of surprise to the face.

The incision follows the upper limit of the eyebrows (Fig. 5.25C). Suturing is done in two planes: 1) deep, to close the subcutaneous tis-sues, and 2) superficial, using 6-0 nylon discon-tinuous stitches (Fig. 5.25D), or 5-0 nylon con-tinuous intradermic stitches. With this techni-que, one can distend the tissue of the upper lids, and the resection there can be more moderate (Fig. 5.25E).

Eyebrow Lifts and Other Orbital Surgeries Used to Improve "Sunken Eyes"

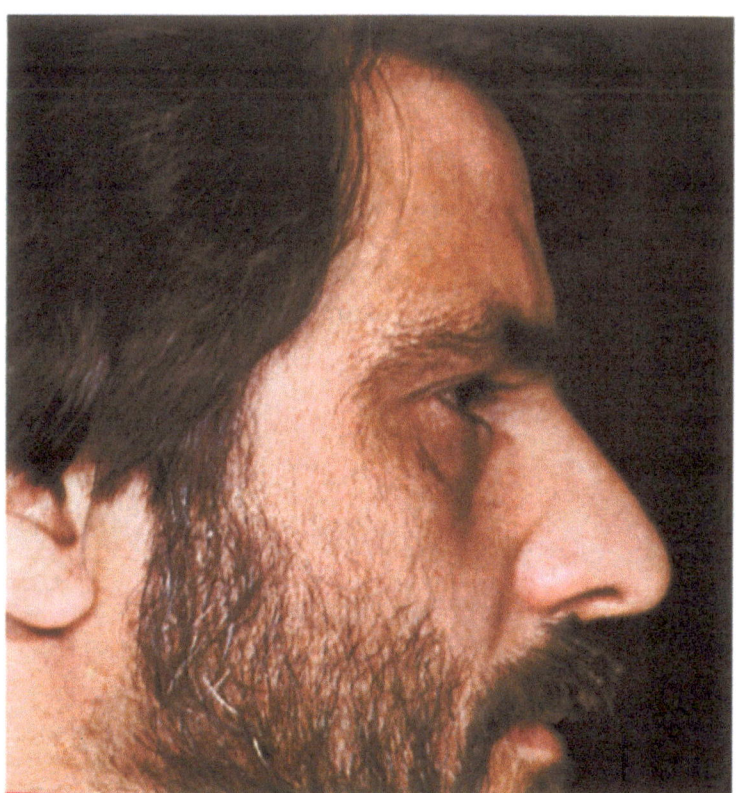

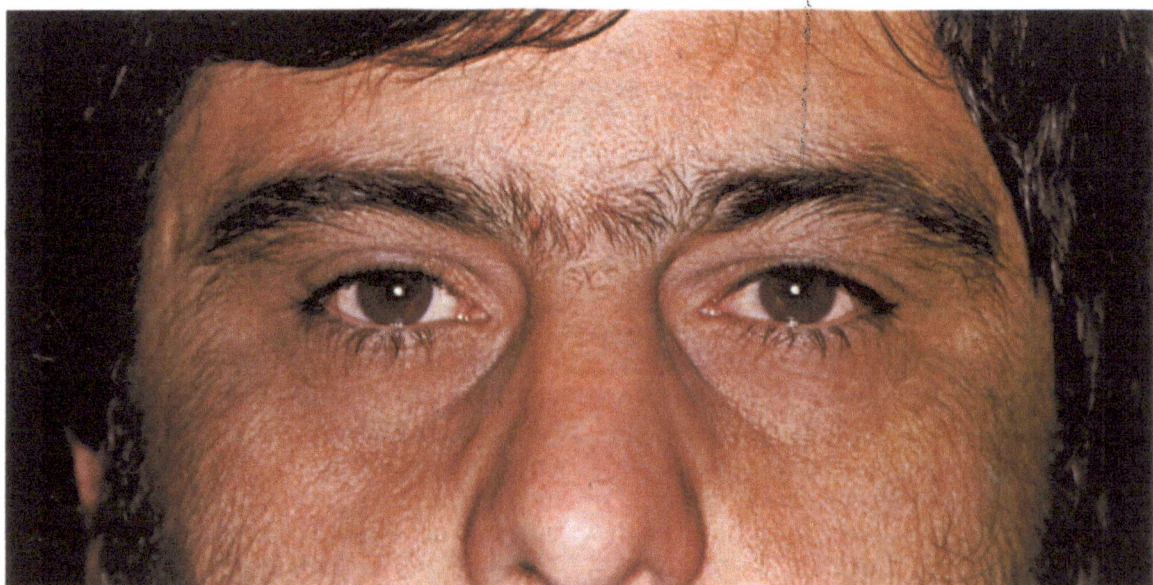

A

FIGURE 5.26. A. Multiple surgeries for the purpose of improving "sunken eyes." A 38-year-old patient with deep-set eyes, ptosis of the eyebrows, excess skin of the upper eyelids, and depressions of the lower lids, which are also heavily pigmented. The total sum of these problems gives him an austere, singularly sad look. The darkness of the palpebral regions is very obvious because of the unusual depth of the orbital regions combined with the pigmentation of the palpebral skin. There is a marked projection of the brow, which is amply covered with thick, black eyebrows. The details of the procedures undertaken to improve his facial expression are illustrated in the figures that follow.

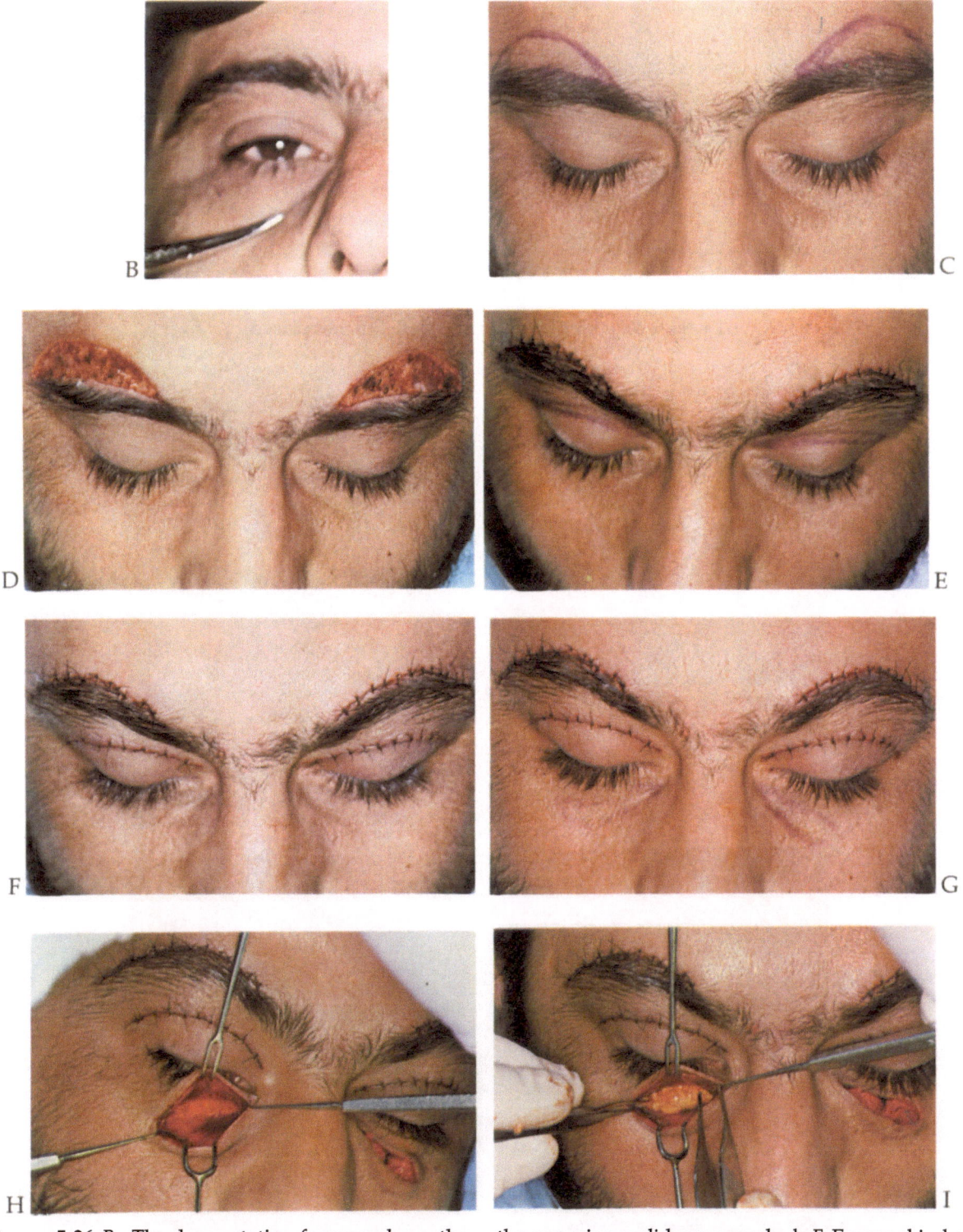

FIGURE 5.26. *B.* The hemostaticc forceps show the depressed region at the level of the nasojugal sulcus. *C.* Markings in the frontal region for an eyebrow lift. *D.* Skin resected and hemostasis accomplished. *E.* Discontinous 6-0 nylon stitches placed. Note that the suture line is at the upper limit of the eyebrows. At the same time the excess of skin to be resected from the superior eyelids was marked. *F.* Excess skin has been resected from upper eyelids and stitches placed. *G.* Markings in the lower eyelids show the depressed areas in which fat grafts will be placed. *H.* Incision and undermining of the lower eyelids. Note the reduced volume of fat tissue. *I.* Introduction of the almond-sized fat graft.

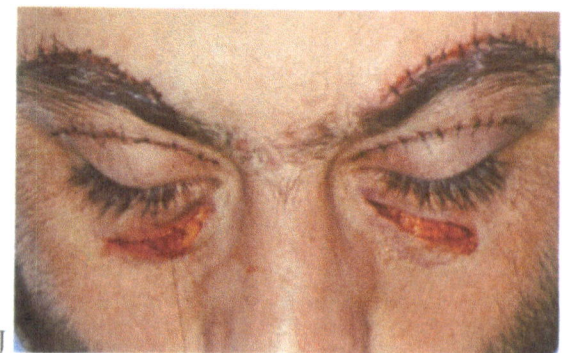
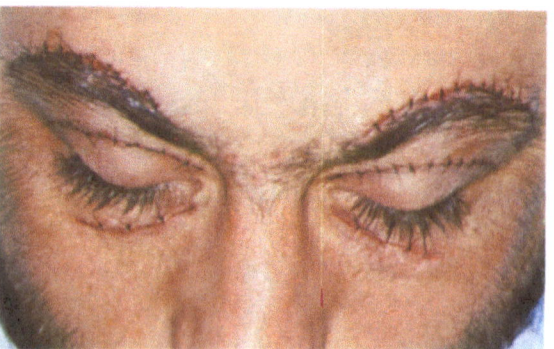

FIGURE 5.26. J. Right eyelid grafted. K. Stitches placed.

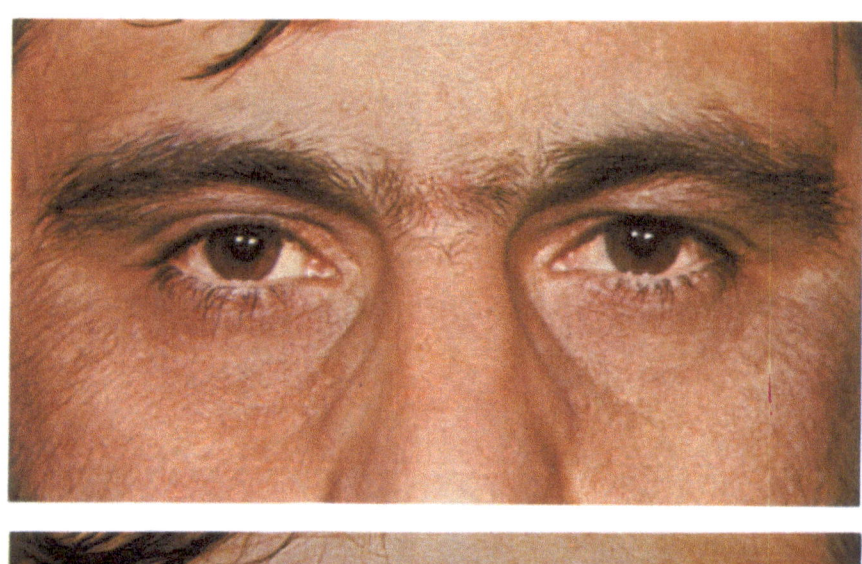
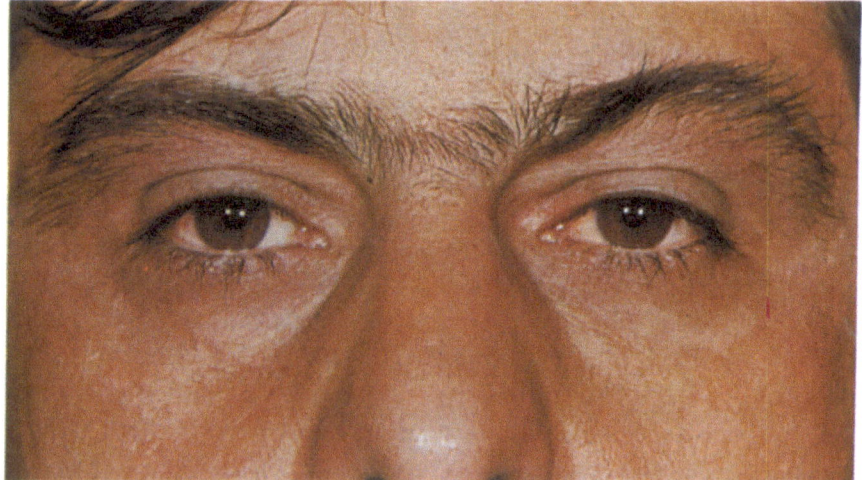

FIGURE 5.26. L. Comparison of preoperative and post-operative appearance. (*Top*) Preoperative view showing the principal defect: sunken eyes. (*Bottom*) Post-operative view after the procedures described above. Note that the eyes do not now appear sunken.

Chemical Peeling

This is widely used for the correction of crow's-feet and skin pigmentation in the palpebral, zygomatic, and cheek regions (Baker and Gordon, 1972).

Correction of Crow's-Feet

Crow's-feet may appear as truly deep sulci or as small superficial wrinkles. Between these two extremes there is a range of intermediate conditions, hence there are many different techniques for their treatment. In incipient cases, peeling alone is sufficient to flatten the area satisfactorily. In more serious cases a temporal lift is frequently necessary before the peeling, since it first improves the deeper wrinkles by the distension of the tissue.

Treatment of Overpigmentation

Some excess pigmentation of the eyelids and neighboring regions may be improved by peeling. These over-pigmentations (Fig. 5.27) should not be confused with the shadows caused by accentuated depressions described on page 40 (See Chapter 4). Before peeling, a test should be made in a small hidden area to ensure that the patient will really benefit from a peel.

The technique of peeling consists of a controlled chemical burn that results in a reduction of the thickness of the treated area. It improves wrinkles by elimination of the epidermis and part of the dermis. The differences of levels between the bulges and the depressions that constitute the wrinkles are lessened, softened or even eliminated by the flattening of the skin. New epithelium forms in the treated areas, reestablishing its integrity and covering the region in six to ten days.

Chemical peeling can be compared to a local second-degree burn. It is, however, aseptic, which greatly benefits the reepithelialization. Chemical peeling is generally done using Baker's caustic solution (1952), which has been well standardized:

USP Phenol, 3 mL
Distilled water, 2 mL
Croton oil, 2 drops
Liquid soap, 8 drops

Technique

The patient is generally sedated with barbiturates the evening before the treatment. In persons with a low threshold to pain, an intramuscular dose of meperidine (Demerol) is given one-half hour before the beginning of treatment. In the treatment of small areas in ambulatory patients, an oral analgesic is sufficient.

The skin is carefully cleaned with an alcohol-ether solution in order to eliminate oils. The phenol solution is applied to the area to be treated with cotton swabs. Obviously, special care should be taken that the phenol is not allowed to come in contact with the palpebral or global conjunctive.

After the application, the skin acquires a whitish appearance, which after some minutes becomes a rosy red. Strips of waterproof adhesive tape approximately 1 cm wide are applied to protect the region and to prevent the evaporation of the phenol solution, so that is reacts more efficiently. Some believe that "strapping" is actually not necessary. The pain is similar to that of a burn; although usually tolerable, it can be more or less intense, depending on the sensitivity of the patient.

The eyelids frequently become edematous; in extreme cases, the patient cannot open the eyes. Approximately 24 hours after the beginning of treatment, a dark-colored serous fluid is secreted, exuding from between the strips of adhesive tape. After 48 hours the tape is carefully removed, generally with the patient sedated. The removal can be earlier, depending on the patient's cutaneous reaction. Upon removal of the tape, the skin surface appears edematous, with some hemorrhaging spots.

The next step is the atraumatic removal of the necrotic tissue. Powdered thymol iodate is applied over the treated skin once or twice a day

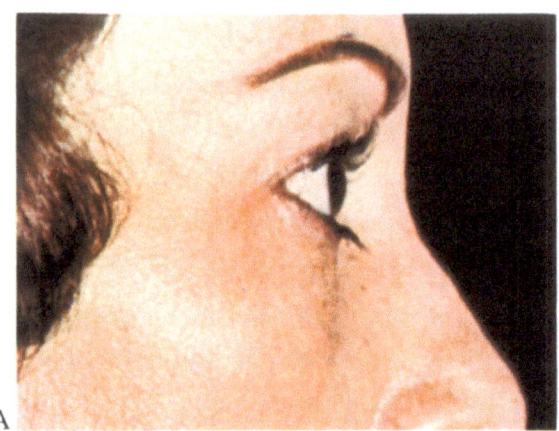

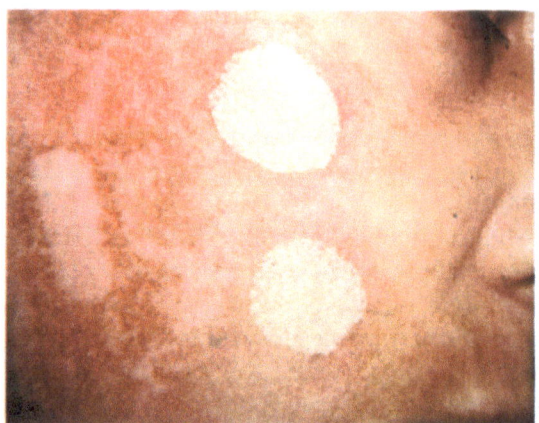

FIGURE 5.27. Complications of peeling. Hyperpigmentation. Some patients show a tendency toward hyperpigmentation. In these cases, before the chemical peeling, a test should be made. *A.* Preoperative view.

B. A phase of the test. (From Loeb, R: in Sucena, RC: Cirurgia Plástica. São Paulo. Livraria Rocca, vol. 2, 1982) (In Portuguese).

for about 36 hours. The crust that forms will be removed, carefully and progressively, with petroleum jelly gauze or an ointment of neomycin and/or cortisone.

The peeled area remains reddish, similar to a second-degree burn, for about 15 days after the removal of the last bandage. After this time the redness deminishes progressively and the skin acquires its normal color 45 to 60 days after the treatment. In a few cases, the erythema takes more time to disappear, sometimes 6 or more months. For at least a month the patient should not use substances that are irritating to the skin, such as strong soaps. He should also follow a strict diet, abstaining from spicy foods that may provoke skin eruptions. For at least 60 days he should also avoid the direct rays of the sun. During this time the skin may show different shades of color. When these differences become small, he can begin exposure to the sun, starting with two to three minutes a day and increasing this progressively. Eventually the action of the solar rays will equalize the differences in the skin color. The use of creams with a solar filter is recommended. Clinical cases of peeling are shown in Figures 5.28 to 5.36.

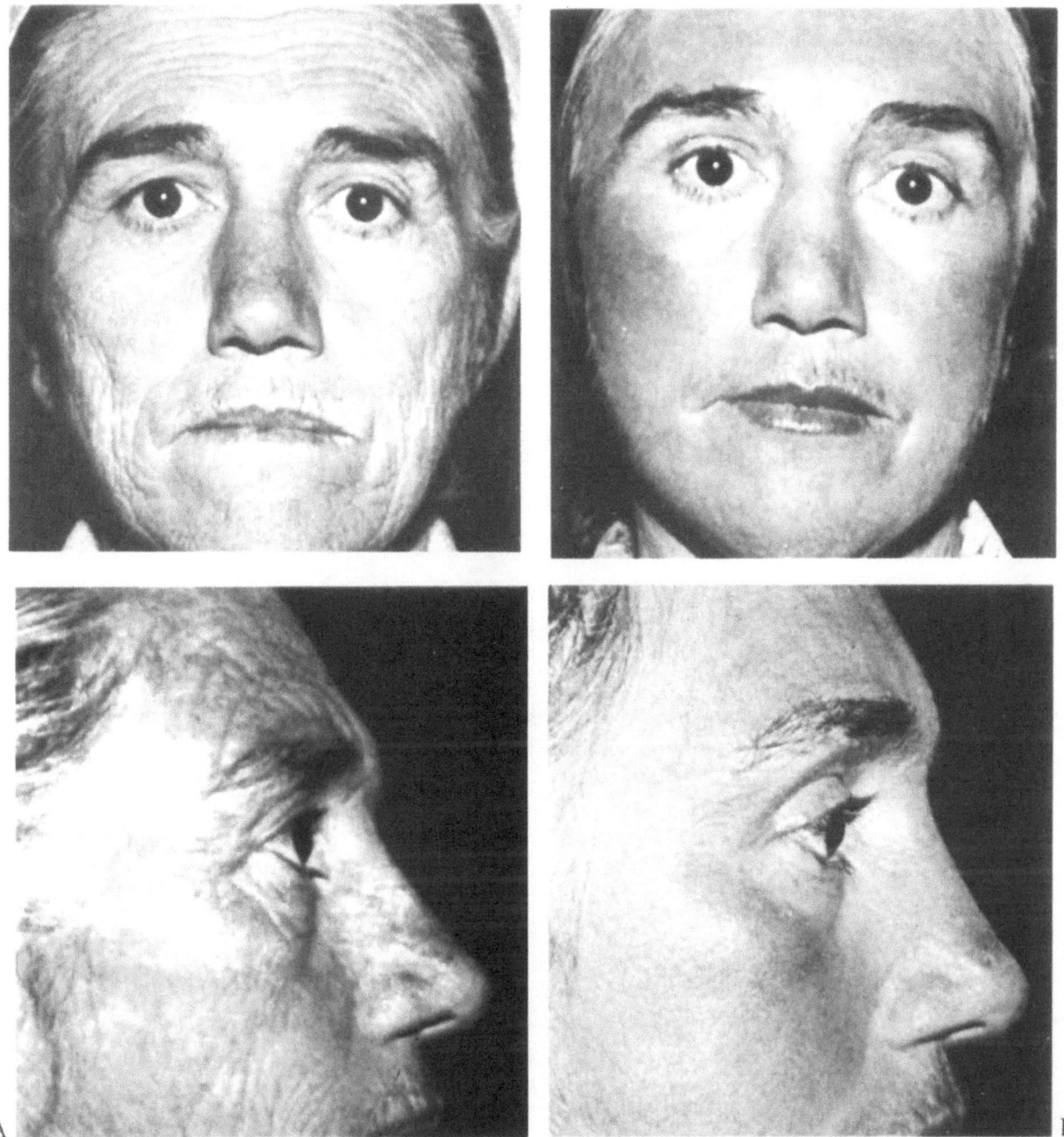

FIGURES 5.28. Blepharoplasty with a face lift and peeling. *A.* Preoperative view showing 50-year-old patient with generalized wrinkling of the face and eyelids, extremely marked crow's-feet, and ptotic eyebrows. *B.* Postoperative view after skin resection in the upper and lower lids, an eyebrow lift, and a complete cervico-facial lift (frontal, cervical and cheek regions), with a subsequent peeling. The skin appears rejuvenated. These procedures bring the patients great aesthetic and emotional benefit, and because of the number of problems corrected, they are among the most rewarding of aesthetic procedures.

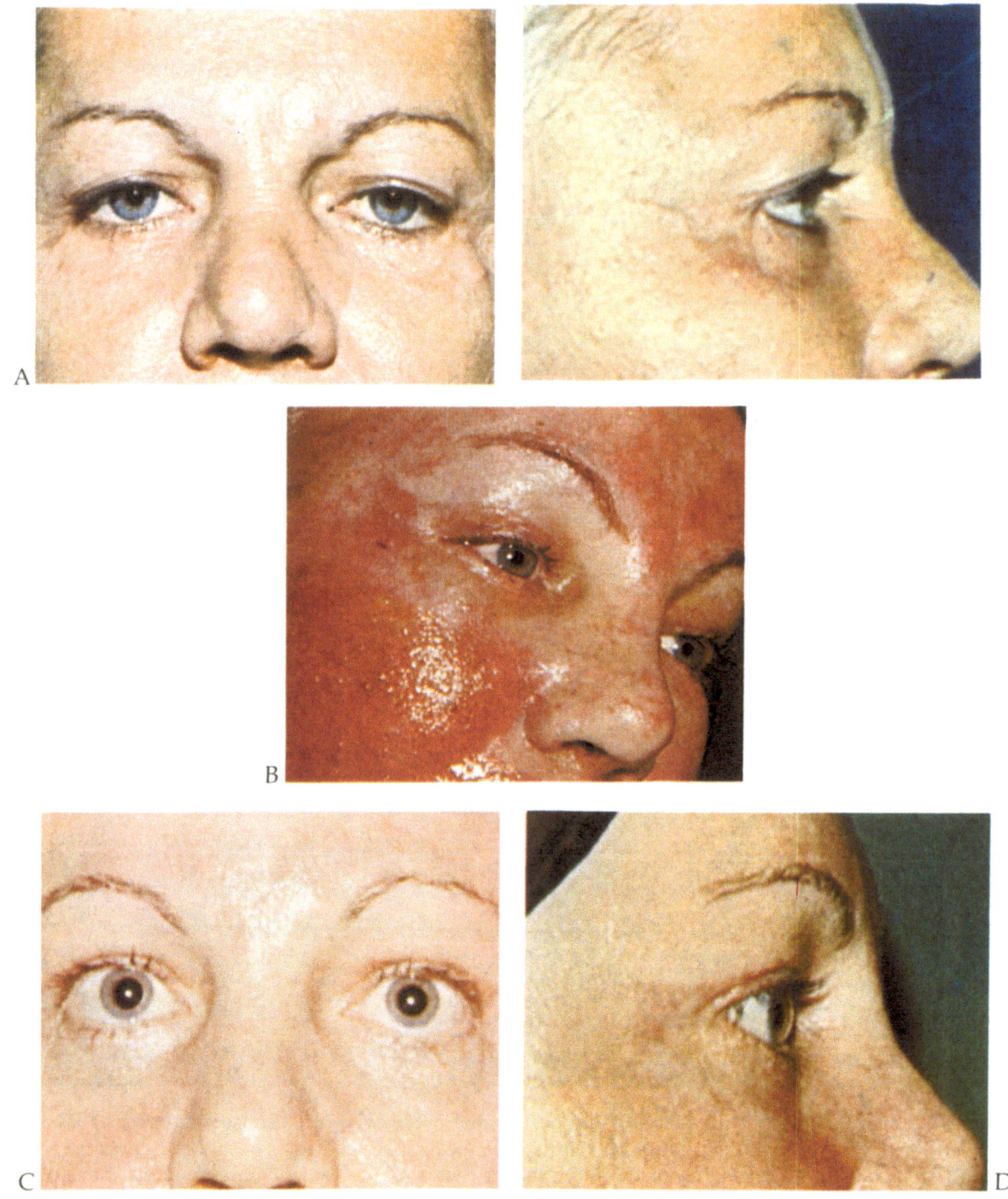

FIGURE 5.29. *A.* Preoperative frontal and profile views showing looseness. *B.* Slight iatrogenic scleral show resulting from a previous blepharoplasty. *C.* Inter-mediate phase of peeling showing the crust partially removed. *D.* Postoperative frontal and profile views showing immediate results obtained. Scleral show.

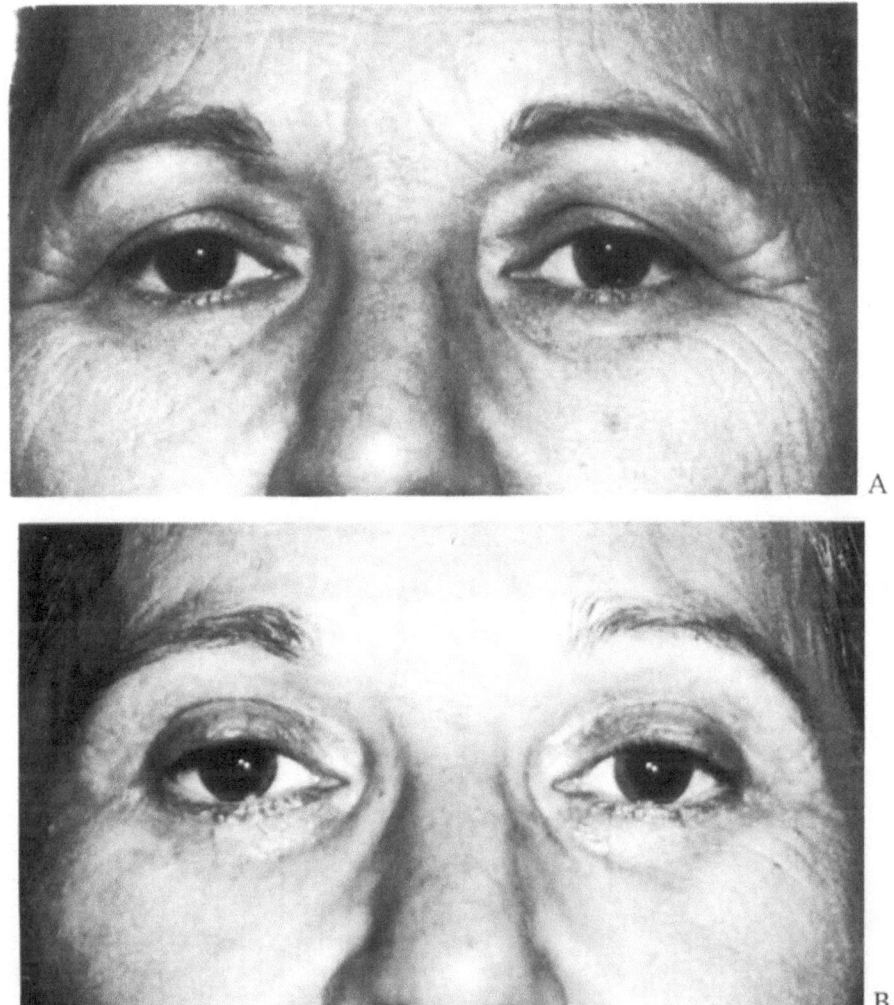

FIGURE 5.30. Blepharoplasty with a cheek-temporal lift and peeling. *A.* Preoperative view showing palpebral looseness and crow's-feet. *B.* Postoperative view after blepharoplasty, cheek-temporal lift, and peeling.

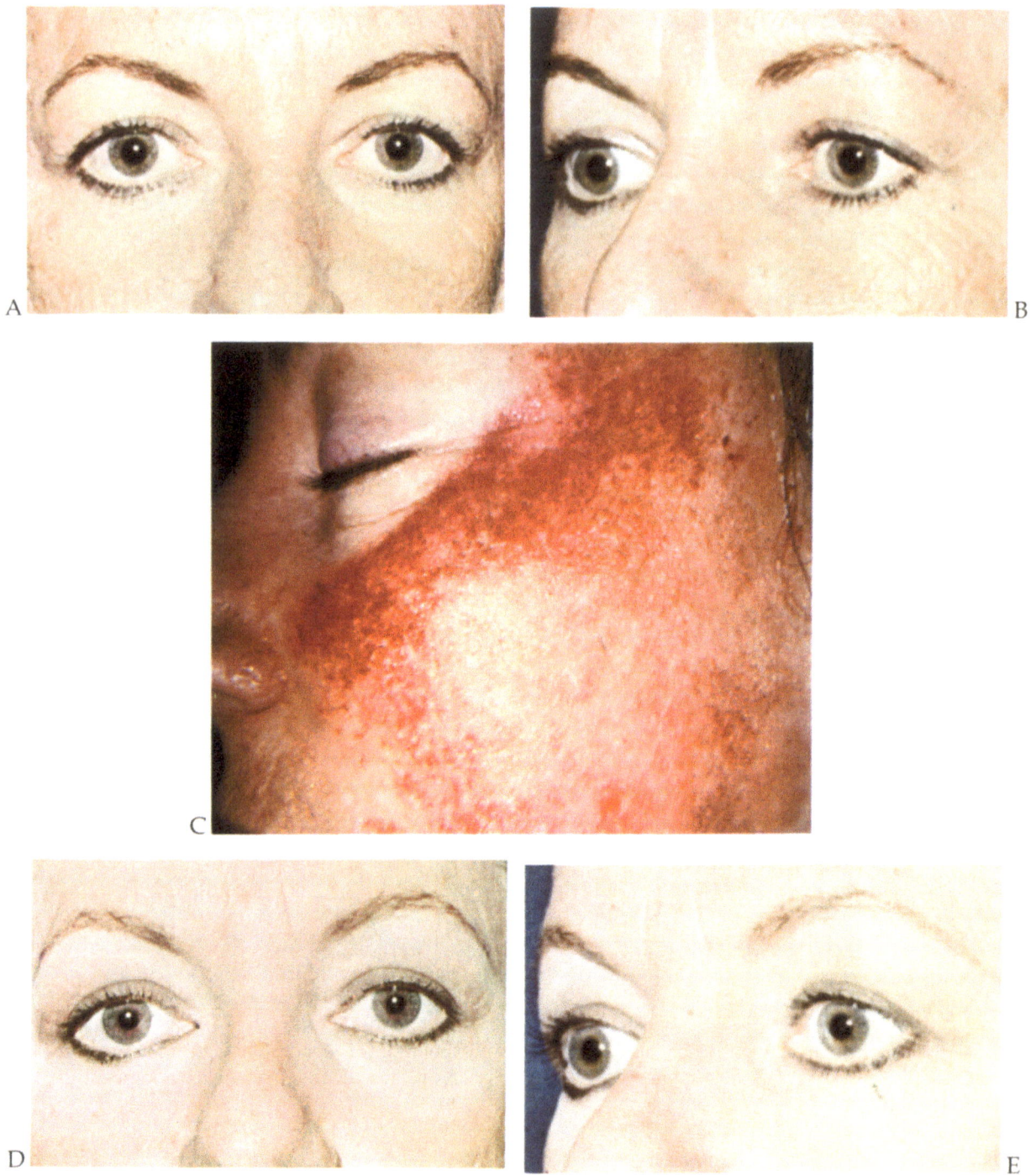

FIGURE 5.31. Crow's-feet corrected by chemical peel. *A.* Preoperative view. *B.* Postoperative view. *C.* Intermediate phase in chemical peeling. The crust that formed is being eliminated. *D, E.* Pre- and postoperative views in half profile. Scleral show.

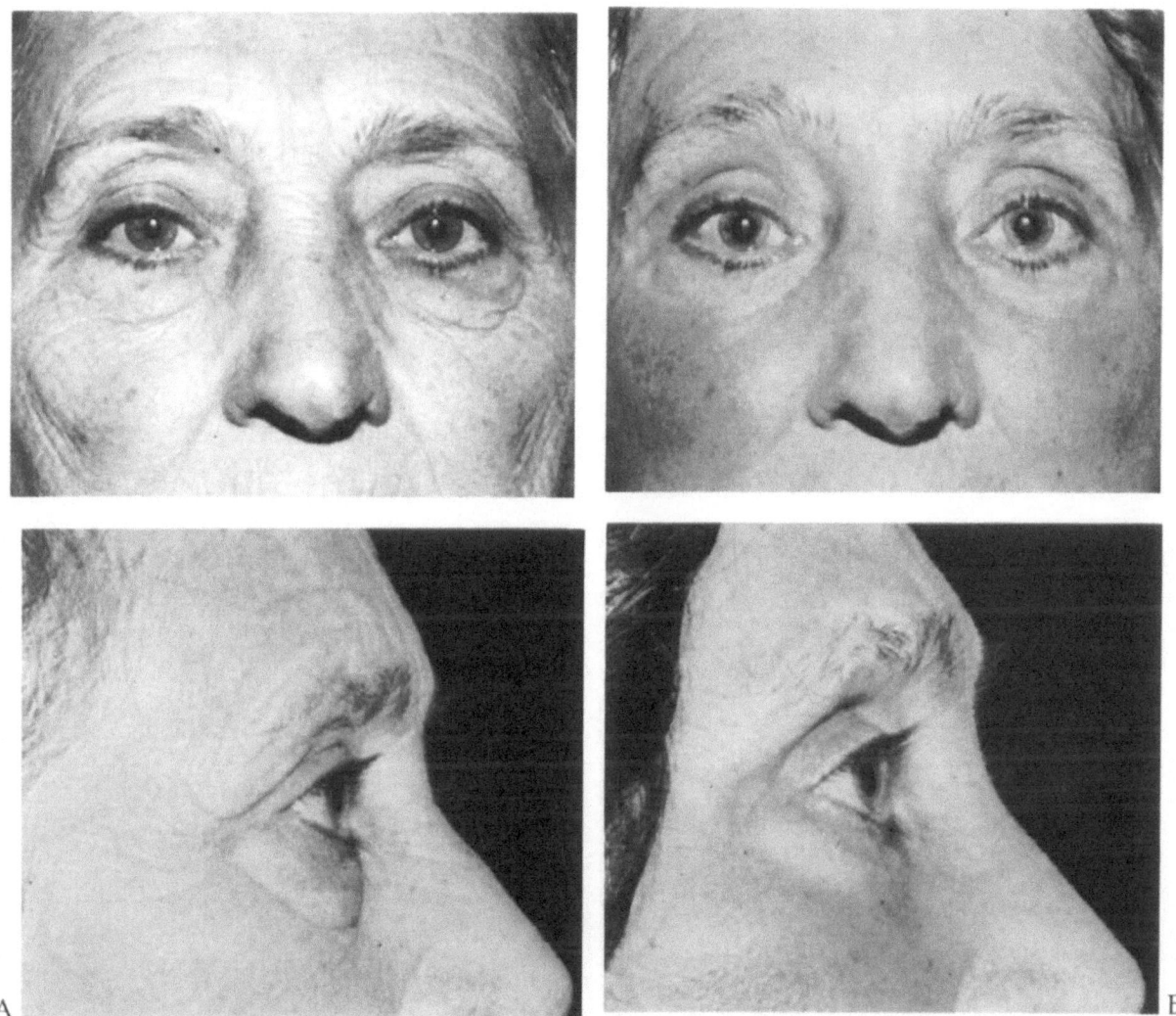

FIGURE 5.32. Blepharoplasty with lift and peeling. *A.* Preoperative view. *B.* Postoperative view.

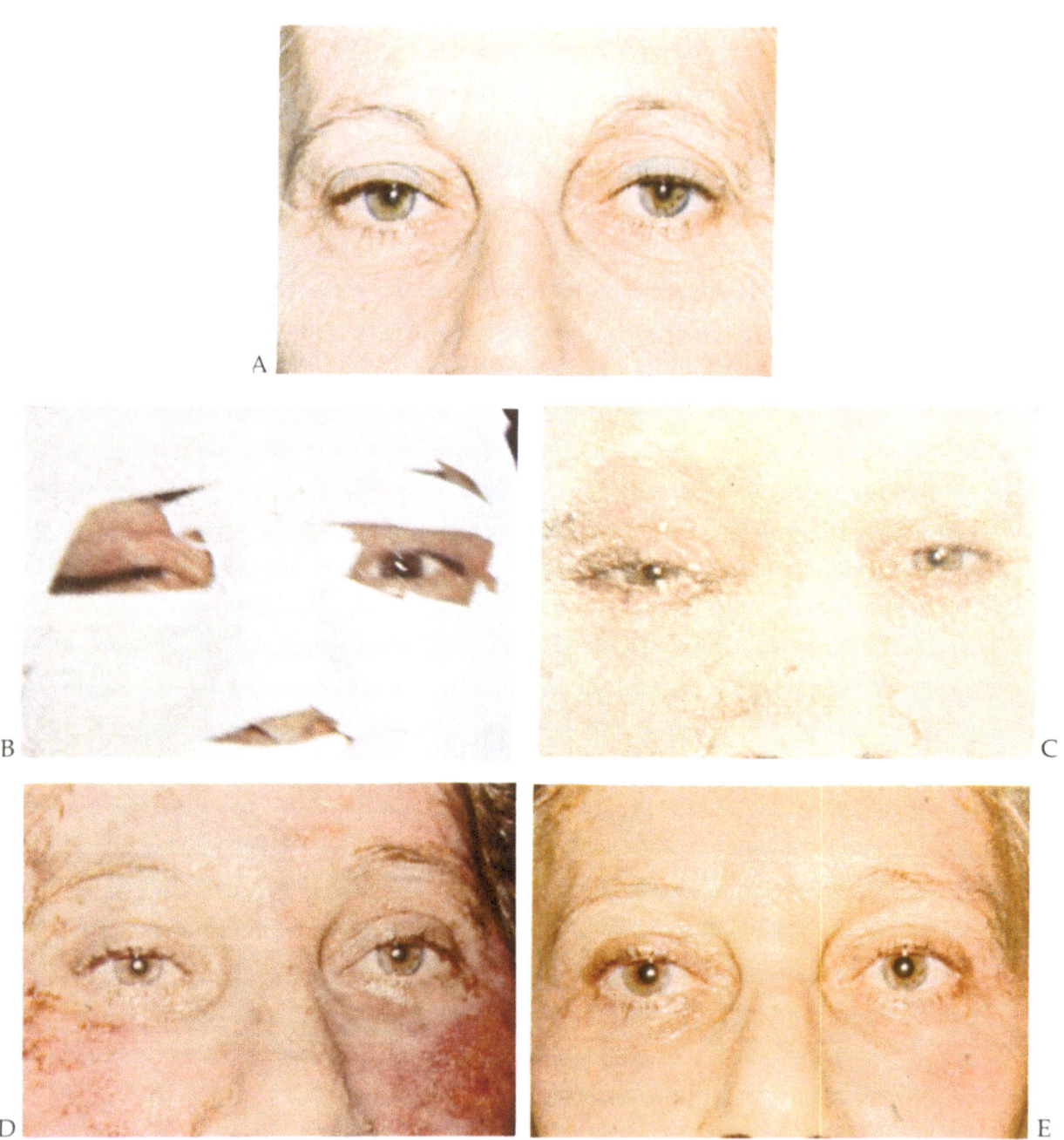

FIGURE 5.33. Blepharoplasty with lift and peeling. *A.* Preoperative view. *B.* Patient with peeled area covered with waterproof adhesive tape. *C.* After the removal of the tape, the skin is powdered with thymol iodate for 48 hours, after which it is greased with a fatty substance to facilitate the elimination of the crust that was formed. *D.* Patient during the elimination of the crust. *E.* Postoperative view.

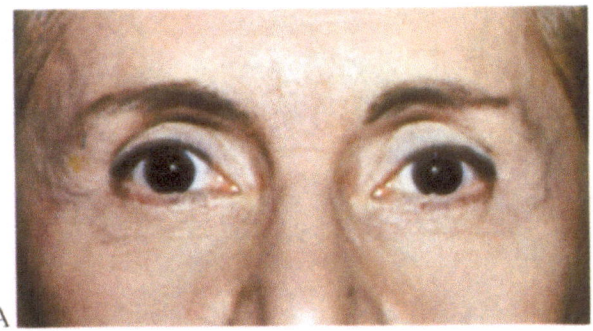 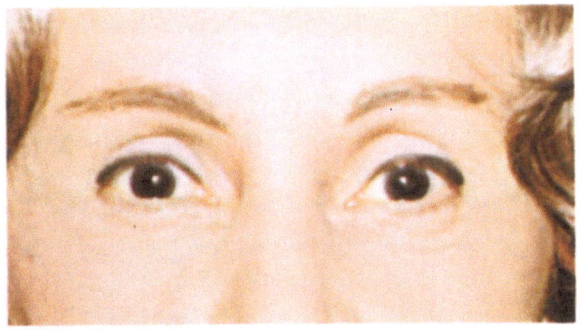

FIGURE 5.34. *A*. Preoperative view of patient with ptosis of the eyebrows and depressed upper palpebral sulcus. *B*. Postoperative view showing improve- ment of the appearance by means of a frontal lift, followed by a peeling.

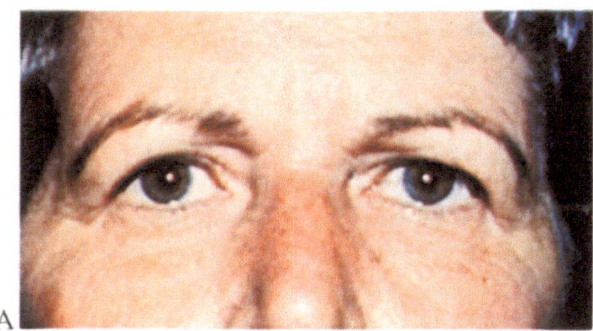 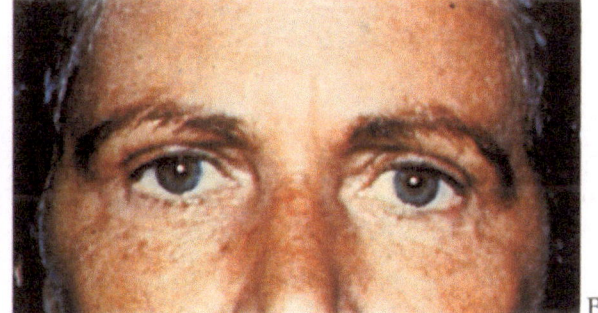

FIGURE 5.35. Blepharoplasty and frontal lift. *A*. Preoperative. *B*. Postoperative.

Division and Suspension of the Orbicularis Oculi Muscle

Another complementary procedure for the correction of crow's-feet is the distending of the orbicularis oculi muscle laterally and superiorly with adequate sutures. The traction and suturing of the muscle bundles cause distension of the tissues of the palpebral, zygomatic, and cheek regions. Great care must be taken not to injure the temporal (zygomatic) branch of the facial nerve. Skoog (1975) proposed the use of this technique under direct vision during a face lift. Aston (1980) modified and improved it for the correction of crow's-feet (Fig. 5.36). We have been using this procedure, very cautiously, to reduce the droop of the lower palpebral border in cases of scleral show.

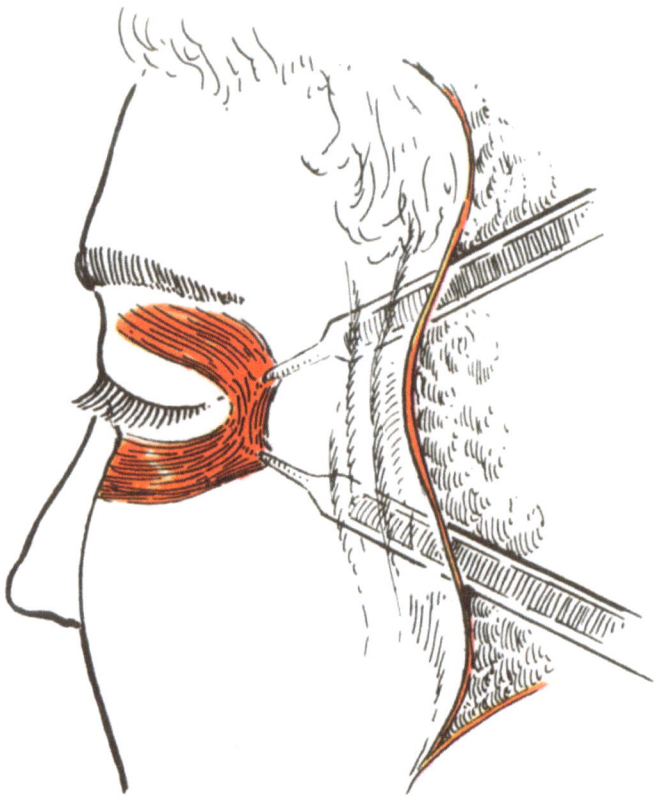

FIGURE 5.36. Under direct view, during face lifting, the distention and suture of the orbicularis muscle is performed.

Liposuction in the Cheek, Near the Nasojugal Sulcus

With aging, the cheek immediately lateral to the nasojugal sulcus may appear excessively voluminous in relation to the septal portion of the eyelid, giving the latter the appearance of being sunken. A detailed analysis shows that the deposit of fat tissue in the cheek region is the determining factor in the difference in level. Controlled liposuction of the region is recommended in these cases. This is easily done through a small incision at the level of the nasojugal sulcus.

Additional Reading

ASTON SJ: Orbicularis Oculi Muscle flaps: A technique to reduce crow's feet and lateral canthal skin folds. *Plast Reconstr Surg* 1980; 65:206.

BAROUDI R: Analitic studie of the incisions for facial ritidoplasties. Annals of the Brazilian Symposium of Facial Contouring. *Soc Bras Cir Plast* São Paulo, 1983. (in Portuguese)

CHRISMAN BB: Blepharoplasty and browlift with surgical variations in non-white patients. *J Dermatol Surg Oncol* 1986; 12:58.

D'ASSUMPÇÃO EA: Simultaneous facelift and chemical peel. *Ann Plast Surg* 1981; 6:470.

DINGMAN RD, PELED I et al: Forehead and brow lifts and their relationship to blepharoplasty. *Ann Plast Surg* 1979; 2:32.

EDWARDS BF: Bilateral temporal neurotomy for frontalis hypermotility. *Plast Reconstr Surg* 1957; 11:341.

ELLENBOGEN R: Transcoronal eyebrow lift with concomitant upper blepharoplasty. *Plast Reconstr Surg* 1983; 71:490.

ELY J: Facial rhitidoplasties, in: Sucena RC: *Cirurgia Plástica*, vol 2. São Paulo, Livraria Roca, 1981. (in Portuguese)

FRANCO T: The face liftings Stigmas. *Ann Plast Surg* 1985; 15:379.

HINDERER U: Blepharocanthoplasty with eyebrow lift. *Plast Reconstr Surg* 1975; 56:402.

KAYE B: The forehead lift. *Plast Reconstr Surg* 1977; 60:161.

LEWIS JR Jr: A method of direct eyebrow lift. *Ann Plast Surg* 1983; 10:115.

LOEB R: The use of abrasion in plastic surgery. *Rev Paul Med* São Paulo, Brasil. 1955; 43:219. (in Portuguese)

MARINO H: Frontal ritidectomies. *Bol Trab Sociedad Cir B Aires* 1963; 47:93. (in Spanish)

MLADICK W: The muscle-suspension lower blepharoplasty. *Plast Reconstr Surg* 1979; 64:171.

OLIVEIRA AR: Proper selection of rhytidoplasty patients. *Transactions of the VII International Congress of Plastic Reconstructive Surgery*. Rio de Janeiro, 1979.

ORTIZ-MONASTERIO F, FARRERA G et al: The coronal incision in rhytidectomy – The brow lift. *Clin Plast Surg* 1978; 5:167.

PITANGUY I: The rhitidoplasty: eclectic solution of the problems. *Minerva Chir* 1967; 22:942. (in Italian)

PSILLAKIS JM: The use of techniques of craneo-facial surgery for rhitidoplasties of the upper third of the face. *Cir Plast Iberolatinoam* 1984; 10:297. (in Spanish)

REBELLO C, FRANCO T: Surgical treatment of facial wrinkles. *Rev Col Bras Cir* 1970; 2:10. (in Portuguese)

REES TD: Rhytidectomy: some observations on variations in technique, in Masters FW, Lewis JR: *Symposium on Aesthetic Surgery of the Face, Eyelid, and Breast*. St. Louis, CV Mosby Co, 1972.

REGNAULT P, DANIEL KR: Eyelids, periorbital region and foreheadlift, in: Regnault P, Daniel RK (eds): *Aesthetic Plastic Surgery*. Little Brown & Company, 1984.

SKOOG T: *Plastic Surgery*. Philadelphia, WB Saunders Co, 1975.

VIÑAS J: Ptosis of the eyebrows and periocular wrinkles simultaneous surgical correction. Transactions of the First Congress of the Latinamerican Society of Plastic Surgery. Buenos Aires, 1962. (in Spanish)

VIÑAS JC, CAVIGLIA C et al: Forehead rhytidoplasty and brow lifting. *Plast Reconstr Surg* 1976; 57:445.

WEBSTER RC, et al: Blepharoplasty: When to combine it with brow, temple, or coronal lift. *J Otolaryngol* 1979; 8:339.

6

Ectropions, Hematomas, and Other Complications

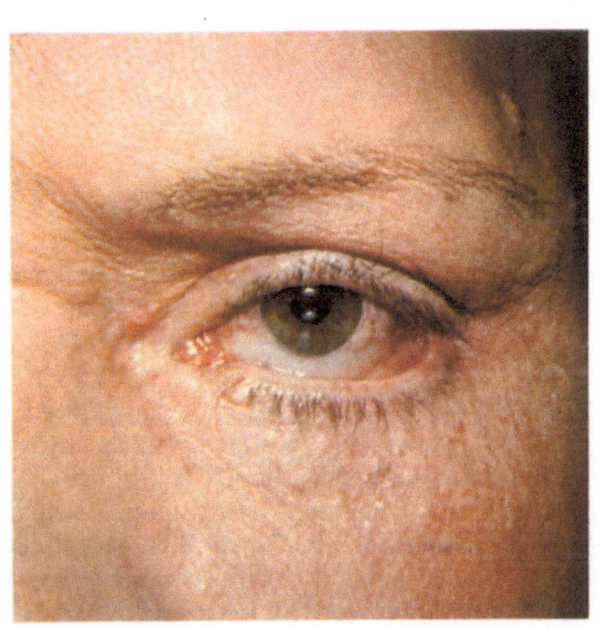

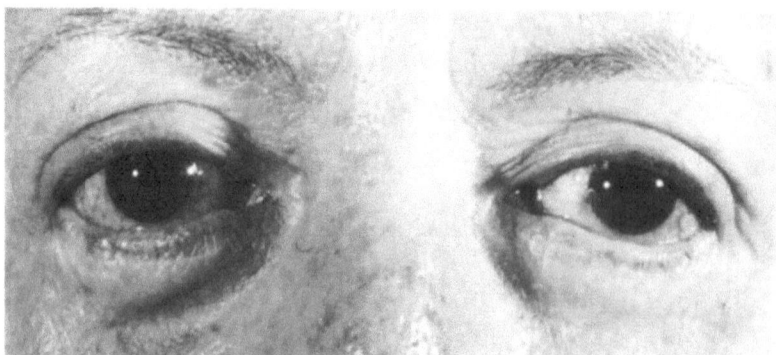

FIGURE 6.1. Incipient ectropion resulting from an unsuccessful blepharoplasty. In addition to the scleral show, observe the eversion of the palpebral border.

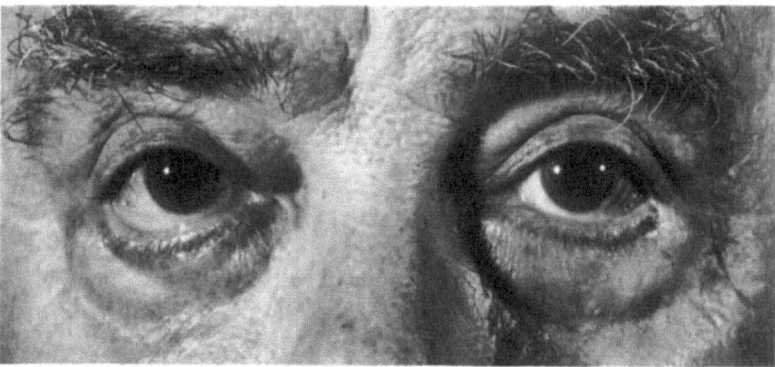

FIGURE 6.2. Bilateral iatrogenic palpebral ectropion, more exacerbated in the right lower lid, deforming the patient's appearance. This defect was consequent to an exaggerated skin resection in the lower lids.

Introduction

In addition to the problems of scleral show (discussed in Chapter 2) and depressions (Chapter 4), there are other serious complications that can beset palpebral surgery: ectropions, hematomas, cicatricial retractions, palpebral asymmetries, exaggerated edemas, overprojection of fat grafts, milias, and others.

Ectropions

Ectropion, or eversion of the ciliary border of the lids, is the most worrisome and frustrating iatrogenic problem occurring after an aesthetic blepharoplasty (Tenzel, 1981). The patient is impressed by the fact that the lid stays separated from the globe, disclosing the pink palpebral conjunctive. He is much more aware of this than

of the exaggerated white portion of "scleral show" which always accompanies the ectropion.

Ectropions occur almost exclusively in the lower lids. Eversion of the ciliary border of the upper lids is rare; what is seen there is an increase of the area of sclera.

The degree of ectropion can vary from an incipient exposition of the palpebral conjunctiva (Fig. 6.1), to a complete presentation of the fornix. In many cases an ectropion can reach the point of deforming the patient's appearance (Fig. 6.2). The patient is emotionally upset because of his appearance and because of the poor functioning of the lids. Generally he blames the surgeon for the results, thinking that the cause was the removal of too much skin. His eyes appear sad, and to this is added an emotional sadness stemming from the unsatisfactory surgery.

The lateral angle of the eye loses its triangular shape and the contact between global and palpebral conjunctivae is reduced. When the defect is localized in the central or medial third, the contact of the punctum with the bulbar conjunctiva can be lost, altering the drainage pattern of the tears and resulting in constant epiphora. Because of the drop of the border of the lateral and central thirds of the lower lid, the major axis of the rim will be directed out and downwards, contrary to its normal, aesthetic direction.

The patient's unhappiness and distress are constant. A solution is necessary but he dreads submitting to more surgery, rebelling against it because this was not contemplated before, much less discussed. In these cases, in addition to the normal attention given to all patients, a solution should be offered as rapidly as possible, along with solid psychological support.

Etiology and Prevention

There are numerous measures that should be taken to prevent ectropion. In general, they are the same measures as those used to prevent the scleral show discussed in Chapter 2. If the ectropion has already occurred, one should carefully look into what caused it: The surgeon asks himself: Could it be a hematoma or an excessive edema that caused the defect? Was there a preexisting tendency toward scleral show? Does an analysis of the surgical notes show that the planning was followed to the letter? Or was it changed in the course of the surgery? Was there too much resection of the skin, fat, or muscle? Were there massive clots that could have produced necrosis and subsequent deep fibrosis? All these questions have answers and are of fundamental importance in the future treatment of the ectropion. An analysis of the patient's history and of the preoperative photographs are crucial for a good documentation of the case.

One should seek to establish the cause of the defect. If there is a depression that is retracting the tissue in the septal portion, the immediate postoperative period is not the time to implant a fat graft. If the orbicular muscle of the eye has been resected excessively in the tarsal portion, it cannot be restored because *it is not possible to replace this muscular tissue:* it would not have the necessary tonicity.

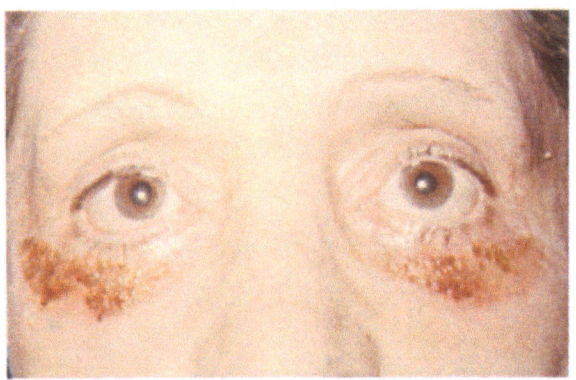

FIGURE 6.3. Ectropion caused by skin retraction consequent to a chemical peel used in the correction of crow's-feet.

Spontaneous improvement of an ectropion usually does not occur, and one must try a temporal lift or an unfolding and distension of the orbicularis oculi muscle (see Chapter 5). A skin graft is one of the most effective therapeutic alternatives, and this and other techniques used are described below.

Ectropion of the Lower Lids

The etiology of ectropion in the lower eyelid is quite variable. It is more likely to occur if the patient demonstrates preoperative scleral show (see Chapter 2). The factors causing ectropion are the same as those that cause iatrogenic scleral show, that is, reckless skin, fat, and/or muscular resections (see pages 39–41, 54–55). Exaggerated tissue resection performed through a periciliary incision can provoke a traction directly on the palpebral border, favoring its eversion. This can also happen when there is an exaggerated shortening of the vertical dimension of the eyelids caused by improper suturing of the orbital fascia and of the orbicularis oculi muscle. It can also occur as a result of skin retraction caused by a palpebral peel (Fig. 6.3).

Senile ectropion takes various forms. In persons of advanced age, it is a normal physiological development caused by progressive looseness of the palpebral tissues (Fig. 6.4).

Treatment

Only after the time necessary for the disappear-

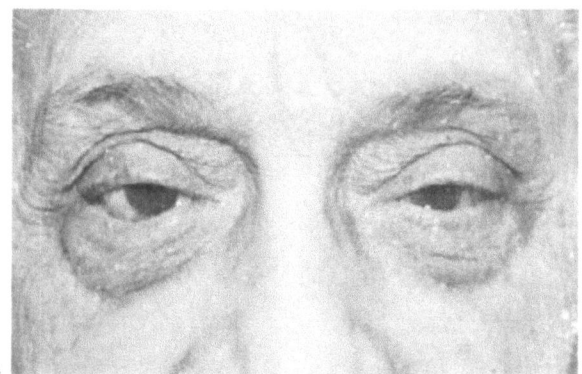

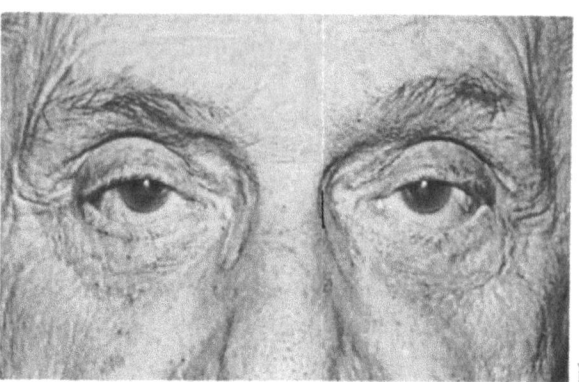

A
B

FIGURE 6.4. Iatrogenic exacerbation of a developmental scleral show, resulting in an ectropion. *A*. Preoperative view showing palpebral looseness and baggy eyelids, with scleral show in the lateral third of the lower right eyelid. *B*. Postoperative view: the tissue looseness and the bagginess were corrected, but the scleral show has exacerbated into an ectropion. (From Loeb R: Esthetic blepharoplasties with special reference to the ectropion of the lateral and central thirds of the lower lid. *Rev Col Bras Cir* Sept-Oct, 1976, pp 177–187. (in Portuguese).)

ance of the edema and the postoperative consolidation of the tissues is the surgeon able to evaluate properly the appearance of the patient. The decision about what to do, never easy, is the surgeon's responsibility. At times, the patient wants immediate action, but it is necessary to wait. At other times, the patient wants to wait, but the surgeon feels that the best solution is to operate. Experience, an ability to persuade, and determination are fundamental. The surgeon alone must decide that the time has arrived. Only then does he make his decision concerning the need for surgical intervention in an attempt to solve the problem of an ectropion.

Some ectropions occur as a result of skin misplacement resulting from an error in suturing. In these cases, one should manipulate the area close to the ectropion; this may sometimes bring about a satisfactory solution. Generally, however, a free skin graft is needed and should be performed. In some cases of exaggerated senility of the orbicularis oculi muscle in aged patients, the Kuhnt-Szimanowsky procedure is indicated (Fig. 6.9).

Correction of Ectropion with Free Skin Transplants

First one must carefully evaluate whether or not there is a loss of skin and if there is, its extension.

To compensate for this loss, the area is grafted, using free skin grafts taken from the opposite eyelid or from the retroauricular region. The technique we generally use in cases that need free skin grafts is described in Figure 6.5A – F.

According to Gonzallez-Ulloa, the lower eyelid should be anchored in the brow region in such a way as to increase the surface of the raw area. Thus one is able to place a large surface area graft, and in so doing, avoid a recurrence of the ectropion. We have rarely used this technique, but in all the cases, the graft has been successful: we have never had a recurrence of the ectropion after a skin graft.

To ensure good integration, the graft must be immobilized in its bed in the receptor area. To do this, the sutures that hold the graft in place are left long and then are tied snugly over a gauze pad (Brown's dressing) (Fig. 6.6). In some cases an occlusive dressing is used, lightly compressing the orbital region. The retraction of the graft can be as great as 30 % of the grafted area; for this reason, the closer the graft is to the palpebral border, the greater the chance of a recurrence of the ectropion. Consequently, the incision for the initiation of the undermining should be far from the palpebral border (Figs. 6.5 and 6.6).

In rare cases, the ectropion is in the mesial third of the lower eyelid. In these circumstances the lacrimal point is separated from the globe and as a result there is epiphora (Fig. 6.7).

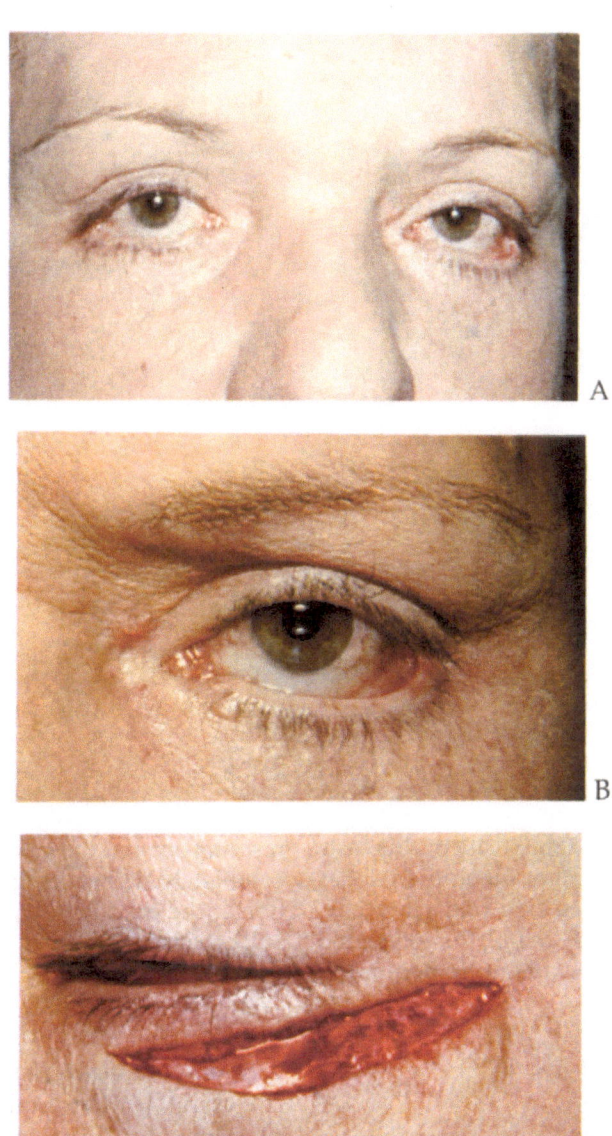

FIGURE 6.5. *A*. Ectropion after an aesthetic blepharo-plasty done elsewhere. The patient's appearance is deformed. The fornix is visible, principally in the left eye. *B*. Close up of the left eye. *C*. The surgery is begun by placing the incision parallel to and about 3 to 4 mm from the palpebral border. In ectropions in the lateral and central thirds of the lower eyelid, this incision should follow the entire length of the lid and extend 1 to 2 cm beyond the lateral angle of the eye. If the ectropion is in the mesial third of the lid, the inci-sion can be limited to the eyelid itself. With fine-pointed scissors, the scar tissue is then liberated by undermining in all directions up to the palpebral border. This maneuver enables the lower palpebral border to return to its normal position, reestablishing contact with the bulbar conjunctiva. Even after this liberation, the elevation of the palpebral border does not always permit the closing of the eye, indicating, as in this case, a retraction of the upper lid.

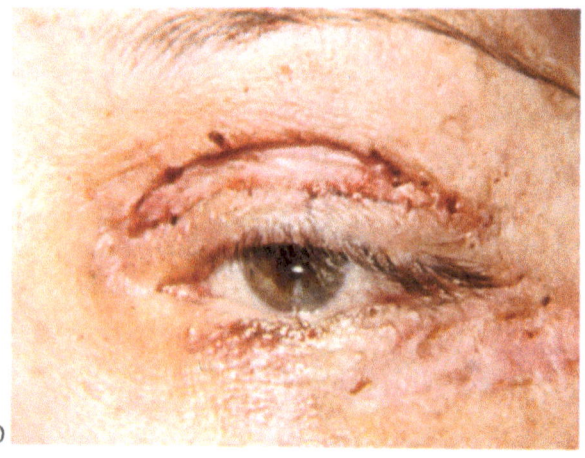
D

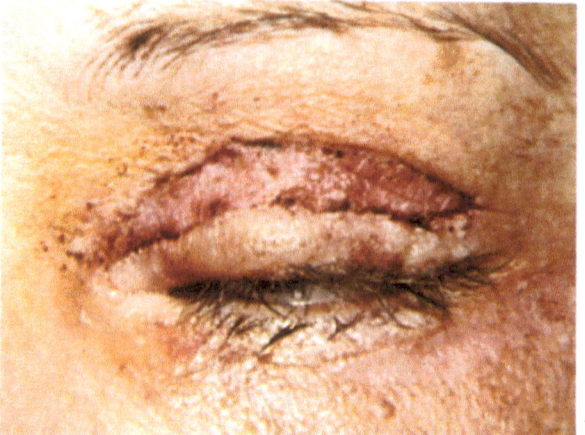
E

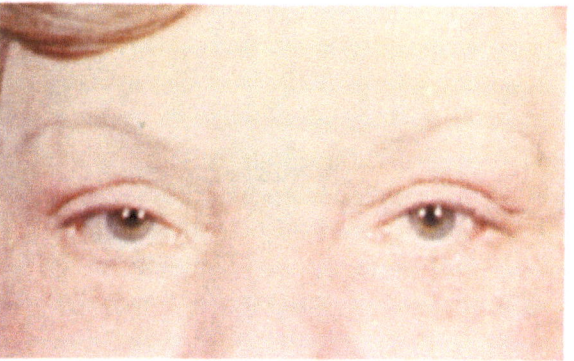
F

FIGURE 6.5. *D*. Because of the complexity of this case, the correction of the retraction of the upper lid was done at a later time. The free skin transplant integrated into the upper lid, as well as the integrated graft in the lower lid, is shown here. *E*. Because of residual edema, the palpebral rim still does not close completely. However, because of the good integration of the graft, it is expected that normal occlusion will occur in the future. *F.* Late result.

Ectropion in the Upper Lids

These are much less frequent than those in the lower eyelid and are seen only when the patient attempts to close the palpebral opening. When the lid is relaxed, the border remains in close contact with the ocular globe by gravity, but the lids are not entirely closed, and sclera is visible above the ciliary margin of the iris. When the patient forces the eyelids down, the palpebral border is everted and, again, the sclera is visible. There are several causes of ectropion in the upper lids:

1. Paralysis of the orbicular muscle of the eye because of damage to a branch of the facial nerve, making it difficult to close the eyes;

2. Exaggerated tension of the frontal tissue owing to a frontal or brow lift, principally when done in association with resection of skin from the upper lid;
3. Excessive reduction of skin in the surface of the upper lid.

When there is excessive skin reduction of the upper eyelid during a blepharoplasty, and there is no eversion of the upper palpebral border, it is classified as a scleral show, not as an ectropion.

In ectropion of the upper eyelid it is necessary to add skin in order to permit the occlusion of the palpebral rim. One must first determine where the original incision was placed. If it was periciliary, it means that the exaggerated skin resection that generated the ectropion was made

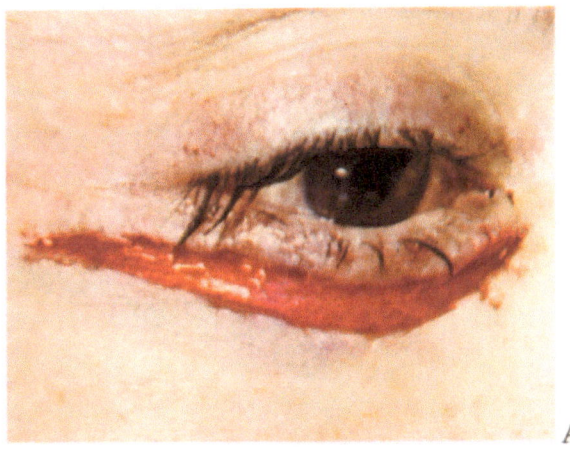

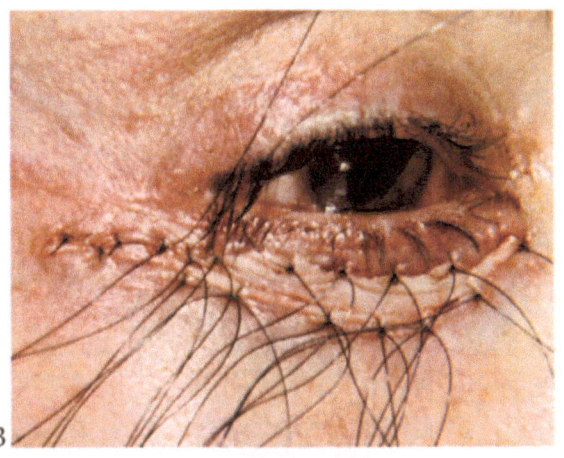

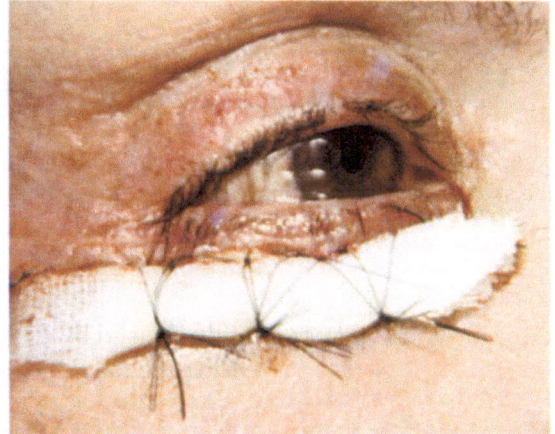

FIGURE 6.6. Brown's dressing. *A.* The raw area shows the loss of cutaneous substance that must be replaced with a graft. *B.* Free skin transplant taken from the retroauricular region. The graft is sutured in place, and the sutures are left long so that they can be tied over the compressive dressing. *C.* The sutures are tied over the dressing. (From Loeb R: Esthetic blepharoplasties with special reference to the ectropion of the lateral and central thirds of the lower lid. *Rev Col Bras Cirurgiões.* Sept-Oct 1976, pp 177–187. (in Portuguese).)

in the lower part of the tarsal portion of the eyelid. In these cases another incision should be made, but lower. Starting from here, the remaining pretarsal skin near the cilia should be totally undermined. The palpebral border then returns to its normal position, permitting complete occlusion of the palpebral rim. The loss of skin that generated the ectropion becomes evident, and it is corrected with a full thickness skin graft taken from the retroauricular region (Fig. 6.8).

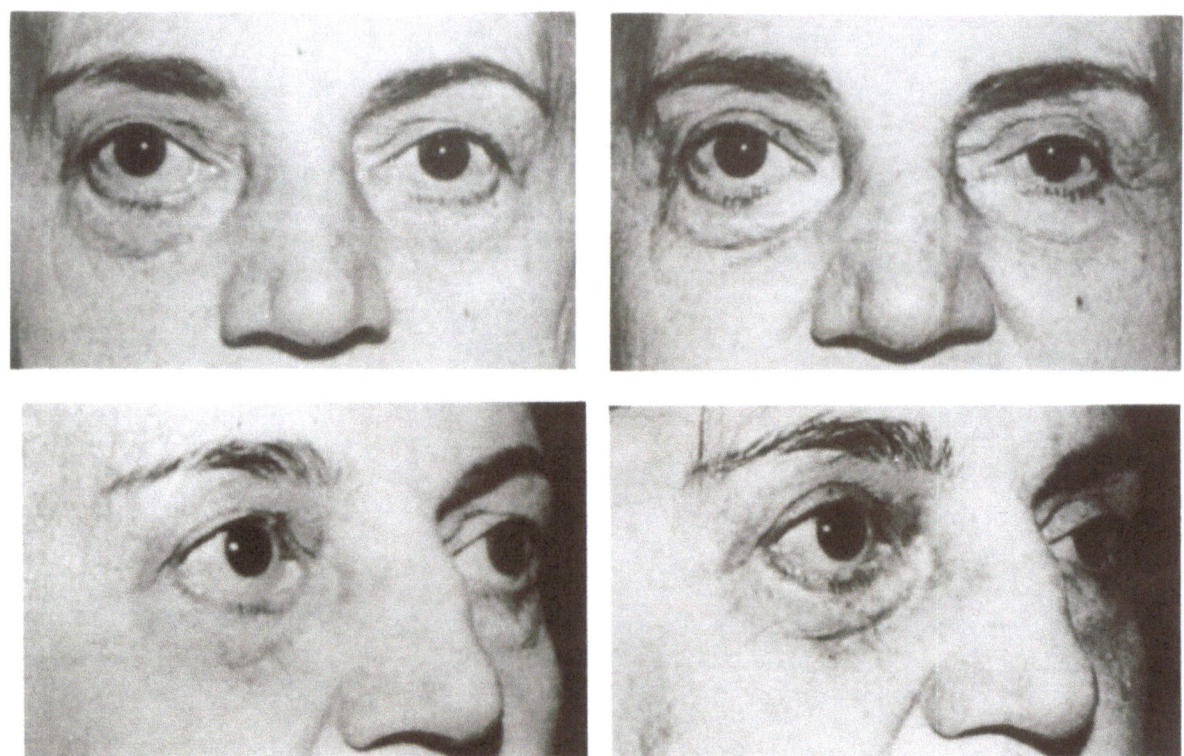

FIGURE 6.7. **Rare** ectropion situated in the medial third of the lower eyelid, with separation of the lacrimal point. After a skin graft, the palpebral border returned to its normal position.

Ectropion of the Upper Eyelids Caused by Erroneous Resection in the Pretarsal Portion with an Erroneous Periciliar Incision (Fig. 6.8)

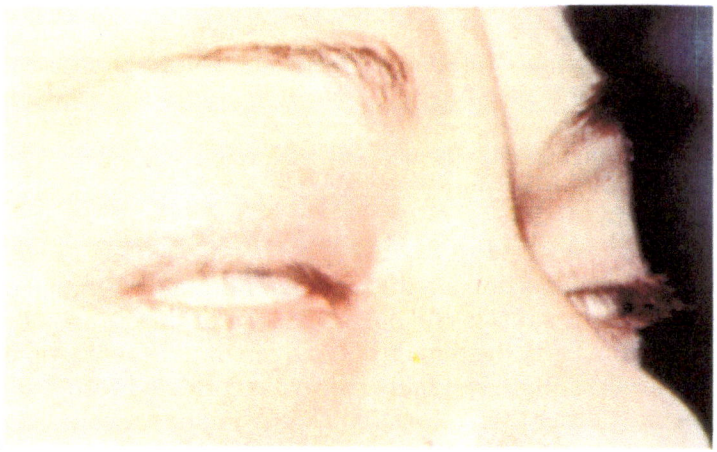

A

FIGURE 6.8. *A.* Lack of occlusion of the palpebral rim due to ectropion of the upper eyelid. This was caused by incorrect skin resection in the pretarsal portion of the lid made through an erroneous periciliary incision.

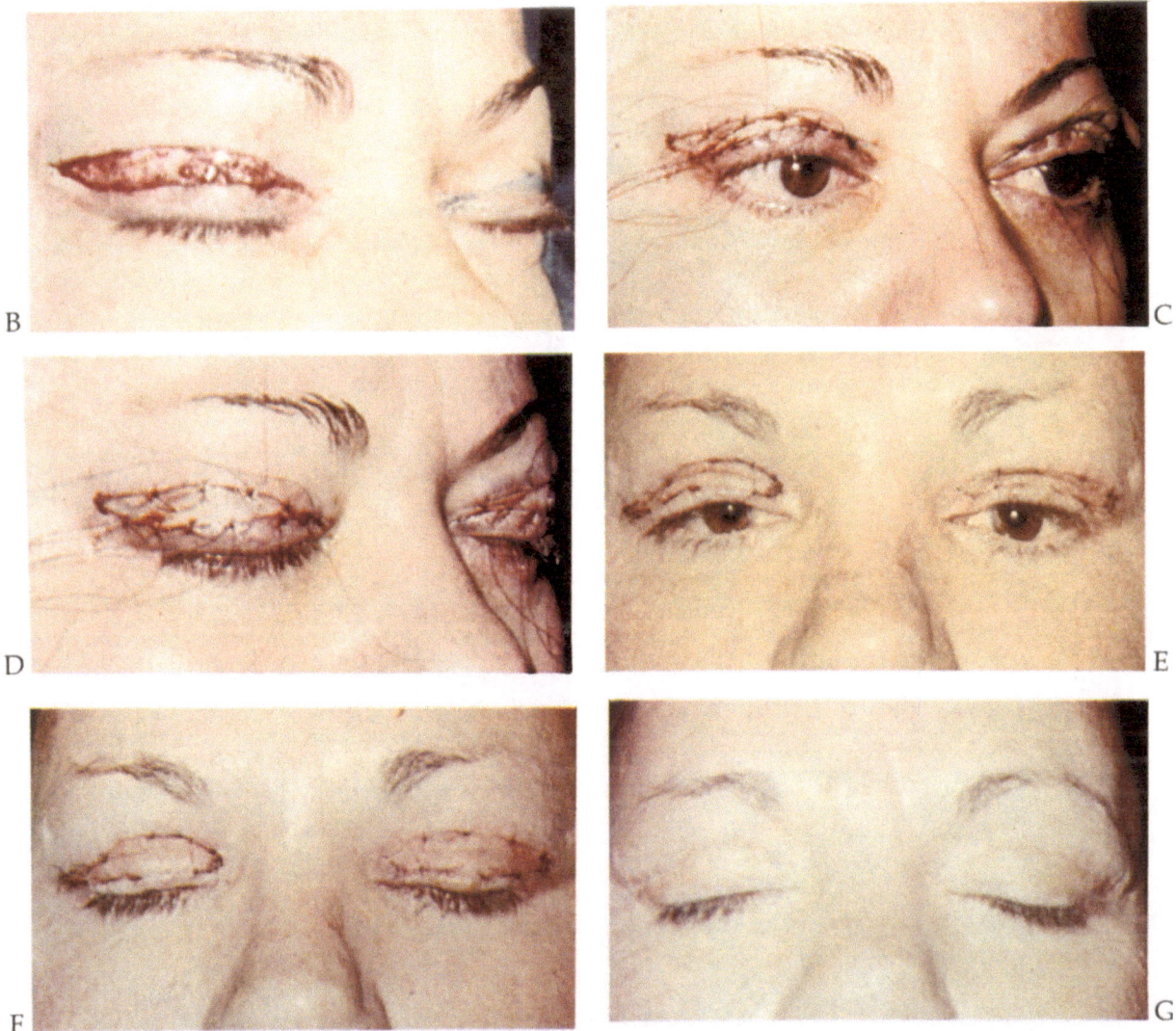

FIGURE 6.8. *B.* Loss of skin. *C.* Free skin graft completed. *D.* The palpebral rim can now be occluded. *E.* Graft integrated. *F.* Palpebral rim occluded. *G.* Graft after 6 months.

Kuhnt-Szimanowsky Technique (Fig. 6.9)

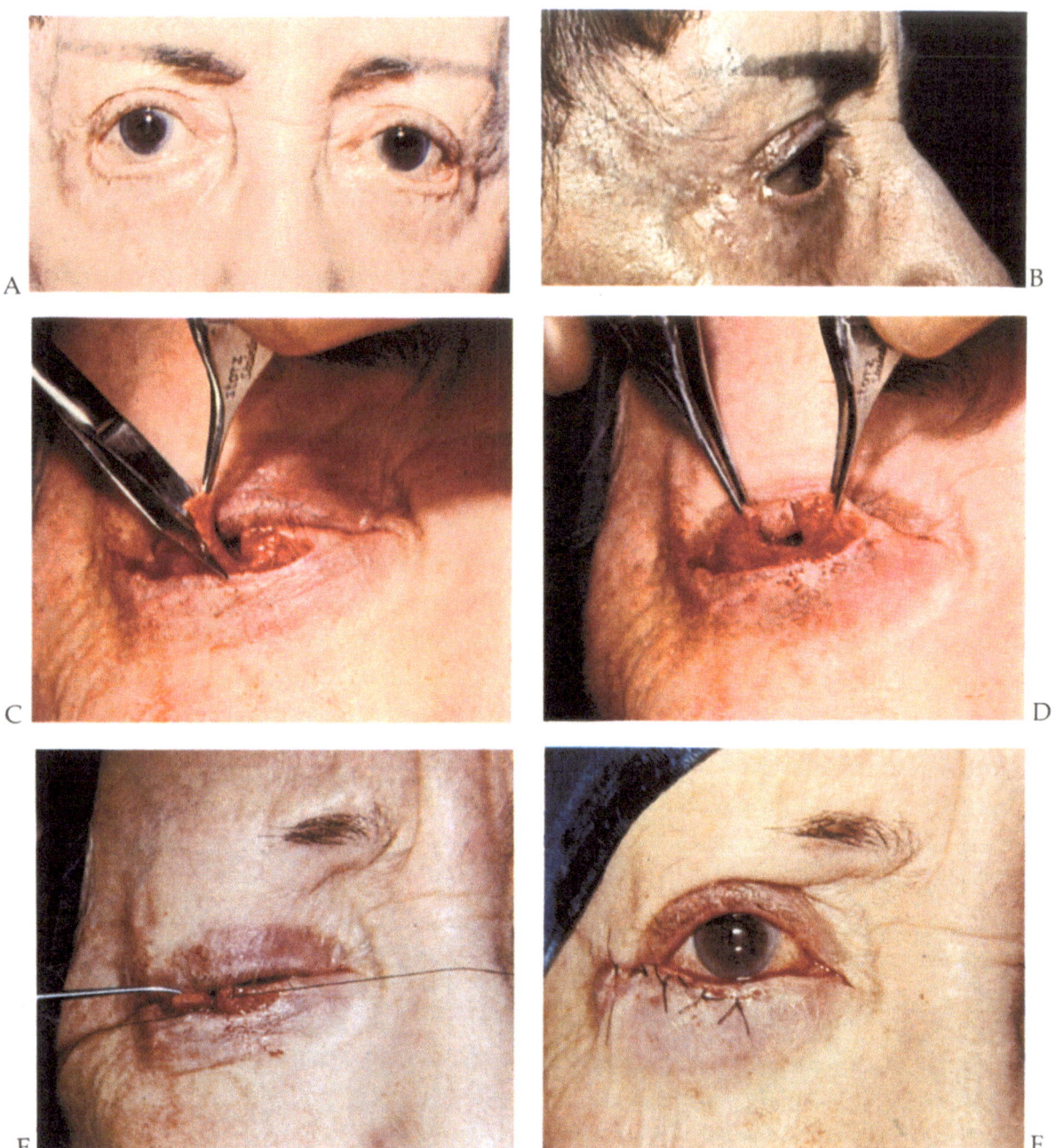

FIGURE 6.9. *A, B.* Patient of advanced age with ectropion consequent to a blepharoplasty done elsewhere. In this case, because of senile reduction of the tonus of the orbicularis oculi muscle, it was decided to use the Kuhnt-Szimanowsky technique as modified by Mustarde. *C.* Separation of the lids accomplished. A wedge-shaped piece of the full thickness of the lid, including the mucosa, the tarsal cartilage, and the orbicularis oculi muscle is being removed. *D.* The wedge has been removed. *E.* Suturing being performed. *F.* Six-O Nylon sutures placed.

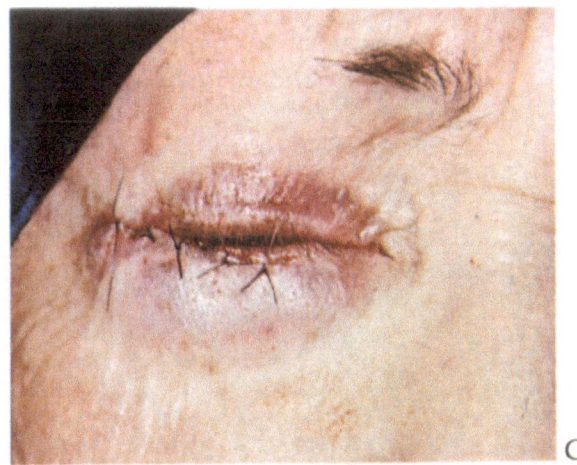

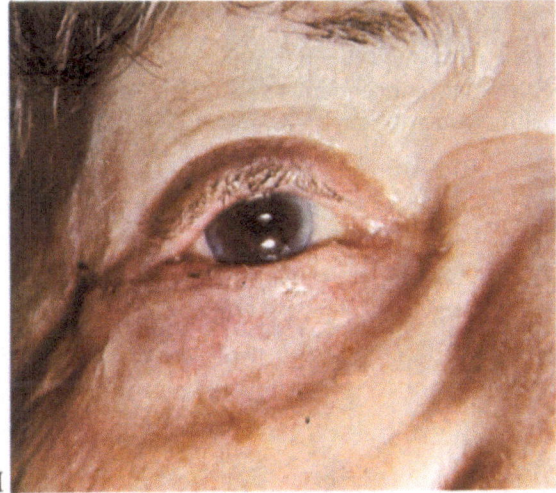
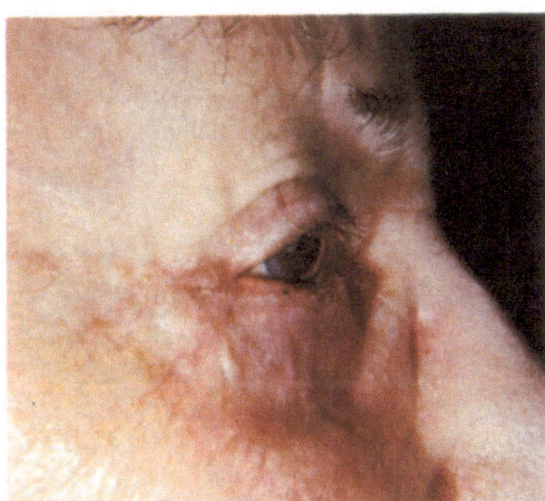

FIGURE 6.9. *G.* Patient occluding the palpebral rim. *H.* Postoperative frontal view after 90 days. *I.* Postoperative profile view.

Hematomas

Hematomas, collections of blood in the eyelids, are always prejudicial to a good prognosis of a blepharoplasty. When they occur during surgery, and there is difficulty in locating the source of the bleeding, it is recommended that one use only a few discontinuous sutures, and not tie them, thus leaving the wound partially open to permit drainage. It is drained for about 24 hours and only then are the sutures tied. Drainage is particularly recommended in patients who are highly unstable emotionally, and thus subject to variations in arterial pressure. Hematomas can originate in the eyelids

being operated on, or from nearby regions, as a consequence of a temporal or frontal lift. We have divided hematomas into superficial, of the fat compartment, and orbital (or retrobulbar).

Superficial hematomas generally have minimal infiltration into the orbicularis oculi muscle, and they hopefully will disappear spontaneously. If surgical intervention is deemed advisable, they can be almost completely eliminated through a small incision followed by digital pressure.

Fat compartment hematomas are those that infiltrate the muscular and fat compartment tissues. They should be drained. Drainage should be maintained for some days so that the blood can extravasate from the orbicular muscle and

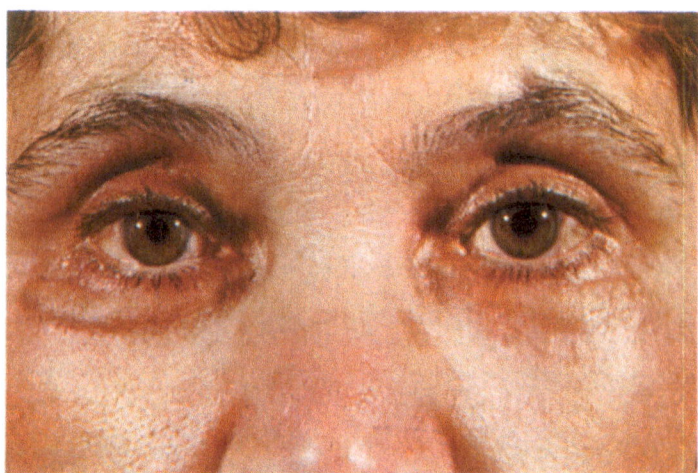

FIGURE 6.10. Patient operated on elsewhere. There is deep fibrosis consequent to an organized hematoma, probably because of inadequate drainage. It was treated with triamcinolone infiltration.

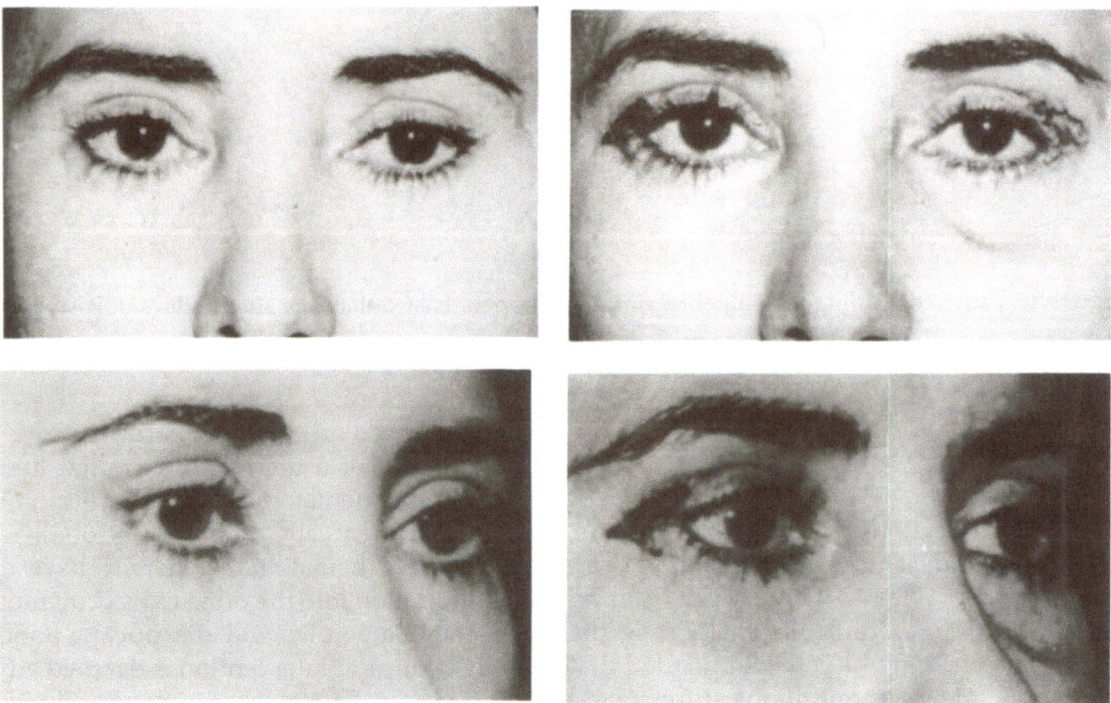

FIGURE 6.11. Rounding of the lateral angle of the eye after a blepharoplasty. After elimination of the scar, the amount of skin lost at the lateral angle of the eye can be gauged. A full thickness skin graft was used to separate the lateral thirds of the upper and lower eyelids.

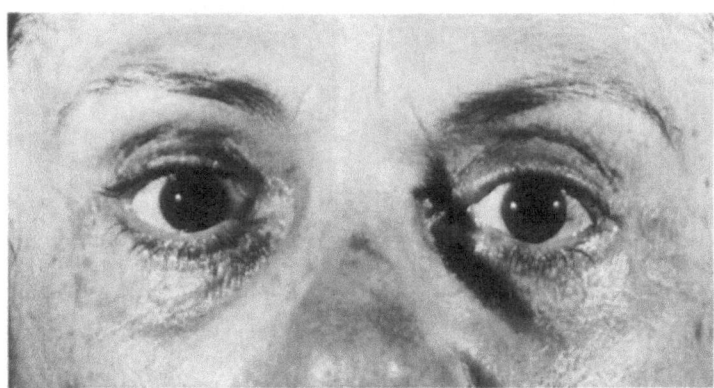

FIGURE 6.12. Typical case of rounding of the lateral angle of the eye.

fat compartments. Spontaneous liquefaction of the clot helps drainage. Hematomas that have not been drained in time can cause complications, since they tend to "organize," and the resultant fibrosis impedes the natural elimination of the retained material. This can then form deep retractions, which can have a variety of consequences. One of these is hardening, which can persist for an indeterminate period (Fig. 6.10). In such cases, infiltration with small doses of triamcinolone (not more than 2 mg) every 20 days is recommended. Hematomas in a fat graft have a bad prognosis, since they make the integration of the implant more difficult.

Orbital (or retrobulbar) hematomas are one of the most dreaded complications of cosmetic blepharoplasty, as described by Tenzel (1981).

Other Complications

Cicatricial Retractions

Adhesions at the lateral angle of the eye can appear when the lateral extremities of the upper and lower incisions meet, or even when they are too close to each other (Figs. 6.11 and 6.12). The fibrous tracts that form between them can exert tension on the lateral angle of the eye, causing it to become rounded. A canthoplasty to prolong the palpebral rim will correct this condition. However this technique can occasionally result in a return of the problem. A Z-plasty or a free skin graft can be used in more serious cases.

Palpebral Asymmetry Consequent to Iatrogenic Paralysis of the Right Frontal Nerve During a
Cheek-Temporal Face Lift

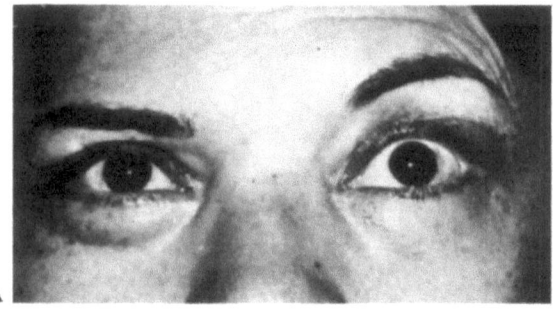

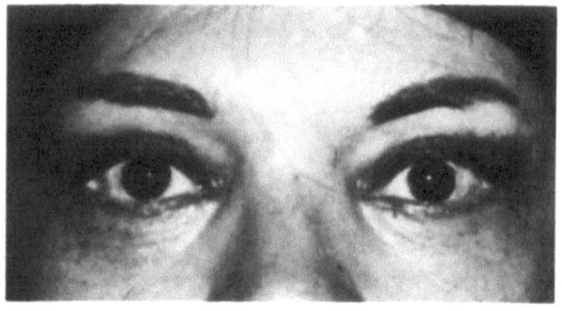

FIGURE 6.13. Iatrogenic paralysis of the right frontal nerve after a face lift. The case was resolved by a selective neurotomy of the left frontal nerve plus a frontal lift. *A.* Patient operated on elsewhere, with a drop of the right eyebrow because of paralysis of the frontal belly of the occipitofrontal muscle. The facial imbalance results from hypermotility of the left contralateral frontal muscle. The left upper eyelid shows more distension because of the normal elevation of the left eyebrow. *B.* Postoperative view after improvement of facial imbalance by selective neurotomy of the left frontal nerve. A frontal lift corrected the drop of the eyebrows. The patient cannot elevate the eyebrows because she has bilateral paralysis of the frontal branch of the facial nerve.

Palpebral Asymmetry Consequent to Paralysis of the Frontal Belly of the Right Occipitofrontal Muscle

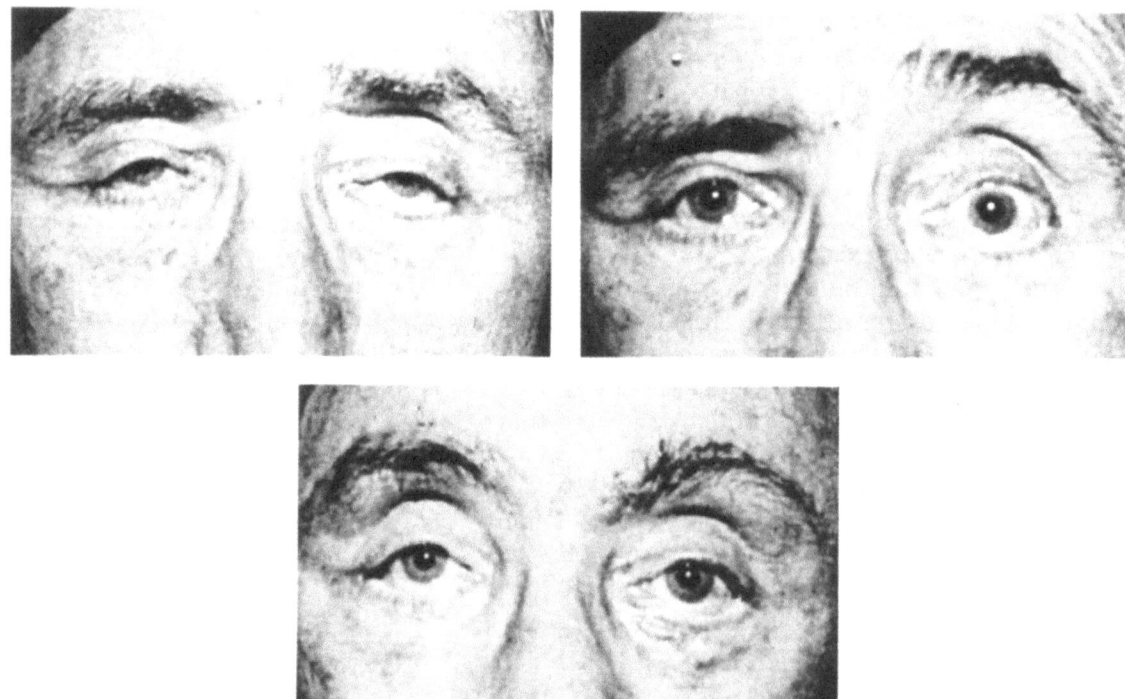

FIGURE 6.14. A 60-year-old patient with face lift elsewhere, presenting with asymmetric upper eyelids resulting from unilateral paralysis of the frontal muscle. This was corrected in our service about 20 years ago by contralateral selective neurotomy and an eyebrow lift. (From Loeb, R. "Ritidoplasties – General Considerations" Monography. Gráfica Saraiva, São Paulo, Brasil, June 1966). (in Portuguese).

Voluminous Post-Blepharoplasty Edema of the Lower Lids Caused by a Reduction of Lymphatic Circulation Due to a Low Incision

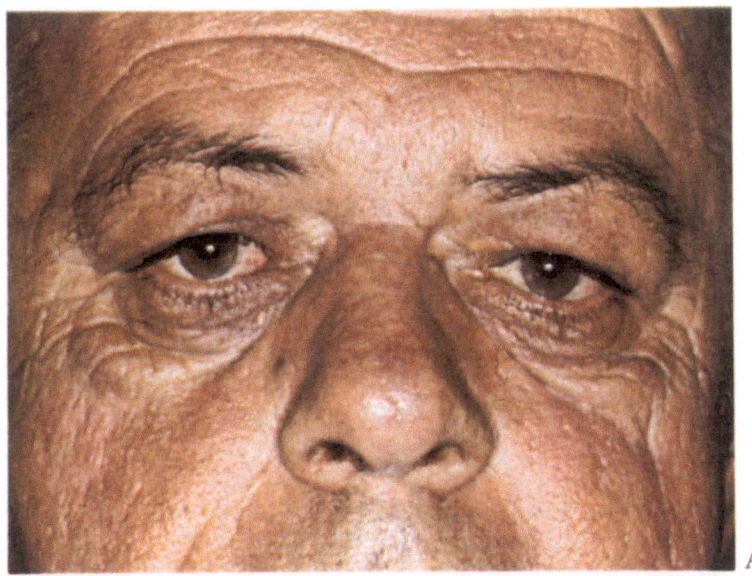

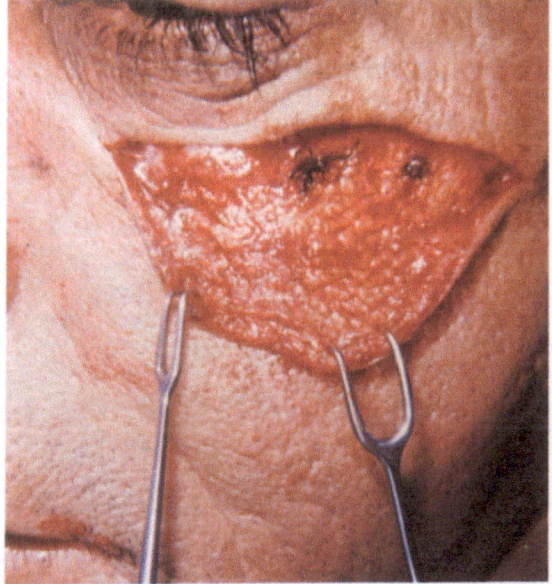

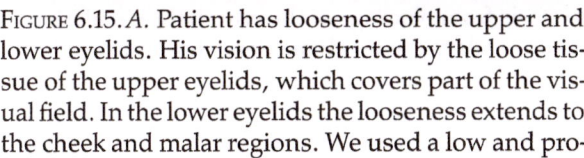

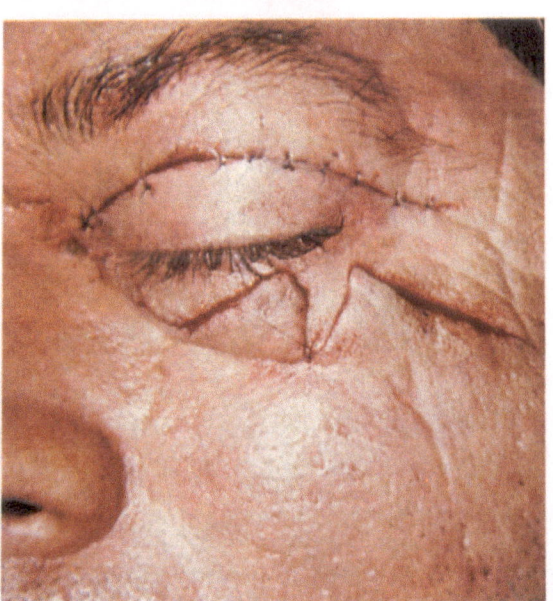

FIGURE 6.15. *A.* Patient has looseness of the upper and lower eyelids. His vision is restricted by the loose tissue of the upper eyelids, which covers part of the visual field. In the lower eyelids the looseness extends to the cheek and malar regions. We used a low and pro-longed incision similar to that in the diagram on page 39. *B.* Ample undermining. *C.* Preliminary evaluation of the resection to be made in accordance with the technique described on page 39.

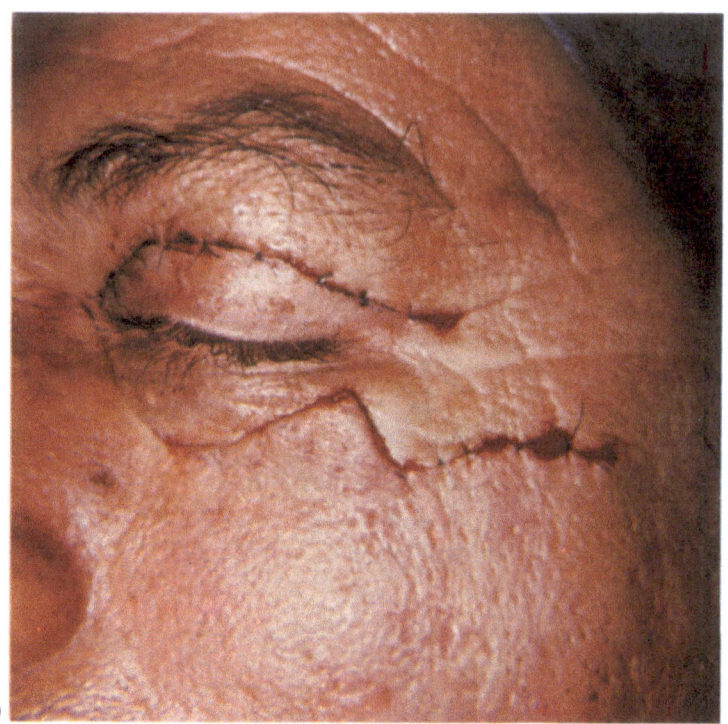

D

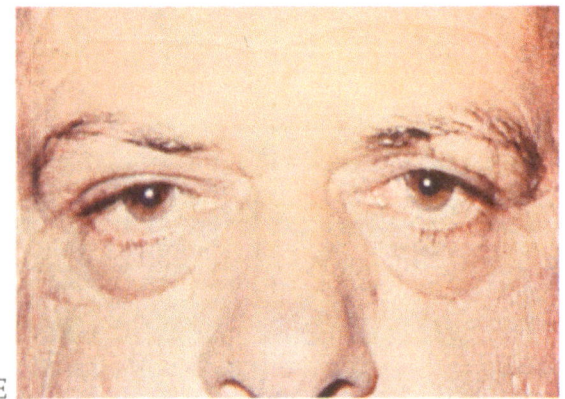

E

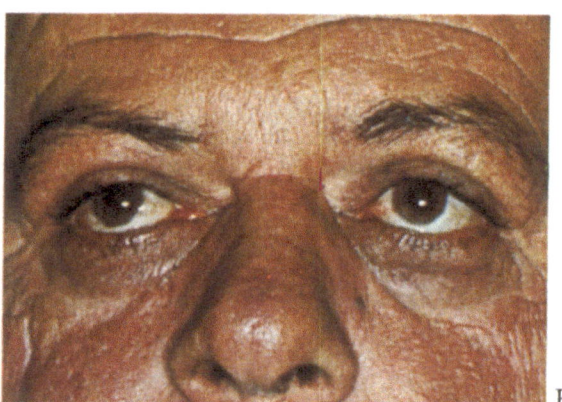

F

FIGURE 6.15. *D.* Test used to prevent ectropion. The head of the patient was elevated to a vertical position. After verification of the absence of ectropion, the excess tissue can be resected. The lateral portion of the excess has already been resected. *E.* Postoperative view after 60 days, showing edema consequent to stasis from blockage of the lymphatic circulation. *F.* After 120 days the residual edema has improved.

Projection of the Fat Graft Due to Persistent Growth of Orbital Fat Tissue

An increase in the projection of a free fat graft in the lids sometimes surprises the surgeon. It is unexpected and is probably due to the fact that the original fat of the orbit has maintained its natural tendency to grow. This tendency, initially the cause of the baggy eyelids, will also cause a projection of the fat implant (Fig. 6.16).

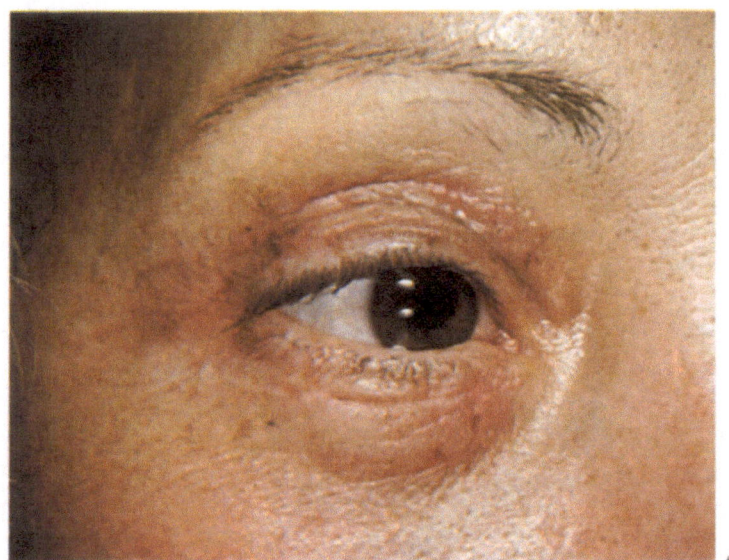

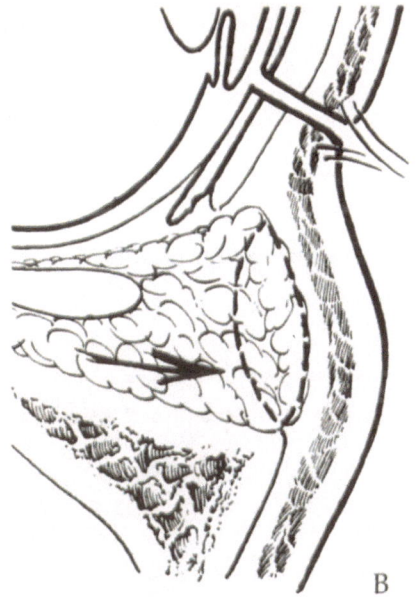

FIGURE 6.16. *A.* For 2 years the patient was satisfied with the results. After this period, to our surprise, we observed exaggerated bulges in the lower eyelids. We believe that the growth tendency of the fat tissue of the orbit, which caused the original bulges, had been maintained. Observe the depression at the level of the nasojugal sulcus below the bulge. (From Loeb R: Free fat grafted under lower lid depressions and sub-sequently slid to level deep naso jugal folds. *Transactions of the VIII International Congress of Plastic Surgery.* Montreal, June-July, 1983, pp 480–481.) *B.* The tendency that had generated the original bulges has continued, projecting the fat graft forward, forming the bulge again. (From Loeb R: Fat pad sliding and fat leveling lid depressions. *Clinics in Plastic Surgery*, v.8, n.4, October 1981.)

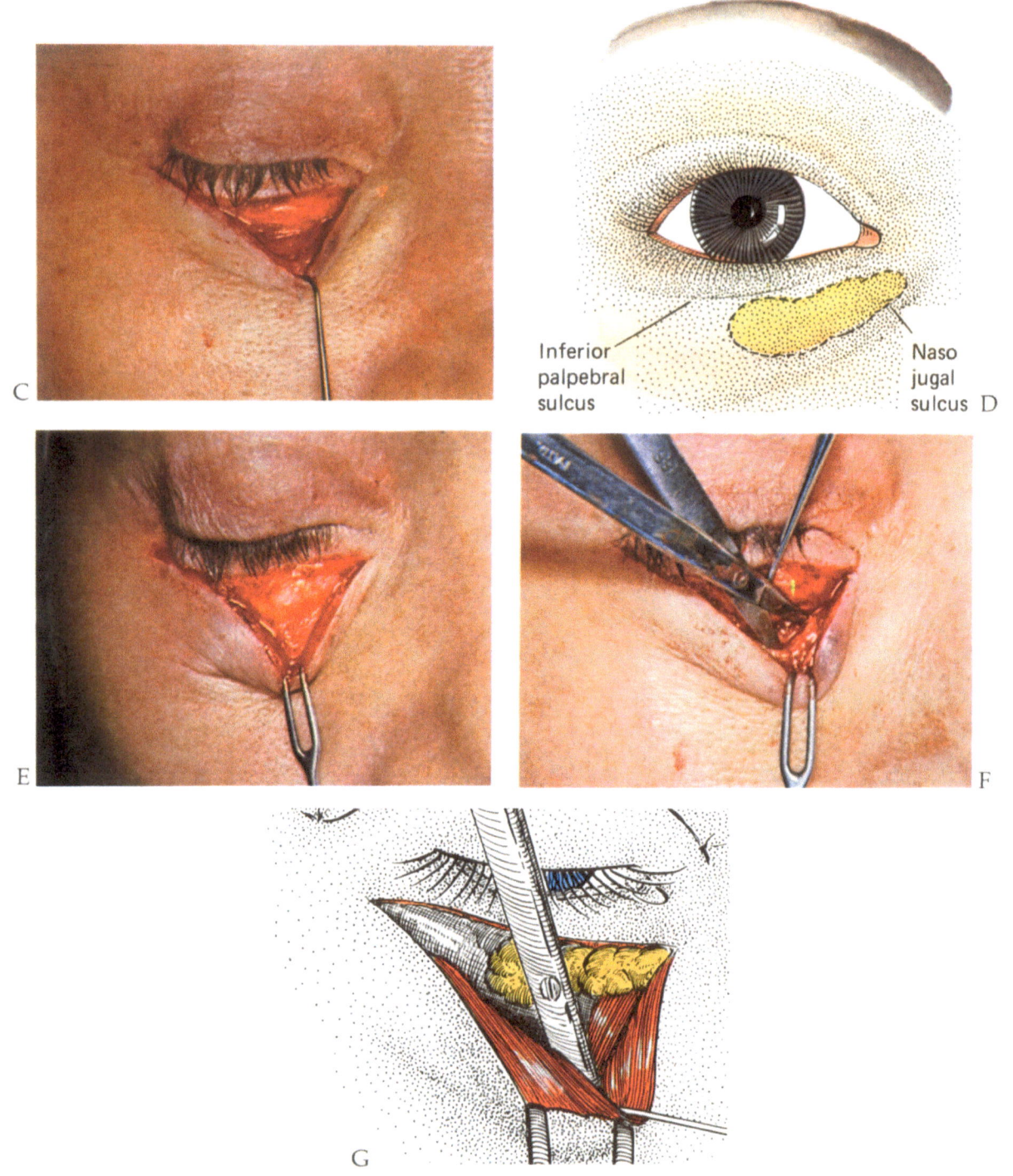

FIGURE 6.16. C. After skin-muscle undermining, a layer of tissue similar to the fascia is seen covering the fat tissue of the fat compartment. It appears normal. D. Projection of the graft that had been placed previously. We decided to slide this fat graft as a flap and use it to level the depression of the nasojugal sulcus. E. After we sectioned the fascia, there was no dif-ferentiation between the grafted and the natural fat; it all seemed to be an integral part of the palpebral pocket. F. Undermining in the direction of the angular muscle is begun. G. Undermining with scissors to section the septum, which separates the orbital region from the nasal and cheek regions.

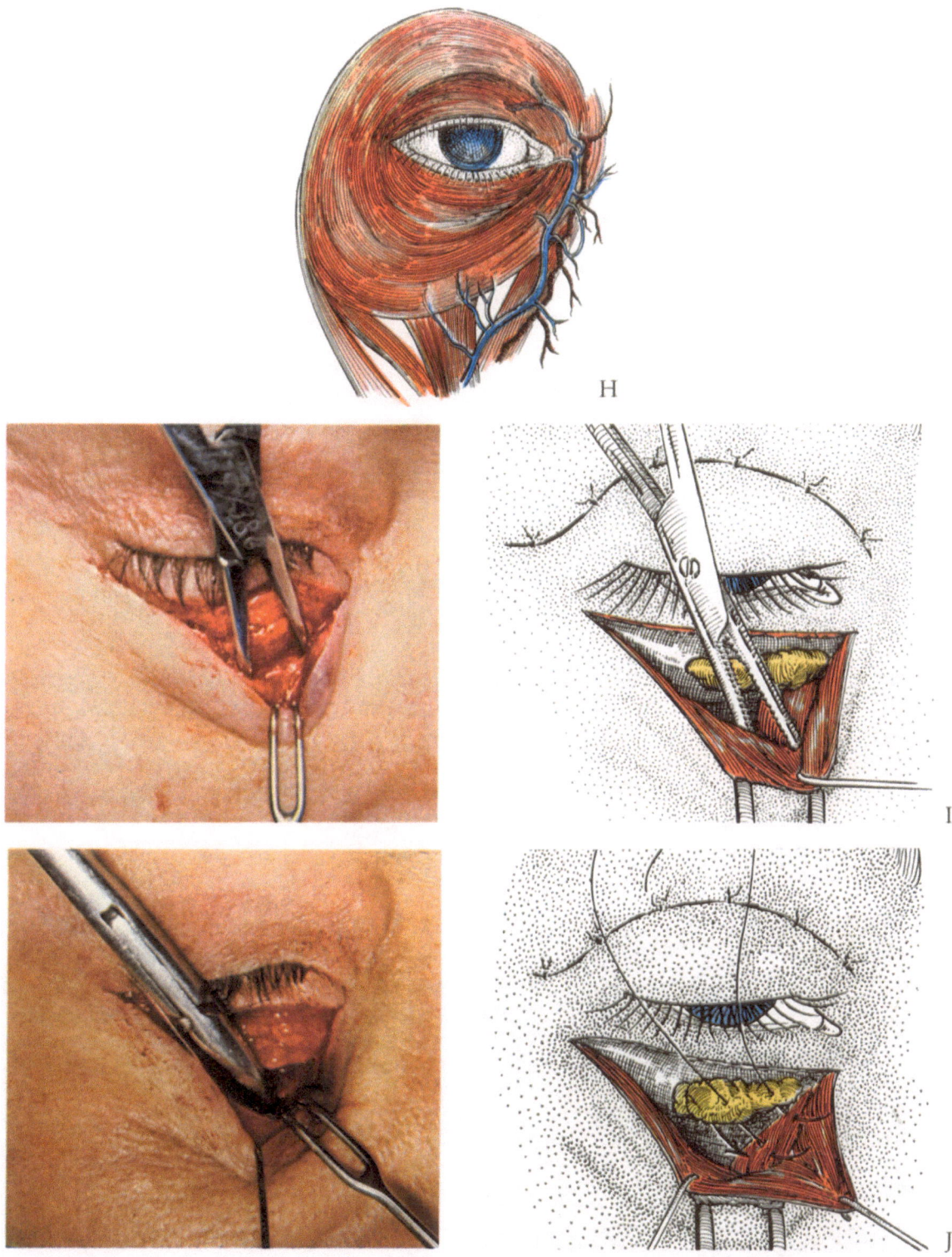

FIGURE 6.16. *H.* Great care should be taken not to injure important arteries and veins. *I.* We continue the undermining, using blunt pointed hemostatic forceps, up to the anterior face of the angular muscle. *J.* Suturing the fat tissue to the anterior face of the angular muscle.

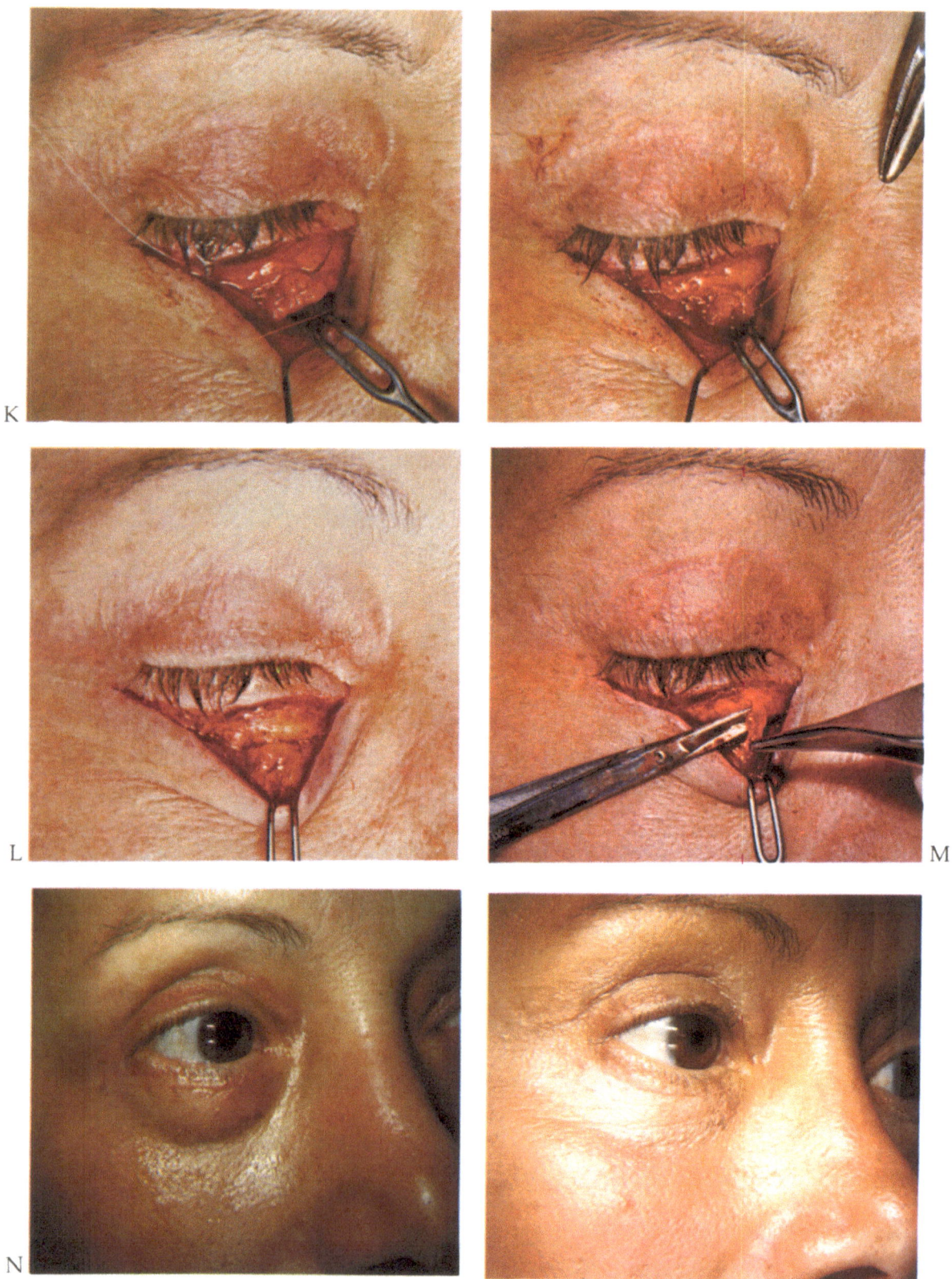

FIGURE 6.16. *K.* Further suturing. *L.* Suturing completed, showing the fat tissue covering the angular muscle. *M.* Biopsy specimen taken. *N.* Comparative pre- and post operative view.

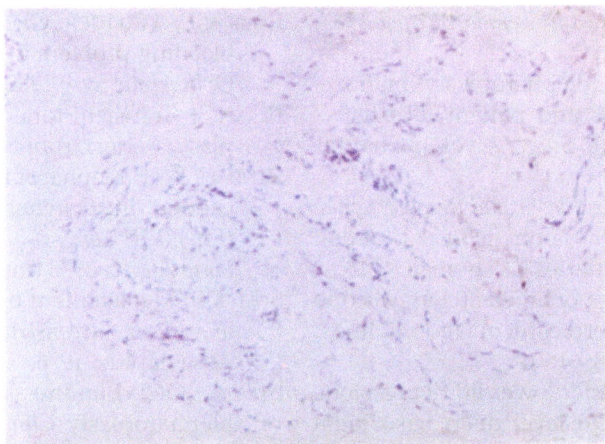

FIGURE 6.16.0. Micro-photograph of the grafted tissue biopsy of this case. Slide showing fat tissue with an adjacent zone of youthful fibrous tissue, and a slight infiltration of lymphocytes (H and E, 200x).

Comment on "Fat Projection"

In cases of congenital depressions, the problem described above does not occur. There is no late development of baggy eyelids, since the potential for growth of the naturally occurring orbital fat is small or nonexistent. This lack of growth potential was possibly the cause of the initial depression.

Milias

The formation of milias, that is, small cysts that arise in the suture line, is a very common complication. Its etiology is as follows: after 48 hours the skin epithelium of the lid penetrates along the suture; unless removed in time, it can tunnelize the entire pathway of the suture. Sebaceous cysts (milias) are then formed in the deep part of the epithelial tunnel. They should be removed with the point of a needle. If they are not removed, they can grow, making removal difficult. They frequently become infected.

Additional Reading

ADAMS BJ, FEURSTEIN SS et al: – Complications of blepharoplasty. *Ear Nose Throat J.*, 1986, 39:395.

BEYER CK et al: Baggy lids: A classification and newer aspects of treatment to avoid complications. *Ophthalmic Surg* 1980; 11:169.

CONVERSE JM: Treatment of ephithelized suture tracts of eyelids by marsupialization. *Plast Reconstr Surg* 1966; 48:477.

CORREIA P de C: Complications of cervico-facial ritidoplasties and their preventions, in: *Annals of the XIII Brazilian Congress of Plastic Surgery and First Brazilian Congress of Aesthetic Surgery*. Porto Alegre, Emma, 1976 (in Portuguese).

DE MERE M, WOOD T et al: Eye complications with blepharoplasty or other eyelid surgery. *Plast Reconstr Surg* 1974; 53:634.

DE MERE M: Blindness and eyelid surgery. *Aesthetic Plast Surg* 1978; 2:41.

FARINA R, MAGALHÃES PB et al: Ectropions and palpebral loss of substance. *Arq Bras Oftalmol* 1964; 27:36. (in Portuguese)

GORMLEY DE: Cutaneous surgery in the infraocular area and ectropion avoidance. *Cutis* 1978; 21:391.

HARLEY RD, NELSON LB et al: Ocular motility disturbances following cosmetic blepharoplasty. *Arch Ophthalmol* 1986; 104:542.

HARTLEY JH, LESTER JC et al: Acute retrobulbar hemorrhage during elective blepharoplasty. *Plast Reconstr Surg* 1973; 52:8.

HUESTON JT, HEINZE JB: Successful early relief of blindness occuring after blepharoplasty. *Plast Reconstr Surg* 1972; 53:588.

JELKS GW, McCORD CD Jr: Dry eye syndrome and other tear film abnormalities. *Clin Plast Surg* 1981; 8:802.

KELLY PW, MAY DR: Central retinal artery occlusion following cosmetic blepharoplasty. *Br J Ophthalmol* 1980, vol 64.

KEPPKE EM, BAROUDI R et al: Severe eye complications after surgery for the corrections of wrinkles and palpebral pouches. *Arq Inst Penido Burnier* 1965; 19:59.

KLATSKY SA, MASON PN: Blepharoplasty management of complications and patient dissatisfaction, in: *Aesthetic Plastic Surgery,* vol 3, Chapter 25, 1986.

KUHNT H, SZYMANOWSKY J: In *Plastic and Reconstructive Surgery,* Padgett EC, Stephenson KL (eds). Springfield, Illinois, Charles C. Thomas, 1948.

LESSA SF, CARREIRÃO SE: Use of an encircling silicone rubber string for the correction of lagophtalmos. *Plast Reconstr Surg* 1978; 61:719.

LOEB R: Free fat grafted under lower lid depressions and subsequent slid to level deep naso jugal folds. *Transactions of the VIII International Congress of Plastic Surgery.* Montreal, June-July, 1983, pp 480–481.

MAHAFFEY PJ, WALLACE AF et al: Blindness following cosmetic blepharoplasty – a review. *Br J Plast Surg* 1986; 39:213.

McCORD CD, SHORE JW: Avoidance of complications in lower lid blepharoplasty. *Ophthalmology (Rochester)* 1983; 90:1039.

MUSTARDE JC, JONES TL et al: Ophtalmic plastic surgery – up to date. Birmingham, Alabama, Aesculapius, 1970.

PARIS GL, WALTUCH GF et al: Salicylate – induced bleeding problem in ophthalmic plastic surgery. *Ophthalmic Surg* 1982; 13:627.

PLANAS J: Transient total blindness during blepharoplasty (letter). *Ann Plast Surg* 1980; 4:526.

SANDALL WH: Blepharoplasties, dangers and complications, in: *Congresso Brasileiro de Cirurgia Plástica, e XIII Congresso Brasileiro de Cirurgia Estética, Porto Alegre, 1976* (in Portuguese).

SOLL DB: Management of complications, in: *Ophthalmic Plastic Reconstructive Surgery.* Birmingham, Aesculapius, 1976.

STASIOR OG: Blindness associated with cosmetic blepharoplasty. *Clin Plast Surg* 1981; 8:793.

TENZEL RR: Surgical treatment of complications of cosmetic blepharoplasty. *Clin Plast Surg* 1978; 5:517.

TENZEL RR: Complications of blepharoplasty. *Clin Plast Surg* 1981; 8:797.

VICTOR WH, HURWITZ JJ et al: Cicatricial ectropion following blepharoplasty: treatment by tissue expansion. *Can J Opthalmol* 1984; 19:317.

WALLER R: Is blindness a realistic complication in blepharoplasty procedures? *Trans Am Acad Ophthalmol Otolaryngol* 1978; 85:730.

Index